AF353005

Artificial Intelligence (AI) and Machine Learning (ML) in Medical Imaging Informatics towards Diagnostic Decision Making

Artificial Intelligence (AI) and Machine Learning (ML) in Medical Imaging Informatics towards Diagnostic Decision Making

Editor

Md Mahmudur Rahman

MDPI • Basel • Beijing • Wuhan • Barcelona • Belgrade • Manchester • Tokyo • Cluj • Tianjin

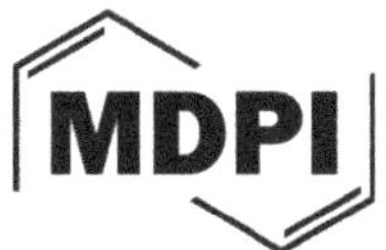

Editor
Md Mahmudur Rahman
Department of Computer Science
Morgan State University
Baltimore
United States

Editorial Office
MDPI
St. Alban-Anlage 66
4052 Basel, Switzerland

This is a reprint of articles from the Special Issue published online in the open access journal *Healthcare* (ISSN 2227-9032) (available at: https://www.mdpi.com/journal/healthcare/special_issues/AIML_medical).

For citation purposes, cite each article independently as indicated on the article page online and as indicated below:

LastName, A.A.; LastName, B.B.; LastName, C.C. Article Title. *Journal Name* **Year**, *Volume Number*, Page Range.

ISBN 978-3-0365-8128-6 (Hbk)
ISBN 978-3-0365-8129-3 (PDF)

Contents

About the Editor . . . . **vii**

Preface to "Artificial Intelligence (AI) and Machine Learning (ML) in Medical Imaging
Informatics towards Diagnostic Decision Making" . . . . **ix**

**Kirill Arzamasov, Yuriy Vasilev, Anton Vladzymyrskyy, Olga Omelyanskaya, Igor Shulkin,
Darya Kozikhina, et al.**
An International Non-Inferiority Study for the Benchmarking of AI for Routine Radiology
Cases: Chest X-ray, Fluorography and Mammography
Reprinted from: *Healthcare* **2023**, *11*, 1684, doi:10.3390/healthcare11121684 . . . . **1**

Ghadah Alwakid, Walaa Gouda and Mamoona Humayun
Deep Learning-Based Prediction of Diabetic Retinopathy Using CLAHE and ESRGAN
for Enhancement
Reprinted from: *Healthcare* **2023**, *11*, 863, doi:10.3390/healthcare11060863 . . . . **17**

**Yurie Kanauchi, Masahiro Hashimoto, Naoki Toda, Saori Okamoto, Hasnine Haque,
Masahiro Jinzaki and Yasubumi Sakakibara**
Automatic Detection and Measurement of Renal Cysts in Ultrasound Images: A Deep
Learning Approach
Reprinted from: *Healthcare* **2023**, *11*, 484, doi:10.3390/healthcare11040484 . . . . **35**

**Mohammad Hamid Asnawi, Anindya Apriliyanti Pravitasari, Gumgum Darmawan,
Triyani Hendrawati, Intan Nurma Yulita, Jadi Suprijadi and Farid Azhar Lutfi Nugraha**
Lung and Infection CT-Scan-Based Segmentation with 3D UNet Architecture and Its
Modification
Reprinted from: *Healthcare* **2023**, *11*, 213, doi:10.3390/healthcare11020213 . . . . **51**

Rana Alabdan, Abdulrahman Alruban, Anwer Mustafa Hilal and Abdelwahed Motwakel
Artificial-Intelligence-Based Decision Making for Oral Potentially Malignant Disorder
Diagnosis in Internet of Medical Things Environment
Reprinted from: *Healthcare* **2023**, *11*, 113, doi:10.3390/healthcare11010113 . . . . **71**

Rasha A. Mansouri and Mahmoud Ragab
Equilibrium Optimization Algorithm with Ensemble Learning Based Cervical Precancerous
Lesion Classification Model
Reprinted from: *Healthcare* **2023**, *11*, 55, doi:10.3390/healthcare11010055 . . . . **87**

Ghadah Alwakid, Walaa Gouda, Mamoona Humayun and Najm Us Sama
Melanoma Detection Using Deep Learning-Based Classifications
Reprinted from: *Healthcare* **2022**, *10*, 2481, doi:10.3390/healthcare10122481 . . . . **103**

Shih-Yen Hsu, Chi-Yuan Wang, Yi-Kai Kao, Kuo-Ying Liu, Ming-Chia Lin, Li-Ren Yeh, et al.
Using Deep Neural Network Approach for Multiple-Class Assessment of Digital
Mammography
Reprinted from: *Healthcare* **2022**, *10*, 2382, doi:10.3390/healthcare10122382 . . . . **121**

Xinzheng Xu, Qiaoyu Guo, Zhongnian Li and Dechun Li
Uncertainty Ordinal Multi-Instance Learning for Breast Cancer Diagnosis
Reprinted from: *Healthcare* **2022**, *10*, 2300, doi:10.3390/healthcare10112300 . . . . **133**

Dong-Her Shih, Ching-Hsien Liao, Ting-Wei Wu, Xiao-Yin Xu and Ming-Hung Shih
Dysarthria Speech Detection Using Convolutional Neural Networks with Gated Recurrent Unit
Reprinted from: *Healthcare* **2022**, *10*, 1956, doi:10.3390/healthcare10101956 . . . . **145**

Niranjana Sampathila, Krishnaraj Chadaga, Neelankit Goswami, Rajagopala P. Chadaga, Mayur Pandya, Srikanth Prabhu, et al.
Customized Deep Learning Classifier for Detection of Acute Lymphoblastic Leukemia Using Blood Smear Images
Reprinted from: *Healthcare* **2022**, *10*, 1812, doi:10.3390/healthcare10101812 . . . . **159**

Chung-Ming Lo, Yu-Hsuan Yeh, Jui-Hsiang Tang, Chun-Chao Chang and Hsing-Jung Yeh
Rapid Polyp Classification in Colonoscopy Using Textural and Convolutional Features
Reprinted from: *Healthcare* **2022**, *10*, 1494, doi:10.3390/healthcare10081494 . . . . **175**

Youngihn Kwon, Juyeon Lee, Joo Hee Park, Yoo Mee Kim, Se Hwa Kim, Young Jun Won and Hyung-Yong Kim
Osteoporosis Pre-Screening Using Ensemble Machine Learning in Postmenopausal Korean Women
Reprinted from: *Healthcare* **2022**, *10*, 1107, doi:10.3390/healthcare10061107 . . . . **185**

Maria Elena Laino, Angela Ammirabile, Ludovica Lofino, Lorenzo Mannelli, Francesco Fiz, Marco Francone, et al.
Artificial Intelligence Applied to Pancreatic Imaging: A Narrative Review
Reprinted from: *Healthcare* **2022**, *10*, 1511, doi:10.3390/healthcare10081511 . . . . **197**

About the Editor

Md Mahmudur Rahman

Dr. Md Mahmudur Rahman is an Associate Professor who is currently serving as the Associate Chair in the Computer Science Department at Morgan State University, Maryland, USA. He received his PhD (2008) in Computer Science from Concordia University, Montreal, Canada with an emphasis on medical informatics and Image Retrieval. Prior to joining as an Assistant Professor at Morgan State University in 2014, Dr. Rahman extensively conducted research at the National Institutes of Health (NIH), USA, for almost six years as a Research Scientist. He has good expertise in the fields of Data Science, AI and Machine Learning, Image Processing and Computer Vision and their application to the classification, annotation, retrieval, and interpretation of biomedical images from large collections. Dr. Rahman has published two books, two book chapters, and more than eighty articles in peer-reviewed journals and conference proceedings. Dr. Rahman's current research is focused on deep learning techniques and their application for automatic captioning and concept generation of medical images, multi-modal retrieval of imaging entities in biomedical literature, and image-based computer-aided diagnostic (CAD) and decision support systems (DSSs).

Preface to "Artificial Intelligence (AI) and Machine Learning (ML) in Medical Imaging Informatics towards Diagnostic Decision Making"

This reprint contains fourteen (14) articles (one review and thirteen research papers) spanning different imaging modalities and techniques (such as radiology, pathology, dermoscopy, mammography, colonoscopy, ultrasound, etc.) to detect different diseases/disorders, including the detection of breast cancer, melanoma, diabetic retinopathy (DR), renal cysts, lung infection, oral cancer, acute lymphoblastic leukemia (ALL), polyp, cervical precancerous lesion, osteoporosis, etc., using advanced Computer Vision and AI/ML/DL-based techniques. We hope articles in this reprint can be valuable resources/references for researchers in medical imaging informatics and will one day find their way into real clinical integration to help healthcare professionals and the healthcare industry as a whole.

Md Mahmudur Rahman
Editor

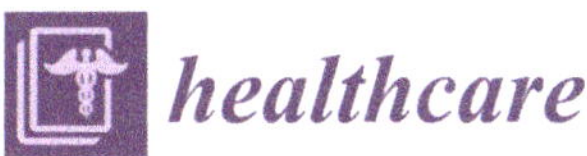

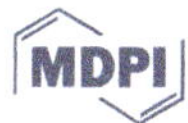

Article

An International Non-Inferiority Study for the Benchmarking of AI for Routine Radiology Cases: Chest X-ray, Fluorography and Mammography

Kirill Arzamasov [1,*], Yuriy Vasilev [1,2], Anton Vladzymyrskyy [1,3], Olga Omelyanskaya [1], Igor Shulkin[1], Darya Kozikhina[1], Inna Goncharova [1], Pavel Gelezhe [1], Yury Kirpichev [1], Tatiana Bobrovskaya [1] and Anna Andreychenko [1]

[1] State Budget-Funded Health Care Institution of the City of Moscow "Research and Practical Clinical Center for Diagnostics and Telemedicine Technologies of the Moscow Health Care Department", Petrovka Street, 24, Building 1, 127051 Moscow, Russia; bobrovskayatm@zdrav.mos.ru (T.B.)

[2] Federal State Budgetary Institution "National Medical and Surgical Center Named after N.I. Pirogov" of the Ministry of Health of the Russian Federation, Nizhnyaya Pervomayskaya Street, 70, 105203 Moscow, Russia

[3] Department of Information and Internet Technologies, I.M. Sechenov First Moscow State Medical University of the Ministry of Health of the Russian Federation (Sechenov University), Trubetskaya Street, 8, Building 2, 119991 Moscow, Russia

[*] Correspondence: arzamasovkm@zdrav.mos.ru; Tel.: +7-9152514838

Abstract: An international reader study was conducted to gauge an average diagnostic accuracy of radiologists interpreting chest X-ray images, including those from fluorography and mammography, and establish requirements for stand-alone radiological artificial intelligence (AI) models. The retrospective studies in the datasets were labelled as containing or not containing target pathological findings based on a consensus of two experienced radiologists, and the results of a laboratory test and follow-up examination, where applicable. A total of 204 radiologists from 11 countries with various experience performed an assessment of the dataset with a 5-point Likert scale via a web platform. Eight commercial radiological AI models analyzed the same dataset. The AI AUROC was 0.87 (95% CI:0.83–0.9) versus 0.96 (95% CI 0.94–0.97) for radiologists. The sensitivity and specificity of AI versus radiologists were 0.71 (95% CI 0.64–0.78) versus 0.91 (95% CI 0.86–0.95) and 0.93 (95% CI 0.89–0.96) versus 0.9 (95% CI 0.85–0.94) for AI. The overall diagnostic accuracy of radiologists was superior to AI for chest X-ray and mammography. However, the accuracy of AI was noninferior to the least experienced radiologists for mammography and fluorography, and to all radiologists for chest X-ray. Therefore, an AI-based first reading could be recommended to reduce the workload burden of radiologists for the most common radiological studies such as chest X-ray and mammography.

Keywords: stand-alone artificial intelligence; radiology; benchmarking; population screening

Citation: Arzamasov, K.; Vasilev, Y.; Vladzymyrskyy, A.; Omelyanskaya, O.; Shulkin, I.; Kozikhina, D.; Goncharova, I.; Gelezhe, P.; Kirpichev, Y.; Bobrovskaya, T.; et al. An International Non-Inferiority Study for the Benchmarking of AI for Routine Radiology Cases: Chest X-ray, Fluorography and Mammography. *Healthcare* **2023**, *11*, 1684. https://doi.org/10.3390/healthcare11121684

Academic Editor: Mahmudur Rahman

Received: 16 April 2023
Revised: 1 June 2023
Accepted: 4 June 2023
Published: 8 June 2023

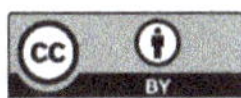

1. Introduction

A steadily increasing volume of prescribed radiological diagnostic examinations and the increasing amount of diagnostic equipment has skyrocketed the workload of radiologists [1]. More than half of all radiology studies are composed of mammography, chest X-ray and chest fluorography [2,3]. The WHO (World Health Organization) guidelines evaluated the reduction in mortality due to mammography screening and consider it to be the most widely used and valuable noninvasive method for early breast cancer detection [4,5]. Chest X-ray (and fluorography in certain countries) is widely used for routine, emergency and screening purposes. During the pandemic, it became even more valuable, as the WHO recommends including chest X-ray into a diagnostic approach for patients suspected of the 2019 novel coronavirus disease (COVID-19) [6,7].

Due to the rapidly increasing number of radiological examinations, the application of artificial Intelligence (AI) models for carrying out a first reading becomes valuable in order to reduce radiologists' workload and improve diagnostic accuracy in the absence of experienced specialists [8,9]. Recent studies have demonstrated that the diagnostic accuracy of AI models for medical imaging approaches the performance of medical experts and even outperforms them in several fields [10]. This has led to a rapid explosion of commercially available and registered AI models for mammography and thoracic radiology (including chest X-ray and fluorography) analysis [11,12]. Thus, AI models are actively integrated into the radiology workflow. However, while the accuracy metrics claimed by the developers are quite high, their real-world performance must be carefully evaluated and compared with the radiologist's performance in order to ensure practical value and safety [3,4,13,14]. Therefore, the WHO warns that, despite obvious benefits, the deployment of AI in medicine is fraught with risks that should be minimized [15].

At the same time, there are controversial opinions on the use of AI models compared to radiologists with various levels of experience. However, studies have demonstrated the ability of AI models to reach the levels of radiologists' performance [13]. On the other hand, the accuracy of mammography interpretation by experienced radiologists varies highly [16] and previous-generation CAD systems have not significantly improved the accuracy of mammography readings [17]. Only several studies [1,7,18] have assessed the accuracy of AI algorithms in relation to the analysis of chest X-rays; there are almost no data for fluorography. The expectations of AI implementation for X-ray imaging thus remain ambiguous. Even promising results of AI models with high accuracy metrics are associated with limited specificity for the classification of the particular findings. Thus, it can barely be a substitute for a radiologist [7,19,20].

Since variations in radiologists' performance are widely observed, they can lead to different results in the comparison between radiologists and AI. This may compromise the objective assessment of a particular AI model, or lead to a misjudgment of the benefits and limitations of AI for the whole field of medical imaging. Therefore, multicenter and international studies with different groups of radiologists are of particular interest for the benchmarking of AI and human readers. A study carried out among 101 radiologists from 7 countries demonstrated that the precision of the AI model accuracy for identifying breast cancer with mammography was comparable to that of an average radiologist [13]. Another major study with more than 1100 participants from 44 countries revealed that none of the AI models could outperform radiologists, but the combination of a single reader evaluation with AI results improved the total accuracy of screening mammography [4]. A recent international study demonstrated that an AI model could exceed the average performance of mammography specialists, but the comparison was performed for a relatively small group of six readers [14]. Undoubtedly, larger international studies are needed in order to establish an unbiased comparison of AI and human readers' performance. This study aimed to determine the average diagnostic accuracy of radiologists interpreting chest X-ray images, including those from fluorography and mammography, on an international scale for benchmarking with the stand-alone AI model's performance metrics for the same cases.

2. Materials and Methods

The retrospective study was conducted according to Standards for Reporting Diagnostic Accuracy Studies (STARD) 2015 guidelines. The overall study design scheme is shown in Figure 1.

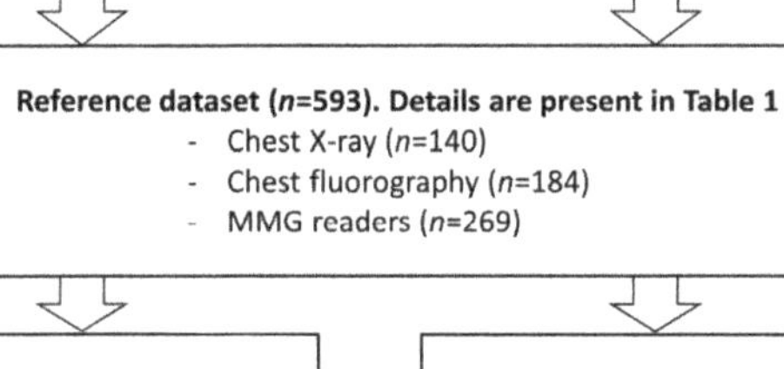

a—amount of ai models; m -amount of human readers; n -amount of studies

Figure 1. The study design scheme.

2.1. Reference Dataset

The reference dataset (local test dataset) was collected retrospectively from the radiological exams performed in outpatient Moscow state medical facilities for screening and diagnostic purposes in 2018–2019. The dataset contained studies marked as 'without (target) pathology' and 'with (target) pathology'. The target pathology was defined based on a list of pathological radiological findings compiled based on their clinical significance and frequency of occurrence in the routine practice of radiologists. All studies were selected based on electronic medical records and then double-checked by radiology experts who had at least 5 years of experience in thoracic radiology or breast imaging. Pathomorphological confirmation for malignancies was derived from electronic medical records. Table 1 contains details on the dataset.

Table 1. Details on the datasets and human readers.

Parameter	X-ray	Fluorography	MMG
Number of cases (cases "with pathology") *	140 (47)	184 (84)	269 (167)
Confirmation of (ab)normality by	Two experts (>5 years of experience)		
Male/female/unknown	59/77/4	94/113/4	0/269/0
Age (years) **	49 ± 18 [15, 89]	53 ± 19 [19, 93]	63 ± 6 [34, 80]
Radiological findings	1. Pleural effusion (9) 2. Pneumothorax (7) 3. Atelectasis (9) 4. Nodules or mass (21) 5. Infiltrate or consolidation (13) 6. Miliary pattern, or dissemination (1) 7. Cavity (1) 8. Pulmonary calcification (7) 9. Fracture (2)	1. Pleural effusion (26) 2. Pneumothorax (7) 3. Nodules or mass (28) 4. Infiltrate or consolidation (26) Pulmonary calcification (14)	BiRADS 0
Number of diagnostic devices	61	69	11
Vendors	(1) GE Medical Systems, LLC (2) Fujifilm (3) Toshiba Medical Systems, Inc (4) RENinMED, LLC	(1) S.P. Gelpik, LLC	(1) Fujifilm
Radiologists (number)	185	28	113 (96 breast imaging specialists)
Years of experience			
0–1	36	6	16 (15)
1–5	60	8	32 (28)
5–10	36	5	28 (24)
10+	53	9	37 (29)
Country ***	AM—1 AZ—1 BY—11 GE—1 KG—2 KZ—6 LV—1 MD—2 RU—141 UA—17 UZ—2	BY—1 GE—1 KZ—1 RU—25	AZ—1 BY—4 GE—1 KG—1 KZ—4 LV—1 MD—1 RU—95 UA—4 UZ—1

* Cases "with pathology" contained at least one of the radiological findings. ** Data are mean ± standard deviation. Data in parentheses are the range. *** Codes for countries from ISO 3166.

The following target pathologies (terminology proposed by the Fleischner society [21]) for digital chest radiography and fluorography were included in this study:

- Pneumothorax;
- Atelectasis;
- Nodules or mass;
- Infiltrate or consolidation;
- Miliary pattern, or dissemination;
- Cavity;
- Pulmonary calcification;
- Pleural effusion;
- Fracture, or rupture of the bone cortical layer.

For digital mammography, a target pathology was defined based on the corresponding malignancy probability classifications of BI-RADS3-5 on the diagnostic scale or BI-RADS0 on the screening scale [22], with the confirmed diagnosis based on biopsy results or a follow-up negative MMG study for BI-RADS1-2. The right and the left breasts were assessed separately; however, the study was marked as pathological if the signs of the pathology were detected in at least one breast.

Inclusion criteria for the study: (1) all studies in the dataset were presented in Digital Imaging and Communications in Medicine (DICOM) format and anonymized; (2) sufficient number and appropriate diagnostic quality of the images was required for every study: a chest X-ray and a digital fluorography study included an anterior–posterior view; mammography studies contained the breasts images in two views (craniocaudal and mediolateral); and (3) for the target pathological findings, the truthing included: (a) histological confirmation of the malignancy presence and a follow-up study without the pathological findings for the absence of the malignancy or (b) a double consensus between two expert radiologists for all other findings.

Exclusion criteria included: (1) lung or breast surgery; (2) additional opacifications from medical devices, clothing or extracorporeal objects; (3) technical defects of the image and/or the positioning; (4) absence of histological or expert confirmation of the pathology; and (5) age < 18 years.

2.2. AI Models

The study included eight AI models that participated in the experiment with the use of innovative computer vision technologies for medical image analysis and subsequent applicability in the healthcare system of Moscow (https://mosmed.ai/en/, accessed on 1 June 2023). This research was registered in ClinicalTrials (NCT04489992). The study included commercial AI models to identify pathological signs on digital chest radiography (4 AI models [23–26]), fluorography (2 AI models [24,27]) and mammography (2 AI models [28,29]). The criterion for inclusion of these models was full compliance with the use cases, i.e., each AI provider declared detection of all radiological findings included in the use case: a list of the lung pathologies for chest X-ray and fluorography, and breast cancer signs corresponding to BI-RADS0 for mammography. As was reported by the AI models' developers, diagnostic accuracy metrics corresponded to those of current state-of-art AI for the use cases [7,13,30–35]. All of the AI models provided responses per study as a general abnormality score (range 0–1) without providing details on the findings. Consequently, this did not allow us to assess the performance per finding. The AI models were deployed as stand-alone systems. The details of AI models are provided in the Supplementary Materials (Table S1).

In the present study, we did not conduct any refinement of the AI models. Instead, we exclusively utilized off-the-shelf commercial solutions as they were provided by the developers. It is important to note that no modifications or alterations were made to the AI models during the course of this study.

2.3. Web Platform for Conducting the Reader Study

For the human reader study, we developed a web-based platform in order to let participants evaluate cases online. A participant could determine a start date for every use case; however, the duration of interpretation was fixed to 3 days from the start date. The participants also chose the number of studies for interpretation—20, 50 or 80 studies. In order to ensure the representativeness of the real practice performance of radiologists, they started the reader study after completing training using the web-based platform for five cases that were not included in the final evaluation.

This study aimed to determine the average accuracy of radiologists to benchmark AI-performed radiological evaluation as a stand-alone service. Therefore, in this study, we compared the diagnostic accuracy metrics of a radiologist without AI, and AI on its own as a first or second independent reading. To create equal conditions for AI models and radiologists, there was no additional information provided, such as complaints or medical history (Figure 2). Patients' age and sex were available to radiologists, but no radiological report or clinical information was provided. Radiologists did not write a detailed clinical report. They only identified findings and rated their confidence in the presence of each case for the presence of any pathological findings using a five-point scale (from 1—definitely without pathology to 5—definitely with pathology) similar to that used in other reader studies [35]. Age and sex were also provided to the AI models as DICOM tags. Whether these data were used by AI models is not known. Providing similar data to radiologists and AI models ensured an objective comparison of their performance in the clinical scenario when AI performed an independent reading.

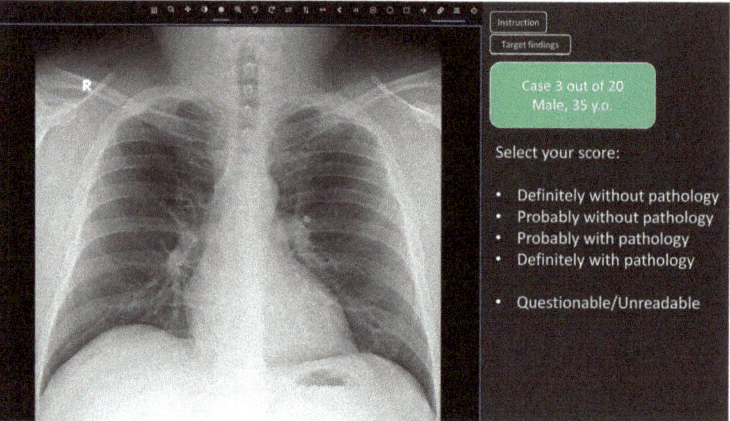

Figure 2. Radiology examination view window of the developed Web platform for the reader study.

In the upper part of the control panel of the Web platform, there were always two buttons that opened dialog boxes containing: (1) the platform user guide and (2) diagnostic criteria, according to which the participant should classify a study as normal ('without pathology') or abnormal ('with pathology')—these corresponded to the AI-based triage. The following options were given for scoring a study on the panel by a human reader:

1. Definitely without pathology (probability of pathology = 0.0);
2. Probably without pathology (probability of pathology = 0.25);
3. Undefined (questionable/unreadable) (probability of pathology = 0.5)
4. Probably with pathology (probability of pathology = 0.75);
5. Definitely with pathology (probability of pathology = 1.0);

2.4. Participating Radiologists

A total of 204 radiologists from 11 countries participated in the study. Some of these participants (n = 96) specialized in breast imaging. Table 1 presents the distribution of radiologists by the use cases with an indication of their experience and country. Each radiologist had access to the reader study datasets of three modalities—chest X-ray, chest fluorography, mammography. The evaluation of studies was conducted by every radiologist independently from 27 November to 13 December 2020. Every radiologist was provided with a set of 20/50/80 cases of the same modality (i.e., chest X-ray, fluorography or mammography) according to his/her choice. Each case and set of cases could be evaluated only once to ensure the uniqueness of responses. A user could complete the interpretation for several modalities. The exclusion criteria for radiologists were as follows: (1) the registration form was not completed (no information regarding experience, employment, preferred modality); and (2) absence of responses.

2.5. Score Analysis: Determination of the Consensus Score for Radiologists and AI Models

Studies in which most scores (>50%) were "undefined" were excluded from further analysis [36]. For the remaining studies, a consensus score was defined based on the median score of the readers. In the case of a tie of frequencies, the higher score was selected. If the case had less than 5 responses it was also excluded from further evaluation with an exception for breast imaging specialists. A consensus score between AI models for each case was reached in the following way: First, the responses for each AI model were calibrated individually in order to combine the probability values of each AI model. Second, an average probability score of all AI models was set as a consensus score for each case.

2.6. Statistical Analysis

The performance of AI and the radiologists was assessed by generating a receiver operating characteristic (ROC) curve. The area under the ROC curve (AUROC) was reported with 95% confidence intervals (95% CI). The Delong method was used to calculate the confidence interval for the AUROC [37]. A smoothing was used to build the ROC curve.

To conduct the ROC analysis, we required a binary estimation (true value) as well as the output from the "classifier". When evaluating AI algorithms, we utilized the pathology probability value as the input, which ranged from 0 to 1, with a precision of 0.01. Similarly, when evaluating a radiologist's performance, we also employed the probability values assigned by the radiologist. However, it is challenging for a radiologist to precisely assign a digital probability value for the presence of pathology. Therefore, we employed a more comprehensible gradient scale that could be easily converted into absolute values: "definitely without pathology" = 0, and "definitely with pathology" = 1. Subsequently, a standard ROC analysis was conducted to determine the diagnostic accuracy indicators.

A p-value for the AUROC was calculated using a permutation test [38]. A p-value less than 0.05 was considered to represent a significant difference. The null hypothesis was that the AUROC of AI and an average human reader were the same. The analysis did not account for the variability between the individual radiologists. A maximum of the Youden Index was used to determine an optimal cut-off value for the radiologists and AI metrics [39,40]. ROC analysis was used to select the cut-off in order to minimize the subjective perception of the probability scales by radiologists.

3. Results

3.1. Chest X-ray

The ROC analysis results for all readers and the AI models are shown in Figure 3a. The threshold for AI was 0.23 (Youden index was 0.75); for human readers, the threshold was 3 (Youden index was 0.84). The AI model achieved an AUROC of 0.92 (0.85–0.98), while for radiologists, the AUROC was 0.97 (0.94–1.0). In most regions of the ROC curve, AI performed a little worse than an average human reader or at the same level, but without a statistically significant difference (Table 2). AI accuracy metrics appeared to be the most similar when radiologists' had less than one year of experience ($p = 0.76$), as shown in Table 2. Examples of the discrepancy between the ground truth and radiologists' opinions and/or AI results are shown in Figure 4a–c.

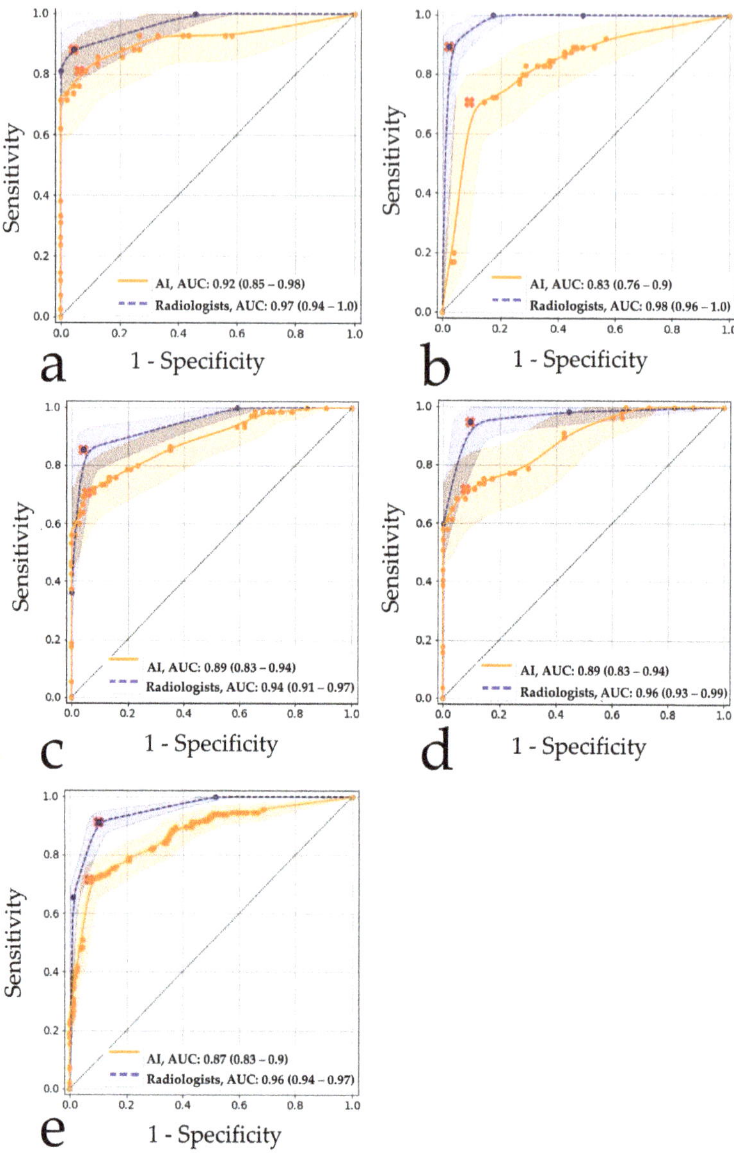

Figure 3. Receiver operator characteristic curves for the human reader study and AI performance on the same datasets: (**a**) Chest X-ray, (**b**) Chest digital fluorography, (**c**) Mammography by all readers, (**d**) Mammography by breast imaging specialists, (**e**) Combined result. Smoothing was used to build the ROC curves. Red markers indicate an operating point determined as the maximum of the Youden index for the readers and AI. The legends display AUC values (95% CI).

Table 2. Human and AI diagnostic performance metrics.

Modality		Diagnostic Performance Metrics				
		AUROC (CI 95%)	Sensitivity * (CI 95%)	Specificity * (CI 95%)	Accuracy * (CI 95%)	*p*-Value (for the AUROC)
X-ray	AI n = 90	0.92 (0.85–0.98)	0.81 (0.66–0.91)	0.94 (0.83–0.99)	0.88 (0.79–0.94)	-
	Radiologists (all) n = 90	0.97 (0.94–1.0)	0.88 (0.74–0.96)	0.96 (0.86–0.99)	0.92 (0.85–0.97)	0.104
	Radiologists (0–1 year) n = 83	0.87 (0.79–0.95)	0.74 (0.57–0.87)	0.96 (0.85–0.99)	0.86 (0.76–0.92)	0.76
	Radiologists (1–5 years) n = 86	0.92 (0.86–0.99)	0.83 (0.69–0.93)	1.00 (0.92–1.00)	0.92 (0.84–0.97)	0.43
	Radiologists (5–10 years) n = 65	0.93 (0.86–1.00)	0.83 (0.65–0.94)	0.97 (0.85–1.00)	0.91 (0.81–0.97)	0.40
	Radiologists (10+ years) n = 84	0.98 (0.96–1.00)	0.92 (0.79–0.98)	0.93 (0.82–0.99)	0.93 (0.85–0.97)	0.08
FLG	AI n = 162	0.83 (0.76–0.9)	0.71 (0.58–0.81)	0.91 (0.83–0.96)	0.83 (0.76–0.88)	-
	Radiologists (all) n = 162	0.98 (0.96–1.00)	0.89 (0.79–0.96)	0.98 (0.93–1.00)	0.94 (0.90–0.97)	0.00 **
	Radiologists (0–1 year) n = 14	0.96 (0.87–1.00)	1.00 (0.63–1.00)	0.83 (0.36–1.00)	0.93 (0.66–1.00)	0.25
	Radiologists (1–5 years) n = 42	0.99 (0.98–1.00)	0.91 (0.72–0.99)	1.00 (0.82–1.00)	0.95 (0.84–0.99)	0.06
	Radiologists (5–10 years) n = 12	1.00 (1.00–1.00)	1.00 (0.48–1.00)	1.00 (0.59–1.00)	1.00 (0.74–1.00)	0.09
	Radiologists (10+ years) n = 27	0.97 (0.90–1.00)	1.00 (0.74–1.00)	0.93 (0.68–1.00)	0.96 (0.81–1.00)	0.04 **
MMG General Radiologists	AI n = 151	0.89 (0.83–0.94)	0.71 (0.59–0.81)	0.95 (0.87–0.99)	0.83 (0.76–0.88)	-
	Radiologists (all) n = 151	0.94 (0.91–0.97)	0.85 (0.75–0.92)	0.96 (0.89–0.99)	0.91 (0.85–0.95)	0.01 **
	Radiologists (0–1 year) n = 15	0.91 (0.77–1.00)	0.88 (0.47–1.00)	0.86 (0.42–1.00)	0.87 (0.60–0.98)	0.33
	Radiologists (1–5 years) n = 62	0.92 (0.87–0.98)	0.77 (0.56–0.91)	0.94 (0.81–0.99)	0.87 (0.76–0.94)	0.15
	Radiologists (5–10 years) n = 35	0.90 (0.78–1.00)	0.83 (0.59–0.96)	0.94 (0.71–1.00)	0.89 (0.73–0.97)	0.26
	Radiologists (10+ years) n = 55	0.97 (0.93–1.00)	0.91 (0.72–0.99)	1.00 (0.89–1.00)	0.96 (0.87–1.00)	0.02 **
MMG Breast Imaging Radiologists	AI n = 120	0.89 (0.83–0.94)	0.72 (0.58–0.83)	0.92 (0.82–0.97)	0.82 (0.75–0.89)	-
	Breast Imaging Radiologists (all) n = 120	0.96 (0.93–0.99)	0.95 (0.85–0.99)	0.90 (0.80–0.96)	0.93 (0.86–0.97)	0.01 **
	Breast Imaging Radiologists (0–1 year) n = 13	0.85 (0.66–1.00)	1.00 (0.63–1.00)	0.60 (0.15–0.95)	0.85 (0.55–0.98)	0.52
	Breast Imaging Radiologists (1–5 years) n = 36	0.88 (0.76–1.00)	0.93 (0.68–1.00)	0.71 (0.48–0.89)	0.81 (0.64–0.92)	0.55
	Breast Imaging Radiologists (5–10 years) n = 58	0.92 (0.85–0.98)	0.88 (0.68–0.97)	0.74 (0.56–0.87)	0.79 (0.67–0.89)	0.10
	Breast Imaging Radiologists (10+ years) n = 109	0.97 (0.94–1.00)	0.91 (0.80–0.97)	0.96 (0.87–1.00)	0.94 (0.87–0.97)	0.001 **
Overall result (X-ray + FLG + MMG)	AI solutions (All) n = 403	0.87 (0.83–0.9)	0.71 (0.64–0.78)	0.93 (0.89–0.96)	0.83 (0.79–0.87)	
	Radiologists and Breast Imaging Radiologists (All) n = 403	0.96 (0.94–0.97)	0.91 (0.86–0.95)	0.90 (0.85–0.94)	0.91 (0.87–0.93)	0.00 **
	Radiologists (0–1 year) n = 112	0.93 (0.89–0.97)	0.93 (0.8–0.98)	0.80 (0.69–0.89)	0.85 (0.77–0.91)	0.65
	Radiologists (1–5 years) n = 190	0.94 (0.91–0.97)	0.89 (0.81–0.94)	0.87 (0.79–0.92)	0.87 (0.83–0.91)	0.02 **
	Radiologists (5–10 years) n = 112	0.95 (0.92–0.98)	0.90 (0.81–0.96)	0.90 (0.82–0.95)	0.90 (0.85–0.94)	0.23
	Radiologists (10+ years) n = 166	0.97 (0.95–0.99)	0.92 (0.86–0.96)	0.91 (0.86–0.95)	0.92 (0.88–0.95)	0.00 **

n, Number of cases. * At the operating point of maximum Youden index. ** Statistically significant difference in AUROC values.

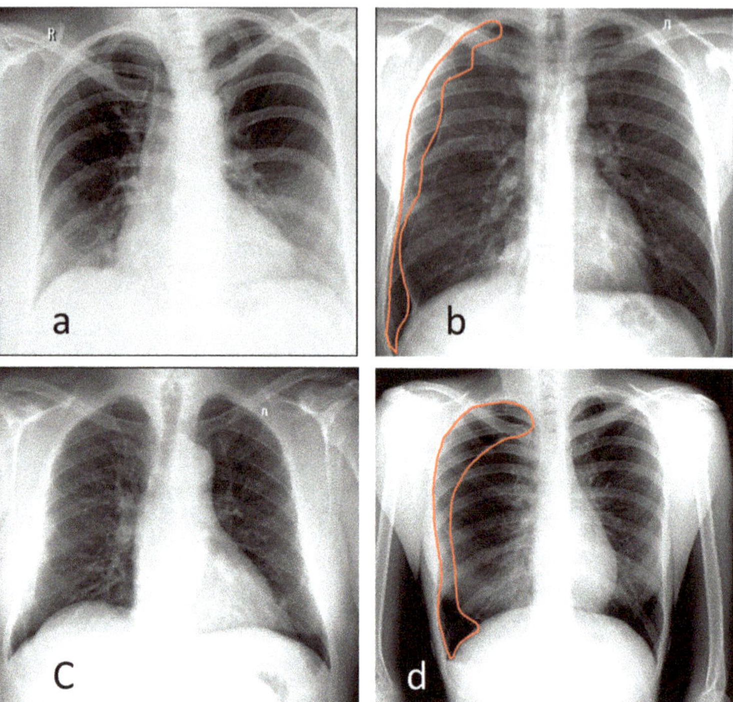

Figure 4. Examples of chest X-rays (**a–c**) and digital fluorography (**d**). (**a**) Radiologists misjudged this case as pathological. Increased opacity in the right- and left-sided lower lobe can be mistakenly interpreted as pneumonia without taking into consideration the patient's suboptimal positioning. The AI models did not detect pathological changes and correctly marked this case as 'without target pathology'. (**b**) AI missed a right-sided pneumothorax (red markup). Radiologists correctly marked this case as pathological. (**c**) Both radiologists and AI misjudged this case as pathological. The only confusing findings included calcified lymph nodes in the right hilum and superposition of anatomical structures. (**d**) AI missed a right-sided pneumothorax (red markup). Radiologists correctly marked this case as pathological.

3.2. Chest Digital Fluorography (FLG)

The ROC analysis results for all readers and the AI models are shown in Figure 3b. The threshold for AI was 0.5 (Youden index was 0.61); for human readers, the threshold was 4 (Youden index was 0.87). A cutoff of 3 (the median of 5-point scale) would reduce the specificity of radiologists to 0.82 (0.79–0.90) but would increase their sensitivity to 1.0 (1.0–1.0). The AI models achieved an AUROC value of 0.83 (0.76–0.9), while radiologists had a higher AUROC of 0.98 (0.96–1.00). The difference between AI and radiologists was statistically significant. Similar to the X-ray use case, AI results were the most comparable to those radiologists with minimal experience ($p = 0.25$) (Table 2). An example of discrepancies in the opinions of AI and radiologists is shown in Figure 4d.

3.3. Mammography (MMG)

The ROC analysis results for all readers and the AI model are illustrated in Figure 3c. The threshold for AI was 0.60 (Youden index was 0.65); for human readers, the threshold it was 3 (Youden index was 0.81). The ROC analysis results for a subgroup of readers, breast imaging specialists and the AI model are shown in Figure 3d. The threshold for breast imaging specialist readers was 3 (Youden index was 0.85). The AI models achieved an AUROC of 0.89 (0.83–0.94) that was lower ($p < 0.05$) than the AUROCs of both general radiologists (0.94 (0.91–0.97)) and breast imaging specialists (0.96 (0.93–0.99)). For both radiologist subgroups, AI models were comparable to the radiologists with less than 5 years of experience. It is worth noting that the dataset used in this study contained an atypical ratio of pathological and normal findings, which could affect the breast imaging specialists' analysis. Therefore, due to their oncological alertness, there was a slight decrease in the average value of specificity. This statement is illustrated by the example in Figure 5.

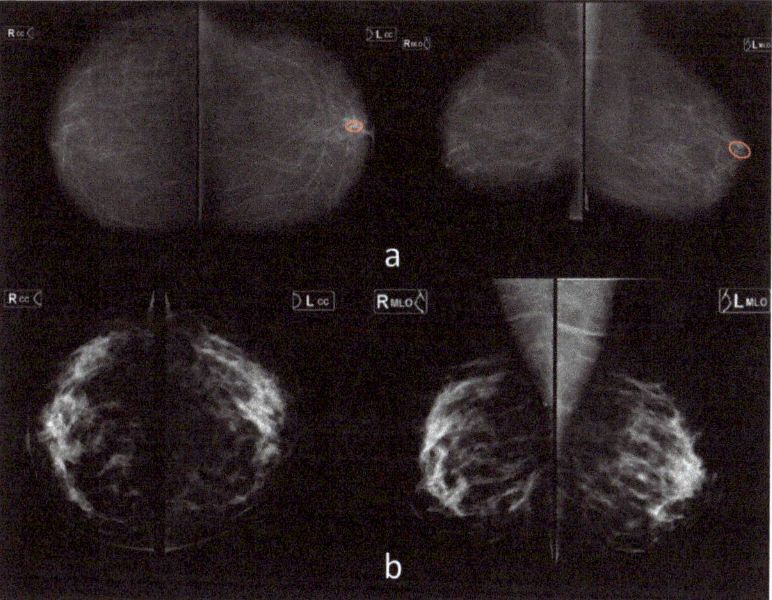

Figure 5. Examples for mammography (**a,b**). (**a**) AI missed a cluster of retroareolar microcalcifications in the left breast (red markup). Radiologists correctly marked this case as pathological. (**b**) Areas of disseminated breast fibroglandular tissue (type C according to ACR) were mistakenly interpreted by breast imaging specialists as suspicious for malignancy. AI did not detect pathological changes.

3.4. Overall

Comparing the average results of the eight AI models, as well as an average assessment of radiologists' performance, the significant differences ($p < 0.05$) in the AUROC values of 0.87 (0.83–0.9) for AI algorithms vs. 0.96 (0.94–0.97) for radiologists were obtained (Figure 3e, Table 2). For the cut-off values calculated by Youden's method, lower values of sensitivity and specificity (95% CIs did not intersect) were detected for AI than for radiologists. Comparison of radiologists' performance with AI revealed the best match with the group of least experienced radiologists ($p = 0.65$) (Table 2). Diagnostic accuracy metrics per AI model are shown in the Supplementary Materials (Table S2).

4. Discussion

The diagnostic accuracy of any method, including an AI model, is a key parameter when making a decision regarding the practical applicability of this method in medicine. Some studies demonstrated an increase in the diagnostic accuracy metrics of a radiologist using an AI model [4,34]. Our work aimed to benchmark radiologists and AI in interpreting images independently. Currently, the question concerning the applicability of AI to interpret screening studies remains open. Several studies have demonstrated the high diagnostic accuracy of AI algorithms for screening studies such as mammography [13,30–32] and chest X-ray [7,18,33]. In a double reading setting, such as in Europe, highly accurate AI models could alleviate the person-power needed for the interpretation, reaching the consensus of two radiologists. However, several studies [4,17,34,40] have indicated a lack of accuracy of AI algorithms. In this study, we compared the average accuracy of AI screening models with the average accuracy of radiologists. This study is important because it not only evaluated the diagnostic accuracy of radiologists in various types of examinations, but also compared the performance of general radiologists with that of mammography specialists.

A collective performance assessment was applied to the groups of radiologists with different levels of experience to estimate the necessary requirements for AI to be able to substitute human readers for mass screening and routine examinations. The collective evaluation of radiologists' responses demonstrated the variability of their accuracy depending on their experience and specialization. A similar calculation was also carried out for all participating AI models to calibrate and combine their responses. The use of the binary criteria 'with pathology' and 'without pathology' allowed the unification of the assessment criteria for radiologists and AI, and ensured their objective comparison for the triage and detection tasks (identifying pathological changes in a study); however, it did not facilitate the comparison of accuracy in solving a classification and differential diagnosis task. It is currently strongly recommended to compare the AI models and healthcare professionals on the same datasets for an objective comparison [41]. In our study, all results were received on the same samples. The values of the diagnostic accuracy metrics obtained in this study could be used as a threshold for a successful validation of adaptive AI models during the acceptance tests [42].

A comparative accuracy assessment of the detection of pathological signs in mammography and fluorographic images between radiologists and AI showed that the diagnostic accuracy metrics of radiologists exceeded those of AI, and this was statistically significant. However, for chest X-ray, our study showed no statistically significant differences between AI and radiologists, which was consistent with the results of Wu et al. [18]. This implies the potential for using AI algorithms for the preliminary interpretation of chest X-ray under conditions of a staff shortage [18]. Regarding mammography, a study by McKinney et al. [14] was indicative, in which the AI model was not inferior in performance to breast imaging specialists and allowed radiologists to reduce the workload on doctors by up to 88%. The other group [4] came to similar conclusions. In contrast to the results of the work of McKinney S.M. [14], in our study, the accuracy metrics of the average radiologists were higher than those of the AI models. None of the AI models surpassed radiologists in this study. However, this study emphasizes the potential of using machine learning techniques to improve the interpretation of screening mammography by radiologists without significant experience in breast imaging.

In the present study, the data obtained clearly demonstrated that AI models exhibited superior diagnostic accuracy compared to novice radiologists. This finding aligns with previous research studies that have also reported the effectiveness of AI models in improving diagnostic accuracy [43] The results suggest that AI models have the potential to serve as decision support systems (DSS) for novice radiologists, assisting them in their training and enhancing the quality of their work. In conclusion, the data from this study support the notion that AI models outperform novice radiologists in terms of diagnostic accuracy, which is consistent with previous research. The potential use of AI models as DSS tools for beginners holds promise in improving their training and improving the quality of their work. More research and implementation efforts are needed to explore the optimal integration of AI models into radiology practice and to assess their long-term impact on patient outcomes.

In this study, we conducted a comparison of diagnostic accuracy between a radiologist and AI algorithms. Our findings clearly demonstrated that, as the radiologist's experience increased, quality indicators also improved. This indicates that with an increasing number of examined studies, the accuracy of the radiologists' work tends to increase. Similarly, the same observation can be made for AI algorithms: the larger the dataset used for training, the higher the quality of the AI model. To provide context, some researchers have used a significant dataset of 108,948 [44] studies when developing AI for chest radiography.

On average, a radiologist interprets 50 examinations per shift. Therefore, over a period of 10 years, a radiologist would review slightly more than 120,000 studies. Consequently, the number of studies evaluated by a radiologist in a 10-year period can be considered comparable to the dataset on which an AI algorithm could be trained.

Due to the lack of radiologists and a continuous increase in the amount of routine radiology examinations, the use of AI will make it possible to revise the healthcare development pathway for radiology [45]. For example, instead of the increase in the number of radiology residents to fulfill primary healthcare needs, one could shift the pathway to the direction of narrower specialization and expertise for the radiologists, while leaving routine screening studies to AI.

5. Conclusions

Benchmarking of AI models and radiologists on a multicenter and multinational level demonstrated that the overall accuracy of AI was lower than the accuracy of the radiologists. The AI and radiologists' performance levels were the most comparable for chest X-ray. In contrast, AI was inferior to human readers for fluorography and mammography. Similar to previous studies, the diagnostic accuracy of AI can be compared with physicians undergoing residency training in radiology. In summary, this study showed that the application of existing AI models for routine and mass screening in radiology is possible as a substitute for residency trainees in their first reading to reduce the workload of radiologists. The diagnostic accuracy metrics for screening methods of the average radiologist obtained in this work can be used as target values in the development, training and fine-tuning of AI algorithms.

6. Limitation

The current study was limited by the relatively small size of the dataset; thus, the diagnostic accuracy metrics of separate pathological findings with sufficient statistical significance could not be calculated.

The limitations of the study from the radiologists' point of view included the lack of clinical information, the limited functionality of the DICOM web viewer, a sample of studies enriched with pathologies that differed from routine practice and a strictly algorithmic probability model for interpreting the studies.

In this work, AI models were used in versions that were relevant at the end of 2021.

Supplementary Materials: The following supporting information can be downloaded at: https://www.mdpi.com/article/10.3390/healthcare11121684/s1, Table S1: Details of AI models; Table S2: Diagnostic performance metrics per AI model.

Author Contributions: Conceptualization, Y.V. and A.V.; methodology, A.A.; software, Y.K.; validation, T.B.; formal analysis, D.K., I.G. and P.G.; investigation, D.K., I.G. and P.G.; resources, O.O.; data curation, A.V.; writing—original draft preparation, K.A.; writing—review and editing K.A. and A.A.; visualization, Y.K.; supervision, A.V. and Y.V.; project administration, I.S.; funding acquisition, O.O. All authors have read and agreed to the published version of the manuscript.

Funding: This paper was prepared by a group of authors as a part of the medical research project No. USIS (in the Unified States Information System for Accounting of Research, Development, and Technological Works): 122112400040–1: "Reference datasets for sustainable development of artificial intelligence-based diagnostics to minimize the long-term impact of the COVID-19 pandemic on the health of the Moscow population".

Institutional Review Board Statement: This study was conducted in accordance with the Declaration of Helsinki and approved by the Independent Ethics Committee of MRO RORR (protocol code 2/2020, date of approval 20 February 2020). Clinical trial: NCT04489992.

Informed Consent Statement: Separate informed consent was not required for this retrospective study.

Data Availability Statement: The data presented in this study are available on request from: [https://mosmed.ai/en/datasets/, accessed on 1 June 2023] or from the corresponding author. The datasets are not publicly available due to them still being used to test AI systems participating in the experiment on the use of innovative computer vision technologies for medical image analysis and their subsequent applicability in the healthcare system of Moscow.

Acknowledgments: We would like to express our great appreciation to Nikolai Pavlov, Victor Gombolevskiy and Ksenia Evteeva for assisting in the multi-reader study, and to Tatiana Logunova for providing radiological image analysis and expert assistance.

Conflicts of Interest: The authors declare no conflict of interest.

References

1. Yu, K.-H.; Lee, T.-L.M.; Yen, M.-H.; Kou, S.C.; Rosen, B.; Chiang, J.-H.; Kohane, I.S. Reproducible Machine Learning Methods for Lung Cancer Detection Using Computed Tomography Images: Algorithm Development and Validation. *J. Med. Internet Res.* **2020**, *22*, e16709. [CrossRef]
2. Herron, J.; Reynolds, J.H. Trends in the on-call workload of radiologists. *Clin. Radiol.* **2006**, *61*, 91–96. [CrossRef]
3. Seibert, J.A. Projection X-ray Imaging: Radiography, Mammography, Fluoroscopy. *Health Phys.* **2019**, *116*, 148–156. [CrossRef]
4. Schaffter, T.; Buist, D.S.M.; Lee, C.I.; Nikulin, Y.; Ribli, D.; Guan, Y.; Lotter, W.; Jie, Z.; Du, H.; Wang, S.; et al. Evaluation of Combined Artificial Intelligence and Radiologist Assessment to Interpret Screening Mammograms. *JAMA Netw. Open* **2020**, *3*, e200265. [CrossRef]
5. *Screening Programmes: A Short Guide. Increase Effectiveness, Maximize Benefits and Minimize Harm*; WHO Regional Office for Europe: Copenhagen, Denmark, 2020. Available online: https://apps.who.int/iris/bitstream/handle/10665/330829/9789289054782-eng.pdf (accessed on 22 July 2021).
6. *Use of Chest Imaging in COVID-19: A Rapid Advice Guide*; World Health Organization: Geneva, Switzerland, 2020. Available online: https://img-cdn.tinkoffjournal.ru/-/who-2019-ncov-clinical-radiology_imaging-20201-eng-1.pdf (accessed on 1 June 2023).
7. Adams, S.J.; Henderson, R.D.E.; Yi, X.; Babyn, P. Artificial Intelligence Solutions for Analysis of X-ray Images. *Can. Assoc. Radiol. J.* **2021**, *72*, 60–72. [CrossRef]
8. Alexander, A.; Jiang, A.; Ferreira, C.; Zurkiya, D. An Intelligent Future for Medical Imaging: A Market Outlook on Artificial Intelligence for Medical Imaging. *J. Am. Coll. Radiol.* **2020**, *17*, 165–170. [CrossRef]
9. Raya-Povedano, J.L.; Romero-Martín, S.; Elías-Cabot, E.; Gubern-Mérida, A.; Rodríguez-Ruiz, A.; Álvarez-Benito, M. AI-based Strategies to Reduce Workload in Breast Cancer Screening with Mammography and Tomosynthesis: A Retrospective Evaluation. *Radiology* **2021**, *300*, 57–65. [CrossRef] [PubMed]
10. Litjens, G.; Kooi, T.; Bejnordi, B.E.; Setio, A.A.A.; Ciompi, F.; Ghafoorian, M.; van der Laak, J.A.W.M.; van Ginneken, B.; Sánchez, C.I. A survey on deep learning in medical image analysis. *Med. Image Anal.* **2017**, *42*, 60–88. [CrossRef] [PubMed]
11. Tadavarthi, Y.; Vey, B.; Krupinski, E.; Prater, A.; Gichoya, J.; Safdar, N.; Trivedi, H. The State of Radiology AI: Considerations for Purchase Decisions and Current Market Offerings. *Radiol. Artif. Intell.* **2020**, *2*, e200004. [CrossRef]
12. Omoumi, P.; Ducarouge, A.; Tournier, A.; Harvey, H.; Kahn, C.E.; Verchère, F.L.-D.; Dos Santos, D.P.; Kober, T.; Richiardi, J. To buy or not to buy—Evaluating commercial AI solutions in radiology (the ECLAIR guidelines). *Eur. Radiol.* **2021**, *31*, 3786–3796. [CrossRef] [PubMed]
13. Rodriguez-Ruiz, A.; Lång, K.; Gubern-Merida, A.; Broeders, M.; Gennaro, G.; Clauser, P.; Helbich, T.H.; Chevalier, M.; Tan, T.; Mertelmeier, T.; et al. Stand-Alone Artificial Intelligence for Breast Cancer Detection in Mammography: Comparison With 101 Radiologists. *JNCI J. Natl. Cancer Inst.* **2019**, *111*, 916–922. [CrossRef] [PubMed]
14. McKinney, S.M.; Sieniek, M.; Godbole, V.; Godwin, J.; Antropova, N.; Ashrafian, H.; Back, T.; Chesus, M.; Corrado, G.S.; Darzi, A.; et al. International evaluation of an AI system for breast cancer screening. *Nature* **2020**, *577*, 89–94. [CrossRef]
15. WHO Issues First Global Report on Artificial Intelligence (AI) in Health and Six Guiding Principles for Its Design and Use. 2021. Available online: https://www.who.int/news/item/28-06-2021-who-issues-first-global-report-on-ai-in-health-and-six-guiding-principles-for-its-design-and-use (accessed on 1 June 2023).
16. Elmore, J.G.; Jackson, S.L.; Abraham, L.; Miglioretti, D.L.; Carney, P.A.; Geller, B.M.; Yankaskas, B.C.; Kerlikowske, K.; Onega, T.; Rosenberg, R.D.; et al. Variability in interpretive performance at screening mammography and radiologists' characteristics associated with accuracy. *Radiology* **2009**, *253*, 641–651. [CrossRef] [PubMed]
17. Lehman, C.D.; Wellman, R.D.; Buist, D.S.M.; Kerlikowske, K.; Tosteson, A.N.A.; Miglioretti, D.L. Diagnostic accuracy of digital screening mammography with and without computer-aided detection. *JAMA Intern. Med.* **2015**, *175*, 1828–1837. [CrossRef] [PubMed]
18. Wu, J.T.; Wong, K.C.L.; Gur, Y.; Ansari, N.; Karargyris, A.; Sharma, A.; Morris, M.; Saboury, B.; Ahmad, H.; Boyko, O.; et al. Comparison of Chest Radiograph Interpretations by Artificial Intelligence Algorithm vs Radiology Residents. *JAMA Netw. Open* **2020**, *3*, e2022779. [CrossRef]

19. Thammarach, P.; Khaengthanyakan, S.; Vongsurakrai, S.; Phienphanich, P.; Pooprasert, P.; Yaemsuk, A.; Vanichvarodom, P.; Munpolsri, N.; Khwayotha, S.; Lertkowit, M.; et al. AI Chest 4 All. In Proceedings of the 2020 42nd Annual International Conference of the IEEE Engineering in Medicine & Biology Society (EMBC), Montreal, QC, Canada, 20–24 July 2020; pp. 1229–1233. [CrossRef]

20. Singh, R.; Kalra, M.K.; Nitiwarangkul, C.; Patti, J.A.; Homayounieh, F.; Padole, A.; Rao, P.; Putha, P.; Muse, V.V.; Sharma, A.; et al. Deep learning in chest radiography: Detection of findings and presence of change. *PLoS ONE* **2018**, *13*, e0204155. [CrossRef]

21. Hansell, D.M.; Bankier, A.A.; MacMahon, H.; McLoud, T.C.; Müller, N.L.; Remy, J. Fleischner Society: Glossary of Terms for Thoracic Imaging. *Radiology* **2008**, *246*, 697–722. [CrossRef]

22. Breast Imaging Reporting & Data System | American College of Radiology [Internet]. Available online: https://www.acr.org/Clinical-Resources/Reporting-and-Data-Systems/Bi-Rads. (accessed on 1 June 2023).

23. Hwang, E.J.; Nam, J.G.; Lim, W.H.; Park, S.J.; Jeong, Y.S.; Kang, J.H.; Hong, E.K.; Kim, T.M.; Goo, J.M.; Park, S.; et al. Deep Learning for Chest Radiograph Diagnosis in the Emergency Department. *Radiology* **2019**, *293*, 573–580. [CrossRef]

24. Ftizisbiomed. Available online: https://ftizisbiomed.ru/#test (accessed on 1 June 2023).

25. Nitris, L.; Zhukov, E.; Blinov, D.; Gavrilov, P.; Blinova, E.; Lobishcheva, A. Advanced neural network solution for detection of lung pathology and foreign body on chest plain radiographs. *Imaging Med.* **2019**, *11*, 57–66. [CrossRef]

26. Sirazitdinov, I.; Kholiavchenko, M.; Mustafaev, T.; Yixuan, Y.; Kuleev, R.; Ibragimov, B. Deep neural network ensemble for pneumonia localization from a large-scale chest x-ray database. *Comput. Electr. Eng.* **2019**, *78*, 388–399. [CrossRef]

27. Celsus - Medical Screening Systems. Available online: https://celsus.ai/en/products-fluorography/ (accessed on 1 June 2023).

28. Kim, H.-E.; Kim, H.H.; Han, B.-K.; Kim, K.H.; Han, K.; Nam, H.; Lee, E.H.; Kim, E.-K. Changes in cancer detection and false-positive recall in mammography using artificial intelligence: A retrospective, multireader study. *Lancet Digit. Health* **2020**, *2*, e138–e148. [CrossRef]

29. Karpov, O.; Bronov, O.; Kapninskiy, A.; Pavlovich, P.; Abovich, Y.; Subbotin, S.; Sokolova, S.; Rychagova, N.; Milova, A.; Nikitin, E. Comparative study of data analysis results of digital mammography AI-based system «CELSUS» and radiologists. *Bull. Pirogov. Natl. Med. Surg. Cent.* **2021**, *16*, 86–92. [CrossRef]

30. Mayo, R.C.; Kent, D.; Sen, L.C.; Kapoor, M.; Leung, J.W.T.; Watanabe, A.T. Reduction of False-Positive Markings on Mammograms: A Retrospective Comparison Study Using an Artificial Intelligence-Based CAD. *J. Digit. Imaging* **2019**, *32*, 618–624. [CrossRef]

31. Rodríguez-Ruiz, A.; Krupinski, E.; Mordang, J.-J.; Schilling, K.; Heywang-Köbrunner, S.H.; Sechopoulos, I.; Mann, R.M. Detection of Breast Cancer with Mammography: Effect of an Artificial Intelligence Support System. *Radiology* **2019**, *290*, 305–314. [CrossRef]

32. Wu, N.; Phang, J.; Park, J.; Shen, Y.; Huang, Z.; Zorin, M.; Jastrzebski, S.; Fevry, T.; Katsnelson, J.; Kim, E.; et al. Deep Neural Networks Improve Radiologists' Performance in Breast Cancer Screening. *IEEE Trans. Med. Imaging* **2019**, *39*, 1184–1194. [CrossRef] [PubMed]

33. Majkowska, A.; Mittal, S.; Steiner, D.F.; Reicher, J.J.; McKinney, S.M.; Duggan, G.E.; Eswaran, K.; Chen, P.-H.C.; Liu, Y.; Kalidindi, S.R.; et al. Chest Radiograph Interpretation with Deep Learning Models: Assessment with Radiologist-adjudicated Reference Standards and Population-adjusted Evaluation. *Radiology* **2020**, *294*, 421–431. [CrossRef] [PubMed]

34. Freeman, K.; Geppert, J.; Stinton, C.; Todkill, D.; Johnson, S.; Clarke, A.; Taylor-Phillips, S. Use of artificial intelligence for image analysis in breast cancer screening programmes: Systematic review of test accuracy. *BMJ* **2021**, *374*, n1872. [CrossRef] [PubMed]

35. Seah, J.C.Y.; Tang, C.H.M.; Buchlak, Q.D.; Holt, X.G.; Wardman, J.B.; Aimoldin, A.; Esmaili, N.; Ahmad, H.; Pham, H.; Lambert, J.F.; et al. Effect of a comprehensive deep-learning model on the accuracy of chest x-ray interpretation by radiologists: A retrospective, multireader multicase study. *Lancet Digit. Health* **2021**, *3*, e496–e506. [CrossRef]

36. Murphy, K.; Smits, H.; Knoops, A.J.G.; Korst, M.B.J.M.; Samson, T.; Scholten, E.T.; Schalekamp, S.; Schaefer-Prokop, C.M.; Philipsen, R.H.H.M.; Meijers, A.; et al. COVID-19 on chest radiographs: A multireader evaluation of an artificial intelligence system. *Radiology* **2020**, *296*, E166–E172. [CrossRef]

37. Sun, X.; Xu, W. Fast Implementation of DeLong's Algorithm for Comparing the Areas Under Correlated Receiver Operating Characteristic Curves. *IEEE Signal Process. Lett.* **2014**, *21*, 1389–1393. [CrossRef]

38. Pauly, M.; Asendorf, T.; Konietschke, F. Permutation-based inference for the AUC: A unified approach for continuous and discontinuous data. *Biom. J.* **2016**, *58*, 1319–1337. [CrossRef] [PubMed]

39. Youden, W.J. Index for rating diagnostic tests. *Cancer* **1950**, *3*, 32–35. [CrossRef] [PubMed]

40. Ruopp, M.D.; Perkins, N.J.; Whitcomb, B.W.; Schisterman, E.F. Youden Index and optimal cut-point estimated from observations affected by a lower limit of detection. *Biom. J.* **2008**, *50*, 419–430. [CrossRef] [PubMed]

41. Liu, X.; Faes, L.; Kale, A.U.; Wagner, S.K.; Fu, D.J.; Bruynseels, A.; Mahendiran, T.; Moraes, G.; Shamdas, M.; Kern, C.; et al. A comparison of deep learning performance against health-care professionals in detecting diseases from medical imaging: A systematic review and meta-analysis. *Lancet Digit. Health* **2019**, *1*, e271–e297. [CrossRef] [PubMed]

42. Zinchenko, V.; Chetverikov, S.; Akhmad, E.; Arzamasov, K.; Vladzymyrskyy, A.; Andreychenko, A.; Morozov, S. Changes in software as a medical device based on artificial intelligence technologies. *Int. J. Comput. Assist. Radiol. Surg.* **2022**, *17*, 1969–1977. [CrossRef] [PubMed]

43. Dratsch, T.; Chen, X.; Rezazade Mehrizi, M.; Kloeckner, R.; Mähringer-Kunz, A.; Püsken, M.; Baeßler, B.; Sauer, S.; Maintz, D.; dos Santos, D.P. Automation Bias in Mammography: The Impact of Artificial Intelligence BI-RADS Suggestions on Reader Performance. *Radiology* **2023**, *307*, e222176. [CrossRef]

44. Wang, X.; Peng, Y.; Lu, L.; Lu, Z.; Bagheri, M.; Summers, R.M. ChestX-Ray8: Hospital-Scale Chest X-Ray Database and Benchmarks on Weakly-Supervised Classification and Localization of Common Thorax Diseases. In Proceedings of the 2017 IEEE Conference on Computer Vision and Pattern Recognition (CVPR), Honolulu, HI, USA, 21–26 July 2017; pp. 3462–3471. [CrossRef]
45. Gusev, A.V.; Vladzymyrskyy, A.V.; Sharova, D.E.; Arzamasov, K.M.; Khramov, A.E. Evolution of research and development in the field of artificial intelligence technologies for healthcare in the Russian Federation: Results of 2021. *Digit. Diagn.* **2022**, *3*, 178–194. [CrossRef]

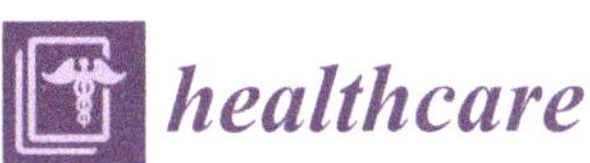

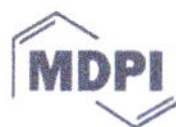

Article

Deep Learning-Based Prediction of Diabetic Retinopathy Using CLAHE and ESRGAN for Enhancement

Ghadah Alwakid [1], Walaa Gouda [2] and Mamoona Humayun [3,*]

[1] Department of Computer Science, College of Computer and Information Sciences, Jouf University, Sakakah 72341, Al Jouf, Saudi Arabia; gnalwakid@ju.edu.sa

[2] Department of Electrical Engineering, Faculty of Engineering at Shoubra, Benha University, Cairo 11672, Egypt; walaa.gouda@feng.bu.edu.eg

[3] Department of Information Systems, College of Computer and Information Sciences, Jouf University, Sakakah 72341, Al Jouf, Saudi Arabia

* Correspondence: mahumayun@ju.edu.sa

Abstract: Vision loss can be avoided if diabetic retinopathy (DR) is diagnosed and treated promptly. The main five DR stages are none, moderate, mild, proliferate, and severe. In this study, a deep learning (DL) model is presented that diagnoses all five stages of DR with more accuracy than previous methods. The suggested method presents two scenarios: case 1 with image enhancement using a contrast limited adaptive histogram equalization (CLAHE) filtering algorithm in conjunction with an enhanced super-resolution generative adversarial network (ESRGAN), and case 2 without image enhancement. Augmentation techniques were then performed to generate a balanced dataset utilizing the same parameters for both cases. Using Inception-V3 applied to the Asia Pacific Tele-Ophthalmology Society (APTOS) datasets, the developed model achieved an accuracy of 98.7% for case 1 and 80.87% for case 2, which is greater than existing methods for detecting the five stages of DR. It was demonstrated that using CLAHE and ESRGAN improves a model's performance and learning ability.

Keywords: vision loss; diabetic retinopathy; image enhancement; APTOS

Citation: Alwakid, G.; Gouda, W.; Humayun, M. Deep Learning-Based Prediction of Diabetic Retinopathy Using CLAHE and ESRGAN for Enhancement. *Healthcare* **2023**, *11*, 863. https://doi.org/10.3390/ healthcare11060863

Academic Editor: Mahmudur Rahman

Received: 1 February 2023
Revised: 11 March 2023
Accepted: 13 March 2023
Published: 15 March 2023

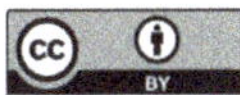

1. Introduction

The progressive eye disease known as DR is a direct result of having mellitus. Increases in blood glucose occur chronically in people with diabetes mellitus where the pancreas does not generate or release enough blood adrenaline [1,2]. Most diabetics go blind from DR, especially those of retirement age in low-income nations. Early identification is crucial for preventing the consequences that can arise from chronic diseases such as diabetes [3,4].

Retinal vasculature abnormalities are the hallmark of DR, which can progress to irreversible vision loss due to scarring or hemorrhage [1,5]. This may cause gradual vision impairment and, in its most severe form, blindness. It is not possible to cure the illness, so treatment focuses on preserving the patient's present level of eyesight [6,7]. In most cases, a patient's sight may be saved if DR is diagnosed and treated as soon as possible. In order to diagnose DR, an ophthalmologist should inspect images of the retina manually, which is an expensive and time-consuming process [8]. The majority of ophthalmologists today still use the tried-and-true method of analyzing retinal pictures for the presence and type of different abnormalities in order to diagnose DR. Microaneurysms (MIA), hemorrhages (HEM), soft exudates (SOX), and hard exudates (HEX) are the four most common forms of lesions identified [1,9], which can be identified as the following:

- In earlier DR, MA appear as tiny, red dots on the retina due to a weakening in the vessel walls. The dots have distinct borders and a dimension of 125 μm or less. There are six subtypes of microaneurysms, but the treatment is the same for all of them [10,11].

- In contrast to MA, HM are characterized by big spots on the retina with uneven edge widths of more than 125 μm. A hemorrhage can be either flame or blot, according to whether the spots are on the surface or deeper in the tissue [12,13].
- The swelling of nerve fibers causes soft exudates, which appear as white ovals on the retina as defined as SX [1,9].
- Yellow spots on the retina, known as EX, are the result of plasma leakage. They extend across the periphery of the retina and have defined borders [1,2].
- Lesions caused by MA and HM tend to be red, while blemishes caused by the two forms of exudates tend to be bright. There are five distinct stages of DR that can be detected: no DR, mild DR, moderate DR, severe DR, and proliferative DR [13], as shown in Figure 1.
- For DR diagnosis to be performed manually, experts in the field are needed, even though the most expert ophthalmologists have problems due to DR variability. Accurate machine learning techniques for automated DR detection have the ability to those defects [2,8].
- Our objective was to develop a quick, fully automated DL based DR categorization that may be used in practice to aid ophthalmologists in assessing DR. DR can be prevented if it is detected and treated quickly after it first appears. To achieve this goal, we trained a model using innovative image preprocessing techniques and an Inception-V3 [14,15] model for diagnosis using the publicly available APTOS dataset [16].

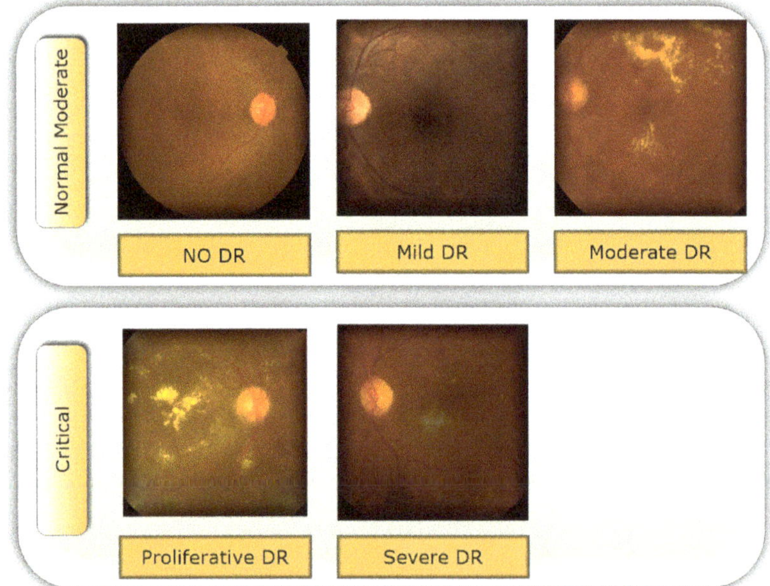

Figure 1. The five phases of diabetic retinopathy, listed by severity.

Below, we highlight the original contributions of our study.

- To generate high-quality images for the APTOS dataset, we used the (CLAHE) [17] filtering algorithm in conjunction with enhanced super-resolution generative adversarial networks (ESRGAN) [18], which is the main contribution of the presented work.
- By employing the technique of augmentation, we ensured that the APTOS dataset contained a consistent amount of data.
- Accuracy (*Acc*), confusion matrix (CM), precision (*Prec*), recall (*Re*), top n accuracy, and the *F1*-score (*F1sc*) were the indicators used in a comprehensive comparative study to determine the viability of the proposed system.

- Pre-trained networks trained on the APTOS data set were fine-tuned with the use of an Inception-V3 weight-tuning algorithm.
- By adopting a varied training procedure backed by various permutations of training strategies, the general reliability of the suggested method was enhanced, and overfitting was avoided (e.g., learning rate, data augmentation, batch size, and validation patience).
- The APTOS dataset was used during both the training and evaluation phases of the model's development. By employing stringent 80:20 hold-out validation, the model achieved a remarkable 98.71% accuracy of classification using enhancement techniques and 80.87% without using enhancement techniques.

This research presents two cases scenarios. In case 1, an optimal technique for DR stage enhancement using CLAHE followed by ESRGAN techniques was developed. In case 2 no enhancement was applied to the images. Due to the class imbalance in the dataset, oversampling was required using augmentation techniques. In addition, we trained the weights of each model using Inception-V3, and the results of the models were compared using APTOS dataset images. Section 2 provides context for the subsequent discussion of the related work. Section 4 presents and analyzes the results of the technique described in Section 3, and Section 5 summarizes the research.

2. Related Work

There are various issues with DR picture detection when done manually. Numerous patients in underdeveloped nations face challenges due to a shortage of competence (trained ophthalmologists) and expensive tests. Because of the importance of timely detection in the fight against blindness, automated processing methods have been devised to facilitate accessibility for accurate and speedy diagnosis and treatment. Automated DR classification accuracy has recently been achieved by Machine Learning (ML) models trained on ocular fundus pictures. A lot of work has gone into developing automatic methods that are both efficient and inexpensive [19–21].

This means that these methods are now universally superior to their traditional counterparts. Following, we present a deeper examination of the two primary schools of thought in DR categorization research: classical, specialist approaches, and state-of-the-art, machine-learning-based approaches. For instance, Kazakh-British et al. [22], performed experimental studies with a relevant processing pipeline that extracted arteries from fundus pictures, and then a CNN model was trained to recognize lesions. Other work presented by Alexandr et al. [23] contrasted two widely-used classic designs (DenseNet and ResNet) with a new, enhanced structure (EfficientNet). Use of the APTOS symposium dataset allowed for the retinal image to be classified into one of five categories. Local binary convolutional neural network (LBCNN) deterministic filter generation was introduced by Macsik et al. [24] which mimicked the successfulness of the CNN with a smaller training set and less memory utilization, making it suitable for systems with limited memory or computing resources. Regarding binary classification of retinal fundus datasets into healthy and diseased groups, they compared their method with traditional CNN and LBCNN that use probabilistic filter sequence.

Al-Antary & Yasmine [19] suggested a multi-scale attention network (MSA-Net) for DR categorization. The encoder network embeds the retina image in a high-level representational space, enriching it with mid- and high-level characteristics. A multi-scale feature pyramid describes the retinal structure in another location. In addition to high-level representation, a multi-scale attention mechanism improves feature representation discrimination. The model classifies DR severity using cross-entropy loss. The model detects healthy and unhealthy retina pictures as an extracurricular assignment using weakly annotations. This surrogate task helps the model recognize non-healthy retina pictures. EyePACS and APTOS datasets performed well with the proposed technique. Medical DR identification was the focus of an investigation by Khalifa et al. [25] on deep transfer learning models. A series of experiments was conducted with the help of the APTOS 2019 dataset. Five different neural network architectures (AlexNet, Res-Net18, SqueezeNet, GoogleNet, VGG16, and VGG19) were used in this research. Selecting models with fewer layers than DenseNet and Inception-Resnet was a key factor. Model stability and overfitting were both enhanced by additional data. Hemanth et al. [26] presented a convolutional neural network–based approach to DR detection and classification. They employed HIST and CLAHE to improve contrast in the images, and the resulting CNN model achieved 97% accuracy in classification and a 94% F-measure. Maqsood et al. [27] introduced a new 3D CNN model to localize hemorrhages, an early indicator of DR, using a pre-trained VGG-19 model to extract characteristics from segmented hemorrhages. Their studies used 1509 photos from HRF, DRIVE, STARE, MESSIDOR, DIARETDB0, and DIARETDB1 databases and averaged 97.71% accuracy. Das et al. [28] suggested a unique CNN for categorizing normal and abnormal patients utilizing the fundus images. The blood arteries were recovered from the images using a maximal principal curvature approach. Adaptive histogram equalization and morphological opening were used to correct improperly segmented regions. The DIARETDB1 dataset was considered, and an accuracy and precision of 98.7% and 97.2%, respectively, was attained.

Wang et al. [29] created Lesion-Net to improve the encoder's representational power by including lesion detection into severity grading. InceptionV3 trained and verified the design. Liu et al. [30] used TL with different models to investigate DR from EyePACS. A new cross-entropy loss function and three hybrid model structures classified DR with 86.34% accuracy.

Table 1 summarizes the many attempts to detect DR anomalies in photos using various DL techniques [19,24,31–37]. According to the results of the research into DR identification and diagnostic methods, there are still a lot of loopholes that need to be investigated. For example, there has been minimal emphasis on constructing and training a bespoke DL model entirely from the beginning because of a lack of a large amount of data, even though numerous researchers have obtained excellent dependability values with pre-trained models using transfer-learning.

Table 1. A review of the literature comparing several DR diagnostic techniques.

Reference	Year	Technique	Total Number of Images	Classes	Dataset	Accuracy	Precision	Recall	Receiver Operating Characteristic ROC
[19]	2021	Multi-scale attention network (MSA-Net)		5	APTOS	84.6%	90.5%	91%	-
					Eyepacs	87.5%	78.7%	90.6%	76.7%
[24]	2022	Local binary convolutional neural network (LBCNN)		2	APTOS	97.41%	96.59%	94.63%	98.71%
[31]	2022	Support vector machine (SVM)	Test: 1928	2	APTOS	94.5%		75.6%	
			Test: 103		IDRiD	93.3%		78.5%	
[32]	2022	CNN		2	APTOS	95.3%			
[33]	2022	Inception-ResNet-v2		5	APTOS	82.18%			
[34]	2021	Squeeze Excitation Densely Connected deep CNN		5	APTOS			96%	
					EyePACS			93%	
[35]	2021	VGG-16	Test = 1728	5	APTOS	74.58%			
[36]	2022	VGG16	13,626	2	APTOS	73.26%	99%	99%	
		DenseNet121				96.11%			
[37]	2022	DenseNet201	3662	5	APTOS	93.85%	90.90%	80.60%	
			2355	3	New Dataset	94.06%	94.74%	94.45%	

Ultimately, training DL models with raw images instead of preprocessed images severely restricts the final classification network's scalability, as was the case in nearly all of these studies. In order to resolve these problems, the current research created a lightweight DR detection system by integrating multiple layers into the architecture of pre-trained models. This leads to a more efficient and effective proposed system that meets users' expectations.

3. Research Methodology

For the DR detection system to operate, as shown in Figure 2, a transfer DL strategy (Inception-V3) was retrained in the image dataset to learn discriminative and usable feature representations. This section offers a concise summary of the method followed when working with the provided dataset. The preprocessing stage is then clearly outlined, and implementation specifics of the proposed system are covered. These include the two cases scenarios used in this context, the preprocessing techniques proposed, the basic design, and the training methodology for the approach that was ultimately chosen.

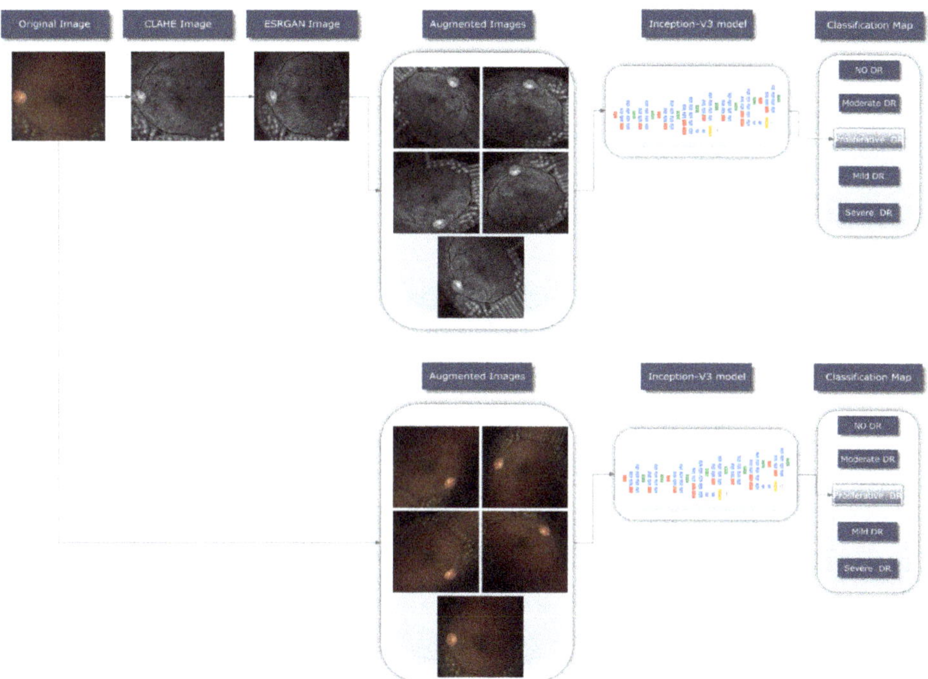

Figure 2. An illustration of the DR detecting system process.

3.1. Data Set Description

Selecting a dataset with a sufficient number of high-quality photos is crucial. This study made use of the APTOS 2019 (Asia Pacific Tele-Ophthalmology Society) Blindness Detection Dataset [16], a publicly available Kaggle dataset that incorporates a huge number of photos. In this collection, high-resolution retinal pictures are provided for the five stages of DR, classified from 0 (none) to 4 (proliferate DR), with labels 1–4 corresponding to the four levels of severity. There are 3662 retinal pictures in total; 1805 are from the "no DR" group, 370 are from the "mild DR" group, 999 are from the "moderate DR" group, 193 are from the "severe DR" group, and 295 are from the "proliferate DR" group, as illustrated in Table 2. Images are 3216 × 2136 pixels in size, and Figure 1 shows some examples of these kind of pictures. There is background noise in the photographs and the labels, much like any real-world data set. It is possible that the provided images will be flawed in some way, be it with artifacts, blurriness, improper exposure, or some other issue. The photos were collected over a long period of time from a number of different clinics using different cameras, all of which contribute to the overall high degree of diversity.

Table 2. Class-Wide Image Distribution.

Class Index	DR Level	# Images
0	No DR	1805
1	Mild DR	370
2	Moderate DR	999
3	Severe DR	193
4	Proliferate DR	295

= number of images.

3.2. Proposed Methodology

An automatic DR classification model was developed using the dataset referenced in this paper; its general process is demonstrated in Figure 1. It demonstrates two different scenarios: case 1 in which the preprocessing step is performed using CLAHE followed by ESRGAN is used, and case 2 in which neither step is performed, while using augmentation of the images to prevent overfitting in both scenarios. Lastly, images were sent into the Inception-V3 model for classification step.

3.2.1. Preprocessing Using CLAHE and ESRGAN

Images of the retinal fundus are often taken from several facilities using various technologies. Consequently, given the high intensity variation in the photographs used by the proposed method, it was crucial to enhance the quality of DR images and get rid of various types of noise. All images in case 1 underwent a preliminary preprocessing phase prior to augmentation, and training necessitated various stages:

1. CLAHE
2. Resize each picture to 224 × 224 × 3 pixels.
3. ESRGAN
4. Normalization

Figure 3 shows that first, CLAHE (shown in Figure 4) was used to improve the DR image's fine details, textures, and low contrast by redistributing the input image's lightness values [38]. Utilizing CLAHE, the input image was first sectioned into four small tiles. Each tile underwent histogram equalization with a clip limit, which involved five steps: computation, excess calculation, distribution, redistribution, and scaling and mapping using a cumulative distribution function (CDF). For each tile, a histogram was calculated, where bins value above the clip limit were aggregated and spread to other bins. Histogram values were then calculated using CDF for the input image pixel scale and then mapped tile to CDF values. To boost contrast, bilinear interpolation stitched the tiles together [39]. This technique improved local contrast enhancement while also making borders and slopes more apparent. Following this, all photos were scaled to suit the input of the learning model, which was 224 × 224 × 3. Figure 3 depicts the subsequent application of ESRGAN on the output of the preceding stage. ESRGAN [40] (shown in Figure 5) pictures can more closely mimic image artifacts' sharp edges [41]. To improve performance, ESRGAN adopted the basic architecture of SRResNet, in which Residual-in-Residual Dense Blocks are substituted for the traditional ESRGAN basic blocks, as shown in Figure 5. Intensity differences between images can be rather large, thus images were normalized so that their intensities fell within the range −1 to 1. This kept the data within acceptable bounds and removed noise. As a result of normalization, the model was less sensitive to variations in weights, making it easier to tune. Since the method shown in Figure 3 improved the image's contrast while simultaneously emphasizing the image's boundaries and arcs, it yielded more accurate findings.

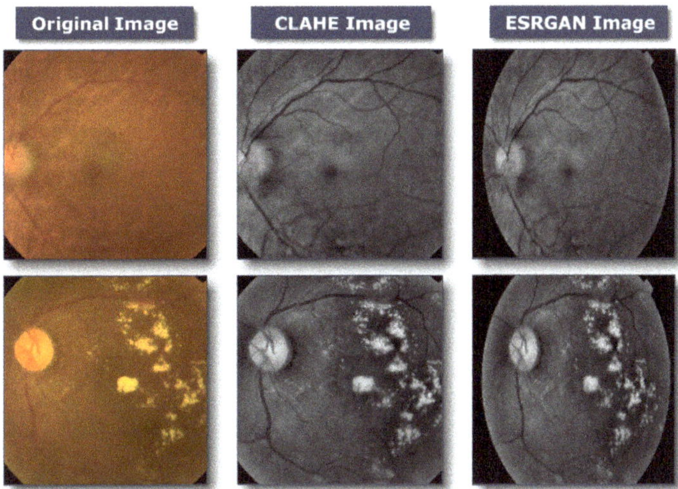

Figure 3. Samples of the proposed image-enhancement techniques: original, unedited image; then rendition of this same image with CLAHE; finally final enhanced image after applying ESRGAN.

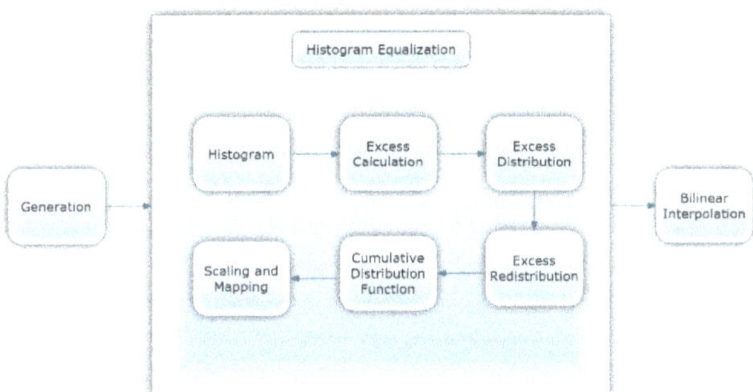

Figure 4. CLAHE architecture.

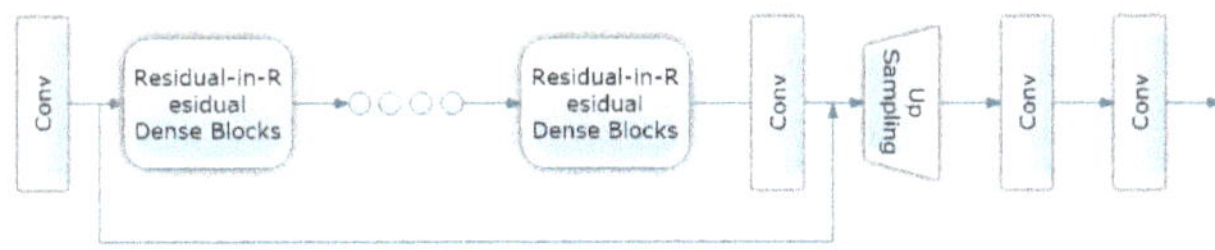

Figure 5. ESRGAN architecture.

3.2.2. Data Augmentation

Data augmentation was implemented on the training set to increase the number of images and alleviate the issue of an imbalanced dataset before exposing Inception-V3 to the dataset images. In most cases, deeper learning models perform better when given more data to learn from. We can utilize the characteristics of DR photos by applying several modifications to each image. A deep neural network (DNN) is unaffected by any changes made to the input image, including scaling it up or down, flipping it horizontally or vertically, or rotating it by a certain number of degrees. Regulating the data, minimizing overfitting, and rectifying imbalances in the dataset are all accomplished through the use of data augmentations (i.e., shifting, rotating, and zooming). One of the transformations used in this investigation was horizontal shift augmentation, which involves shifting the pixels of an image horizontally while maintaining the image's aspect ratio, with the step size being specified by an integer between 0 and 1. Another kind of transformation is rotation, in which the image is arbitrarily rotated by an angle between 0 and 180 degrees. To create fresh samples for the network, all prior alterations to the training set's images were applied.

In this study, two scenarios were utilized to train Inception-V3. The first was to apply augmentation to the enhanced images, as depicted in Figure 6, and the second was to apply augmentation to the raw images, as depicted in Figure 7. Both Figures 4 and 5 are attempts to expand data volume by making slightly modified copies of current data or by synthesizing data generated from existing data while keeping all other parameters constant (Figures 4 and 5), with the same total number of images in both cases.

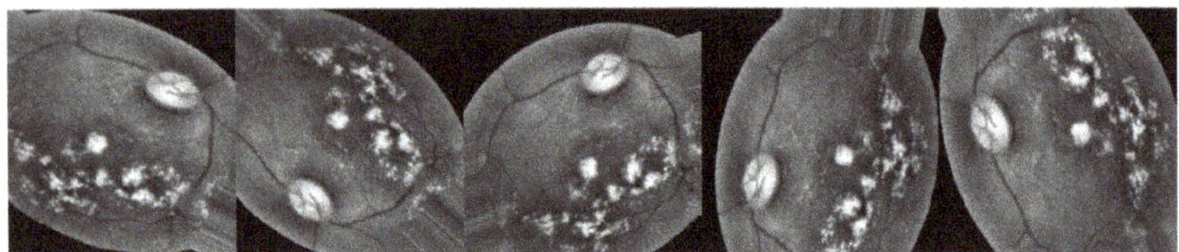

Figure 6. Illustrations of the same image, augmented with enhancement.

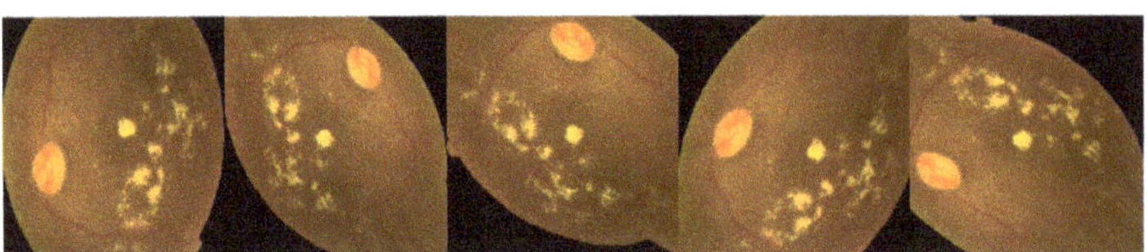

Figure 7. Illustrations of the same image augmented without enhancement.

In a second use of data augmentation techniques, the issues of inconsistent sample sizes and complicated classifications were resolved. As seen in Table 2, the APTOS dataset exemplifies the "imbalanced class" because the samples are not distributed evenly throughout the several classes. After applying augmentation techniques to the dataset, the classes are obviously balanced for both scenarios, as depicted in Figure 8.

3.2.3. Learning Model (Inception-V3)

In this section, the approach's fundamental theory is outlined and explained. Inception-v3 [11,12] is among transfer learning pretrained models, superseding the original architecture for Inception-v1 [42] and Inception-v2 [43]. The Inception-v3 model is trained using the ImageNet datasets [44,45], which contain the information required for identifying one thousand classes. The error rate for the top five in ImageNet is 3.5%, while the error rate for the top one was lowered to 17.3%.

Inception was influenced in particular by technique of Serre et al. [46], which processes information in several stages. By adopting the Lin et al. [47] method, the developers of Inception were able to improve the model precision of the neural networks, making them a significant design requirement. As a result of the dimension reduction to 1*1 convolutions, this also protected them from computing constraints. Researchers were able to significantly reduce the amount of time and effort spent on DL picture classification using Inception [48]. Using only the theoretical explanations offered by Arora et al. [49], they emphasized discovering an optimal spot between the typical technique of improving performance—increasing both depth and size—and layer separability. When utilized independently, both procedures are computationally expensive. This was the fundamental goal of the 22-layer architecture employed by the Inception DL system, in which all filters are learned. On the basis of research by Arora et al. [49], a correlation statistical analysis was developed to generate highly associated categories that were input into the subsequent layer. The 1×1 layer, the 3×3 layer, and the 5×5 convolution layer were all inspired by the concept of multiscale processing of visual data. Each of these layers eventually becomes a set of 1×1 convolutions [48] following a process of dimension reduction.

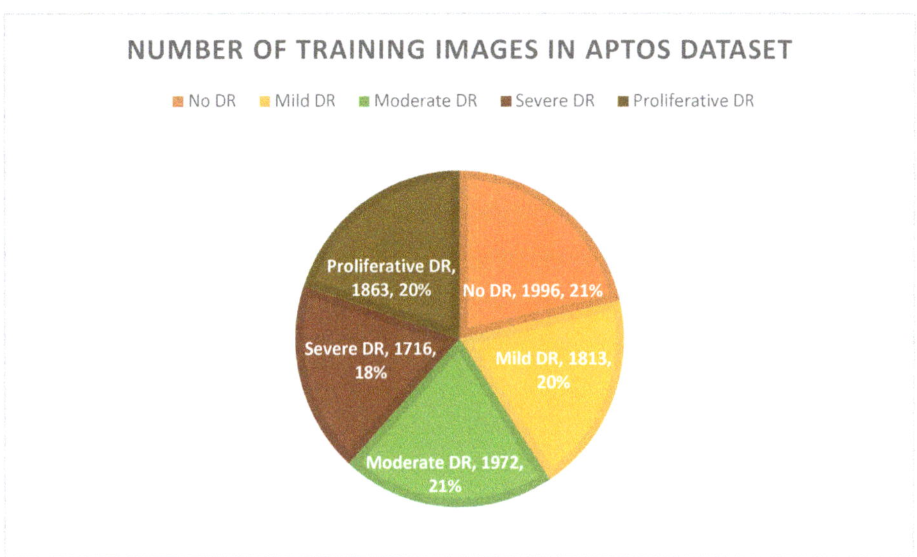

Figure 8. Number of training images after using augmentation techniques.

4. Experimental Results

4.1. Instruction and Setup of Inception-V3

To demonstrate the effectiveness of the deployed DL system and to compare results to industry standards, tests were carried out on the APTOS dataset. The dataset was divided into three categories in accordance with the suggested training method. Eighty percent of the data was utilized for training (9952 photographs), ten percent for testing (1012 photos), and the remaining ten percent was randomly selected and used as a validation set (1025 photos) to evaluate performance and save the best weight combinations. All photographs were reduced in size during the training process to $224 \times 224 \times 3$ pixel resolution. We tested the proposed system's TensorFlow Keras implementation on a Linux desktop equipped with a GPU RTX3060 and 8 GB of RAM.

Using the Adam optimizer and a method that slows down training when learning has stalled for too long, the proposed framework was first trained on the APTOS dataset (i.e., validation patience). Throughout the entirety of the training process, hyperparameters were input into the Adam optimizer. We used a range of 1×10^3 to 1×10^5 for the learning rate, 2–64 for the batch size (with an increase of $2 \times$ the previous value), 50 epochs, 10 for patience, and 0.90 for momentum. Our arsenal of anti-infectious measures was completed by a method known as "batching" for the dissemination of infectious forms.

4.2. Evaluative Parameters

This section describes the evaluation methods and their results. Classifier accuracy (*Acc*) is a standard performance measure. It is determined by dividing the number of successfully categorized instances (images) by the total number of examples in the dataset (Equation (1)). Picture categorization systems are often evaluated using precision (*Prec*) and recall (*Re*). As demonstrated in Equation (2), precision improves with the number of accurately labeled photos, whereas recall is the ratio of properly categorized images in the dataset to those related numerically (3). The higher the *F1*-score, the more reliable the system is at making predictions about the future. The *F1*-score can be determined using Equation (4), (*F1sc*). With respect to the study's last criterion, top N accuracy, it was found that the highest probability answers from model N should coincide with the expected softmax distribution. An accurate classification is made if at least one of N predictions corresponds to the target label.

$$Accuracy = \frac{T^p + T^n}{T^p + T^n + F^p + F^n} \tag{1}$$

$$Precision = \frac{T^p}{T^p + F^p} \tag{2}$$

$$Recall = \frac{T^p}{T^p + F^n} \tag{3}$$

$$F1\text{-}score = 2 * \left(\frac{Prec * Re}{Prec + Re} \right) \tag{4}$$

True positives, represented by the symbol (T^p), are successfully anticipated positive cases, and true negatives (T^n) are effectively predicted negative scenarios. False positives (F^p) are falsely predicted positive situations, whereas false negatives (F^n) are falsely projected negative situations.

4.3. Performance of Inception-V3 Model Outcomes

Considering the APTOS dataset, two distinct cases sets were investigated, in which Inception-V3 was applied to our dataset in two distinct scenarios, the first with enhancement (CLAHE + ESRGAN) and the second without enhancement (CLAHE + ESRGAN), as depicted in Figure 2. We split it up this way to cut down on the total amount of time needed to conduct the project. To train a model, 50 epochs were used, with learning rates ranging from 1×10^3 to 1×10^5, and batch sizes varying from 2 to 64. To achieve the highest possible level of precision, Inception-V3 was further tweaked by freezing between 140 and 160 layers. Several iterations of the same model with the same parameters were used to generate a model ensemble, since random weights were generated for each iteration, the precision fluctuated from iteration to iteration. Mean and standard deviation statistics for this procedure are displayed in Tables 3 and 4, respectively, for the cases where the first 143 layers were frozen with CLAHE + ESRGAN and the cases where they were not.

Table 3. Average and standard deviation accuracy with enhancement (CLAHE + ESRGAN).

Batch Size	Learning Rate	Accuracy	Mean	Standard Deviation
	0.00001	0.983202		
2	0.0001	0.983202	0.982543	0.001140989
	0.001	0.981225		
	0.00001	0.982213		
4	0.0001	0.982213	0.982213	0
	0.001	0.982213		
	0.00001	0.982213		
8	0.0001	0.987154	0.980237	0.008088282
	0.001	0.971344		

Table 3. *Cont.*

Batch Size	Learning Rate	Accuracy	Mean	Standard Deviation
	0.00001	0.980237		
16	0.0001	0.982213	0.980896	0.001141024
	0.001	0.980237		
	0.00001	0.979249		
32	0.0001	0.978261	0.979249	0.000988126
	0.001	0.980237		
	0.00001	0.978261		
64	0.0001	0.978261	0.977931	0.000570495
	0.001	0.977273		

Table 4. Average and standard deviation accuracy without enhancement (CLAHE + ESRGAN).

Freeze	Batch Size	Learning Rate	Accuracy	Mean	Standard Deviation
		0.00001	0.779599		
	2	0.0001	0.76867	0.761992	0.021731047
		0.001	0.737705		
		0.00001	0.783242		
	4	0.0001	0.785064	0.780814	0.005855271
		0.00001	0.774135		
		0.00001	0.777778		
	8	0.0001	0.781421	0.780814	0.002782382
		0.001	0.783242		
140		0.00001	0.790528		
	16	0.0001	0.783242	0.7881	0.004206547
		0.001	0.790528		
		0.00001	0.786885		
	32	0.0001	0.799636	0.788707	0.01014166
		0.001	0.779599		
		0.00001	0.794171		
	64	0.0001	0.808743	0.798421	0.008985212
		0.001	0.79235		

The top performance from each iteration was saved and is shown in Tables 5 and 6, for case 1 and case 2, respectively, revealing that the best results produced with and without preprocessing using CLAHE + ESRGAN were 98.7% and 80.87%, respectively. Figure 9 depicts the optimal outcome for the two scenarios based on the utilized evaluation metrics case 1 using CLAHE and ESRGAN, and case 2 without using them.

Table 5. Best accuracy with enhancement (CLAHE + ESRGAN).

Acc	Prec	Re	F1sc	Top-2 Accuracy	Top-3 Accuracy
0.9872	0.99	0.99	0.99	0.996	0.999

Table 6. Best accuracy without enhancement (CLAHE + ESRGAN).

Acc	*Prec*	*Re*	*F1sc*	**Top-2 Accuracy**	**Top-3 Accuracy**
0.8087	0.80	0.81	0.80	0.9144	0.9800

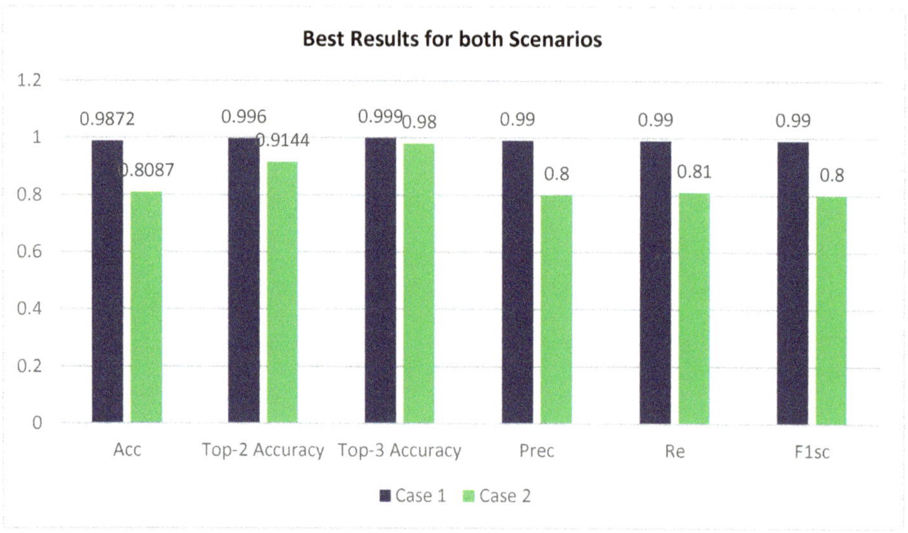

Figure 9. Best results for both scenarios.

Figures 10 and 11 show the confusion matrix with and without using CLAHE + ESRGAN, respectively.

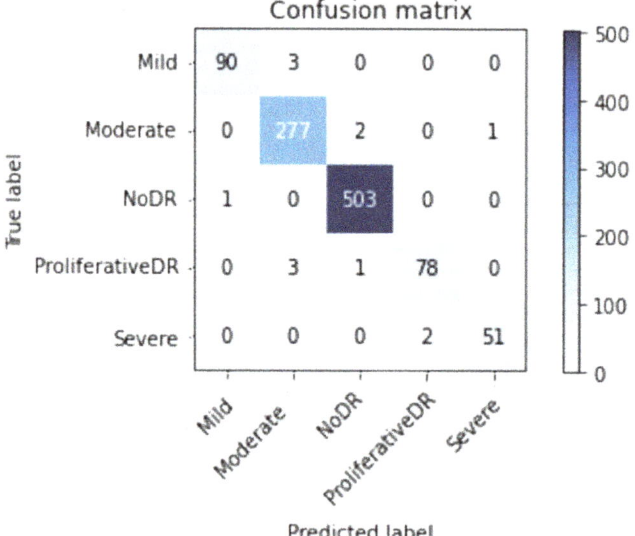

Figure 10. Best confusion matrix of Inception-V3 with enhancement (with CLAHE + ESRGAN).

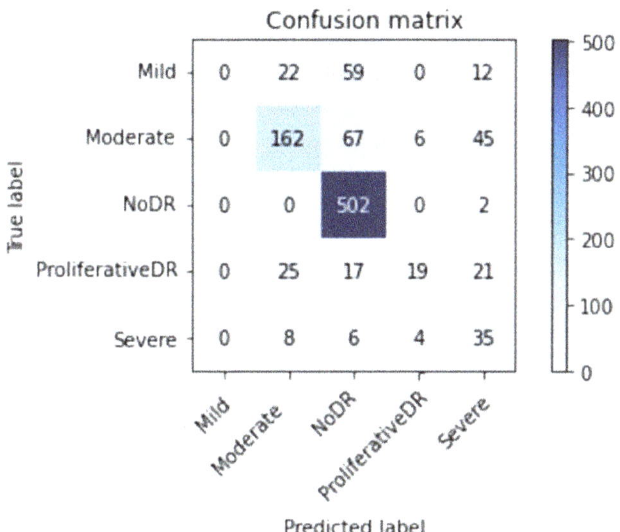

Figure 11. Best confusion matrix of Inception-V3 without enhancement (without CLAHE + ESRGAN).

Tables 7 and 8 show the total number of photos utilized for testing in each class for the APTOS dataset. According to the data, it is clear that the No DR class has the most images with 504, and its *Prec*, *Re*, and *F1sc* give the highest values of 99 100 and 100% for case 1, and 97, 97, and 97% for case 2.

Table 7. Detailed results for each class using CLAHE + ESRGAN.

	Prec	*Re*	*F1sc*	**Total Images**
Mild DR	0.99	0.97	0.98	93
Moderate DR	0.98	0.99	0.98	280
No DR	0.99	1.00	1.00	504
Proliferative DR	0.97	0.95	0.96	82
Severe DR	0.98	0.96	0.97	53
Average	0.99	0.99	0.99	1012

Table 8. Detailed results for each class without using CLAHE + ESRGAN.

	Prec	*Re*	*F1sc*	**Total Images**
Mild DR	0.58	0.62	0.60	93
Moderate DR	0.70	0.78	0.74	280
No DR	0.97	0.97	0.97	504
Proliferative DR	0.68	0.48	0.56	82
Severe DR	0.43	0.31	0.36	53
Average	0.80	0.81	0.80	1012

Using retinal pictures to improve the accuracy with which ophthalmologists identify infections, while reducing their effort, was demonstrated to be practical in real-world scenarios.

4.4. Evaluation Considering a Variety of Other Methodologies

Effectiveness was compared to that of other methods. According to Table 9, our method exceeds other alternatives in terms of effectiveness and performance. The proposed inception model achieved an overall accuracy rate of 98.7%, surpassing the present methods.

Table 9. Comparison of system performance to previous research using the APTOS Dataset.

Reference	Technique	Accuracy
[19]	MSA-Net	84.6%
[24]	*LBCNN*	97.41%
[31]	SVM	94.5%
[32]	CNN	95.3%
[33]	Inception-ResNet-v2	97.0%,
[35]	VGG-16	74.58%
[36]	VGG16	73.26%
	DenseNet121	96.11%
[37]	DenseNet201	93.85%
[50]	Vision Transformer, Bidirectional Encoder representation for image Transformer, Class-Attention in Image Transformers, Data efficient image Transformers	94.63%
[51]	EfficientNet-B6	86.03%
[52]	SVM classifier and MobileNet_V2 for feature extraction	88.80%
[53]	Densenet-121, Xception, Inception-v3, Resnet-50	85.28%
[54]	Inception-ResNet-v2	72.33%
[55]	MobileNet_V2	93.09%
[56]	EfficientNet and DenseNet	96.32%
[57]	VGG16	96.86%
[58]	Resnet-50	77.22%
[59]	Hybrid Residual U-Net	94%
[60]	Inception-v3	88.1%
Proposed Methodology	Inception-V3 (without using CLAHE + ESRGAN) Case 2	80.87%
	Inception-V3 (using CLAHE + ESRGAN) Case 1	98.7%

5. Discussion

Based on CLAHE and ESRGAN, a novel DR categorization scheme is presented in this research. The developed model was tested on the DR images founded in the APTOS 2019 dataset. There were two training scenarios: case 1 with CLAHE + ESRGAN applied to the APTOS dataset, and case 2 without CLAHE + ESRGAN. Through 80:20 hold-out validation, the model attained a five-class accuracy rate of 98.7% for case 1 and 80.87% for case 2. The proposed method classified both cases scenarios using the pretrained Inception-V3 infrastructure. Throughout model construction, we evaluated the classification performance of two distinct scenarios and found that enhancement techniques produced the best results (Figure 9). The main contributing element in our methodology was the general resolution enhancement of CLAHE + ESRGAN, which we proved, with evidence, is responsible for the great improvement in the accuracy.

6. Conclusions

By identifying retinal images displayed in the APTOS dataset, we established a strategy for quickly and accurately diagnosing five distinct forms of cancer. The proposed method employs case 1 with images enhanced with CLAHE and ESRGAN, and case 2 with original images. The case 1 scenario employs four-stage picture enhancement techniques to increase the image's luminance and eliminate noise. CLAHE and ESRGAN were the two stages with the best impact on accuracy, as demonstrated by experimental results. State-of-the-art techniques in preprocessed medical imagery were employed to train Inception-V3 with augmentation techniques that helped reduce overfitting and raised the entire competencies of the suggested methodology. This solution showed that when using Inception-V3, the conception model achieved a correctness of 98.7% $\approx$ 99% for the case 1 scenario and 80.87% $\approx$ 81% for the case 2 scenario, both of which are in line with the accuracy of trained ophthalmologists. The use of CLAHE and ESRGAN in the preprocessing step further contributed to the study's novelty and significance. The proposed methodology outperformed established models, as evidenced by a comparison of their respective strengths and weaknesses. To prove the effectiveness of the proposed method, it must be tested on a sizable and intricate dataset, ideally consisting of a significant number of potential DR instances. In the future, new datasets may be analyzed using DenseNet, VGG, or ResNet, as well as additional augmentation approaches. Additionally, ESRGAN and CLAHE can be conducted independently to determine their impact on the classification procedure.

Author Contributions: Conceptualization, W.G.; Data curation, W.G.; Formal analysis, G.A. and W.G.; Funding acquisition, G.A.; Methodology, W.G. and M.H.; Project administration, M.H.; Supervision, W.G. and M.H.; Writing—original draft, W.G.; Writing—review & editing, W.G. and M.H. All authors have read and agreed to the published version of the manuscript.

Funding: The authors extend their appreciation to the Deputyship for Research & Innovation, Ministry of Education in Saudi Arabia for funding this research work through the project number 223202.

Institutional Review Board Statement: Not Applicable.

Informed Consent Statement: Not Applicable.

Data Availability Statement: Will be furnished on request.

Acknowledgments: The authors extend their appreciation to the Deputyship for Research & Innovation, Ministry of Education in Saudi Arabia for funding this research work through the project number 223202.

Conflicts of Interest: The authors declare no conflict of interest.

References

1. Atwany, M.Z.; Sahyoun, A.H.; Yaqub, M. Deep learning techniques for diabetic retinopathy classification: A survey. *IEEE Access* **2022**, *10*, 28642–28655. [CrossRef]
2. Amin, J.; Sharif, M.; Yasmin, M. A review on recent developments for detection of diabetic retinopathy. *Scientifica* **2016**, *2016*, 6838976. [CrossRef] [PubMed]
3. Kharroubi, A.T.; Darwish, H.M. Diabetes mellitus: The epidemic of the century. *World J. Diabetes* **2015**, *6*, 850. [CrossRef] [PubMed]
4. Alwakid, G.; Gouda, W.; Humayun, M. Enhancement of Diabetic Retinopathy Prognostication Utilizing Deep Learning, CLAHE, and ESRGAN. *Preprints* **2023**, 2023020218. [CrossRef]
5. Mamtora, S.; Wong, Y.; Bell, D.; Sandinha, T. Bilateral birdshot retinochoroiditis and retinal astrocytoma. *Case Rep. Ophthalmol. Med.* **2017**, *2017*, 6586157. [CrossRef]
6. Taylor, R.; Batey, D. *Handbook of Retinal Screening in Diabetes: Diagnosis and Management*; John Wiley & Sons: Hoboken, NJ, USA, 2012.
7. Imran, M.; Ullah, A.; Arif, M.; Noor, R. A unified technique for entropy enhancement based diabetic retinopathy detection using hybrid neural network. *Comput. Biol. Med.* **2022**, *145*, 105424.
8. Alyoubi, W.L.; Shalash, W.M.; Abulkhair, M.F. Diabetic retinopathy detection through deep learning techniques: A review. *Inform. Med. Unlocked* **2020**, *20*, 100377. [CrossRef]
9. Dubow, M.; Pinhas, A.; Shah, N.; Cooper, R.F.; Gan, A.; Gentile, R.C.; Hendrix, V.; Sulai, Y.N.; Carroll, J.; Chui, T.Y. Classification of human retinal microaneurysms using adaptive optics scanning light ophthalmoscope fluorescein angiography. *Investig. Ophthalmol. Vis. Sci.* **2014**, *55*, 1299–1309. [CrossRef]
10. Mazhar, K.; Varma, R.; Choudhury, F.; McKean-Cowdin, R.; Shtir, C.J.; Azen, S.P.; Group, L.A.L.E.S. Severity of diabetic retinopathy and health-related quality of life: The Los Angeles Latino Eye Study. *Ophthalmology* **2011**, *118*, 649–655. [CrossRef]

11. Willis, J.R.; Doan, Q.V.; Gleeson, M.; Haskova, Z.; Ramulu, P.; Morse, L.; Cantrell, R.A. Vision-related functional burden of diabetic retinopathy across severity levels in the United States. *JAMA Ophthalmol.* **2017**, *135*, 926–932. [CrossRef]
12. Vora, P.; Shrestha, S. Detecting diabetic retinopathy using embedded computer vision. *Appl. Sci.* **2020**, *10*, 7274. [CrossRef]
13. Murugesan, N.; Üstunkaya, T.; Feener, E.P. Thrombosis and hemorrhage in diabetic retinopathy: A perspective from an inflammatory standpoint. *Semin. Thromb. Hemost.* **2015**, *41*, 659–664. [CrossRef]
14. Szegedy, C.; Ioffe, S.; Vanhoucke, V.; Alemi, A.A. Inception-v4, inception-resnet and the impact of residual connections on learning. In Proceedings of the Thirty-First AAAI Conference on Artificial Intelligence, San Francisco, CA, USA, 4–9 February 2017; Association for the Advancement of Artificial Intelligence: Washington, DC, USA, 2017.
15. Xia, X.; Xu, C.; Nan, B. Inception-v3 for flower classification. In Proceedings of the 2017 2nd International Conference on Image, Vision and Computing (ICIVC), Chengdu, China, 2–4 June 2017; pp. 783–787.
16. APTOS 2019 Blindness Detection Detect Diabetic Retinopathy to Stop Blindness before It's too Late. 2019. Available online: https://www.kaggle.com/c/aptos2019-blindnessdetection/data (accessed on 28 August 2022).
17. Pizer, S.M.; Amburn, E.P.; Austin, J.D.; Cromartie, R.; Geselowitz, A.; Greer, T.; ter Haar Romeny, B.; Zimmerman, J.B.; Zuiderveld, K. Adaptive histogram equalization and its variations. *Comput. Vis. Graph. Image Process.* **1987**, *39*, 355–368. [CrossRef]
18. Ledig, C.; Theis, L.; Huszár, F.; Caballero, J.; Cunningham, A.; Acosta, A.; Aitken, A.; Tejani, A.; Totz, J.; Wang, Z. Photo-realistic single image super-resolution using a generative adversarial network. In Proceedings of the IEEE Conference on Computer Vision and Pattern Recognition, Honolulu, HI, USA, 21–26 July 2017; pp. 4681–4690.
19. Al-Antary, M.T.; Arafa, Y. Multi-scale attention network for diabetic retinopathy classification. *IEEE Access* **2021**, *9*, 54190–54200. [CrossRef]
20. Gargeya, R.; Leng, T. Automated identification of diabetic retinopathy using deep learning. *Ophthalmology* **2017**, *124*, 962–969. [CrossRef]
21. Ali, R.; Hardie, R.C.; Narayanan, B.N.; Kebede, T.M. IMNets: Deep learning using an incremental modular network synthesis approach for medical imaging applications. *Appl. Sci.* **2022**, *12*, 5500. [CrossRef]
22. Kazakh-British, N.P.; Pak, A.; Abdullina, D. Automatic detection of blood vessels and classification in retinal images for diabetic retinopathy diagnosis with application of convolution neural network. In Proceedings of the 2018 International Conference on Sensors, Signal and Image Processing, Prague, Czech Republic, 12–14 October 2018; pp. 60–63.
23. Pak, A.; Ziyaden, A.; Tukeshev, K.; Jaxylykova, A.; Abdullina, D. Comparative analysis of deep learning methods of detection of diabetic retinopathy. *Cogent Eng.* **2020**, *7*, 1805144. [CrossRef]
24. Macsik, P.; Pavlovicova, J.; Goga, J.; Kajan, S. Local Binary CNN for Diabetic Retinopathy Classification on Fundus Images. *Acta Polytech. Hung.* **2022**, *19*, 27–45.
25. Khalifa, N.E.M.; Loey, M.; Taha, M.H.N.; Mohamed, H.N.E.T. Deep transfer learning models for medical diabetic retinopathy detection. *Acta Inform. Med.* **2019**, *27*, 327. [CrossRef]
26. Hemanth, D.J.; Deperlioglu, O.; Kose, U. An enhanced diabetic retinopathy detection and classification approach using deep convolutional neural network. *Neural Comput. Appl.* **2020**, *32*, 707–721. [CrossRef]
27. Maqsood, S.; Damaševičius, R.; Maskeliūnas, R. Hemorrhage detection based on 3D CNN deep learning framework and feature fusion for evaluating retinal abnormality in diabetic patients. *Sensors* **2021**, *21*, 3865. [CrossRef] [PubMed]
28. Das, S.; Kharbanda, K.; Suchetha, M.; Raman, R.; Dhas, E. Deep learning architecture based on segmented fundus image features for classification of diabetic retinopathy. *Biomed. Signal Process. Control* **2021**, *68*, 102600. [CrossRef]
29. Wang, Y.; Yu, M.; Hu, B.; Jin, X.; Li, Y.; Zhang, X.; Zhang, Y.; Gong, D.; Wu, C.; Zhang, B. Deep learning-based detection and stage grading for optimising diagnosis of diabetic retinopathy. *Diabetes/Metab. Res. Rev.* **2021**, *37*, e3445. [CrossRef] [PubMed]
30. Liu, H.; Yue, K.; Cheng, S.; Pan, C.; Sun, J.; Li, W. Hybrid model structure for diabetic retinopathy classification. *J. Healthc. Eng.* **2020**, *2020*, 8840174. [CrossRef]
31. Saranya, P.; Umamaheswari, K.; Patnaik, S.C.; Patyal, J.S. Red Lesion Detection in Color Fundus Images for Diabetic Retinopathy Detection. In Proceedings of the International Conference on Deep Learning, Computing and Intelligence, Chennai, India, 7–8 January 2021; pp. 561–569.
32. Thomas, N.M.; Albert Jerome, S. Grading and Classification of Retinal Images for Detecting Diabetic Retinopathy Using Convolutional Neural Network. In *Advances in Electrical and Computer Technologies*; Springer: Singapore, 2022; pp. 607–614.
33. Crane, A.; Dastjerdi, M. Effect of Simulated Cataract on the Accuracy of an Artificial Intelligence Algorithm in Detecting Diabetic Retinopathy in Color Fundus Photos. *Investig. Ophthalmol. Vis. Sci.* **2022**, *63*, 2100–F0089.
34. Majumder, S.; Kehtarnavaz, N. Multitasking deep learning model for detection of five stages of diabetic retinopathy. *IEEE Access* **2021**, *9*, 123220–123230. [CrossRef]
35. Deshpande, A.; Pardhi, J. Automated detection of Diabetic Retinopathy using VGG-16 architecture. *Int. Res. J. Eng. Technol.* **2021**, *8*, 3790–3794.
36. Yadav, S.; Awasthi, P.; Pathak, S. Retina Image and Diabetic Retinopathy: A Deep Learning Based Approach. Available online: https://www.irjmets.com/uploadedfiles/paper/issue_6_june_2022/26368/final/fin_irjmets1656163002.pdf (accessed on 28 July 2022).
37. Kobat, S.G.; Baygin, N.; Yusufoglu, E.; Baygin, M.; Barua, P.D.; Dogan, S.; Yaman, O.; Celiker, U.; Yildirim, H.; Tan, R.-S. Automated Diabetic Retinopathy Detection Using Horizontal and Vertical Patch Division-Based Pre-Trained DenseNET with Digital Fundus Images. *Diagnostics* **2022**, *12*, 1975. [CrossRef]

38. Reza, A.M. Realization of the contrast limited adaptive histogram equalization (CLAHE) for real-time image enhancement. *J. VLSI Signal Process. Syst. Signal Image Video Technol.* **2004**, *38*, 35–44. [CrossRef]
39. Tondin, B.; Barth, A.; Sanches, P.; Júnior, D.; Müller, A.; Thomé, P.; Wink, P.; Martins, A.; Susin, A. Development of an Automatic Antibiogram Reader System Using Circular Hough Transform and Radial Profile Analysis. In Proceedings of the XXVII Brazilian Congress on Biomedical Engineering: CBEB 2020, Vitória, Brazil, 26–30 October 2020; pp. 1837–1842.
40. Wang, X.; Yu, K.; Wu, S.; Gu, J.; Liu, Y.; Dong, C.; Qiao, Y.; Change Loy, C. Esrgan: Enhanced super-resolution generative adversarial networks. In Proceedings of the European Conference on Computer Vision (ECCV) Workshops, Munich, Germany, 8–14 September 2018; Springer: Cham, Switzerland.
41. Jolicoeur-Martineau, A. The relativistic discriminator: A key element missing from standard GAN. *arXiv* **2018**, arXiv:1807.00734.
42. Ioffe, S.; Szegedy, C. Batch normalization: Accelerating deep network training by reducing internal covariate shift. In Proceedings of the International Conference on Machine Learning, Lille, France, 7–9 July 2015; pp. 448–456.
43. Krause, J.; Sapp, B.; Howard, A.; Zhou, H.; Toshev, A.; Duerig, T.; Philbin, J.; Fei-Fei, L. The unreasonable effectiveness of noisy data for fine-grained recognition. In Proceedings of the 14th European Conference on Computer Vision, Amsterdam, The Netherlands, 11–14 October 2016; pp. 301–320.
44. Krizhevsky, A.; Sutskever, I.; Hinton, G.E. Imagenet classification with deep convolutional neural networks. In Proceedings of the 25th International Conference on Neural Information Processing Systems, Lake Tahoe, NV, USA, 3–6 December 2012; Volume 25.
45. Simonyan, K.; Zisserman, A. Very deep convolutional networks for large-scale image recognition. *arXiv* **2014**, arXiv:1409.1556.
46. Serre, T.; Wolf, L.; Bileschi, S.; Riesenhuber, M.; Poggio, T. Robust object recognition with cortex-like mechanisms. *IEEE Trans. Pattern Anal. Mach. Intell.* **2007**, *29*, 411–426. [CrossRef]
47. Lin, M.; Chen, Q.; Yan, S. Network in network. *arXiv* **2013**, arXiv:1312.4400.
48. Szegedy, C.; Liu, W.; Jia, Y.; Sermanet, P.; Reed, S.; Anguelov, D.; Erhan, D.; Vanhoucke, V.; Rabinovich, A. Going deeper with convolutions. In Proceedings of the IEEE Conference on Computer Vision and Pattern Recognition, Boston, MA, USA, 7–12 June 2015; pp. 1–9.
49. Arora, S.; Bhaskara, A.; Ge, R.; Ma, T. Provable bounds for learning some deep representations. In Proceedings of the International Conference on Machine Learning, Beijing, China, 21–26 June 2014; pp. 584–592.
50. Adak, C.; Karkera, T.; Chattopadhyay, S.; Saqib, M. Detecting Severity of Diabetic Retinopathy from Fundus Images using Ensembled Transformers. *arXiv* **2023**, arXiv:2301.00973.
51. Maqsood, Z.; Gupta, M.K. Automatic Detection of Diabetic Retinopathy on the Edge. In *Cyber Security, Privacy and Networking*; Springer: Singapore, 2022; pp. 129–139.
52. Lahmar, C.; Idri, A. Deep hybrid architectures for diabetic retinopathy classification. *Comput. Methods Biomech. Biomed. Eng. Imaging Vis.* **2022**, *11*, 166–184. [CrossRef]
53. Oulhadj, M.; Riffi, J.; Chaimae, K.; Mahraz, A.M.; Ahmed, B.; Yahyaouy, A.; Fouad, C.; Meriem, A.; Idriss, B.A.; Tairi, H. Diabetic retinopathy prediction based on deep learning and deformable registration. *Multimed. Tools Appl.* **2022**, *81*, 28709–28727. [CrossRef]
54. Gangwar, A.K.; Ravi, V. Diabetic retinopathy detection using transfer learning and deep learning. In *Evolution in Computational Intelligence*; Springer: Singapore, 2021; pp. 679–689.
55. Lahmar, C.; Idri, A. On the value of deep learning for diagnosing diabetic retinopathy. *Health Technol.* **2022**, *12*, 89–105. [CrossRef]
56. Canayaz, M. Classification of diabetic retinopathy with feature selection over deep features using nature-inspired wrapper methods. *Appl. Soft Comput.* **2022**, *128*, 109462. [CrossRef]
57. Escorcia-Gutierrez, J.; Cuello, J.; Barraza, C.; Gamarra, M.; Romero-Aroca, P.; Caicedo, E.; Valls, A.; Puig, D. Analysis of Pre-trained Convolutional Neural Network Models in Diabetic Retinopathy Detection through Retinal Fundus Images. In Proceedings of the 21st International Conference on Computer Information Systems and Industrial Management, Barranquilla, Colombia, 15–17 July 2022; Springer International Publishing: Cham, Switzerland; pp. 202–213.
58. Lin, C.-L.; Wu, K.-C. Development of Revised ResNet-50 for Diabetic Retinopathy Detection. *Res. Sq.* **2023**. [CrossRef]
59. Salluri, D.K.; Sistla, V.; Kolli, V.K.K. HRUNET: Hybrid Residual U-Net for automatic severity prediction of Diabetic Retinopathy. *Comput. Methods Biomech. Biomed. Eng. Imaging Vis.* **2022**, 1–12. [CrossRef]
60. Yadav, S.; Awasthi, P. Diabetic retinopathy detection using deep learning and inception-v3 model. *Int. Res. J. Mod. Eng. Technol. Sci.* **2022**, *4*, 1731–1735.

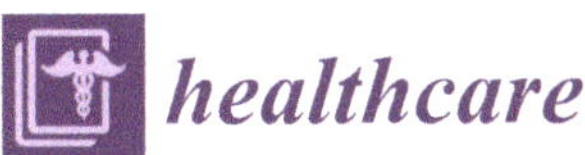

healthcare

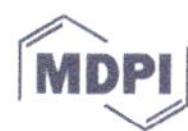

Article

Automatic Detection and Measurement of Renal Cysts in Ultrasound Images: A Deep Learning Approach

Yurie Kanauchi [1], Masahiro Hashimoto [2], Naoki Toda [2], Saori Okamoto [2], Hasnine Haque [3], Masahiro Jinzaki [2] and Yasubumi Sakakibara [1,*]

1   Department of Biosciences and Informatics, Keio University, Yokohama 2238522, Japan
2   Department of Radiology, Keio University School of Medicine, Tokyo 1608582, Japan
3   GE HealthCare Japan, Tokyo 1918503, Japan
*   Correspondence: yasu@bio.keio.ac.jp

Abstract: Ultrasonography is widely used for diagnosis of diseases in internal organs because it is nonradioactive, noninvasive, real-time, and inexpensive. In ultrasonography, a set of measurement markers is placed at two points to measure organs and tumors, then the position and size of the target finding are measured on this basis. Among the measurement targets of abdominal ultrasonography, renal cysts occur in 20–50% of the population regardless of age. Therefore, the frequency of measurement of renal cysts in ultrasound images is high, and the effect of automating measurement would be high as well. The aim of this study was to develop a deep learning model that can automatically detect renal cysts in ultrasound images and predict the appropriate position of a pair of salient anatomical landmarks to measure their size. The deep learning model adopted fine-tuned YOLOv5 for detection of renal cysts and fine-tuned UNet++ for prediction of saliency maps, representing the position of salient landmarks. Ultrasound images were input to YOLOv5, and images cropped inside the bounding box and detected from the input image by YOLOv5 were input to UNet++. For comparison with human performance, three sonographers manually placed salient landmarks on 100 unseen items of the test data. These salient landmark positions annotated by a board-certified radiologist were used as the ground truth. We then evaluated and compared the accuracy of the sonographers and the deep learning model. Their performances were evaluated using precision–recall metrics and the measurement error. The evaluation results show that the precision and recall of our deep learning model for detection of renal cysts are comparable to standard radiologists; the positions of the salient landmarks were predicted with an accuracy close to that of the radiologists, and in a shorter time.

Keywords: deep learning; ultrasonic imaging; kidney; object detection

Citation: Kanauchi, Y.; Hashimoto, M.; Toda, N.; Okamoto, S.; Haque, H.; Jinzaki, M.; Sakakibara, Y. Automatic Detection and Measurement of Renal Cysts in Ultrasound Images: A Deep Learning Approach. *Healthcare* **2023**, *11*, 484. https://doi.org/10.3390/healthcare11040484

Academic Editor: Mahmudur Rahman

Received: 28 December 2022
Revised: 29 January 2023
Accepted: 1 February 2023
Published: 7 February 2023

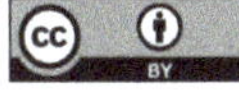

1. Introduction

Ultrasonography is widely used for diagnosis of diseases in internal organs, such as the abdomen, heart, and thyroid gland, as well as for prenatal diagnosis. This is because it is nonradioactive, noninvasive, real-time, and inexpensive. In ultrasonography, a set of measurement markers is placed at two points to measure organs and tumors, and the position and size of the target finding are measured based on these. While the markers play an important role in diagnosis, they must be manually positioned, which places a burden on the sonographer. Furthermore, because of the absence of fixed rules on the placement of markers, differences between individuals with different levels of experience create an additional problem [1]. Therefore, we believe that automating the placement of markers using deep learning would lead to a reduced burden on sonographers, shorten the test duration, and promote the elimination of inter-operator variability.

Studies have been conducted to automate measurement in ultrasonography using deep learning. In ultrasonic image analysis, deep learning systems for detection and classification of thyroid nodules, breast lesions, and liver lesions have been developed [2].

Ma et al. [3] developed a system to automatically detect thyroid nodules from ultrasound B-mode images using a cascade model containing two CNN models, achieving an area under the curve (AUC) of 98.51%. Li et al. [4] employed a CNN model consisting of ResNet 50 and Darknet pre-trained with ImageNet [5] for the diagnosis of thyroid cancer. Using large datasets collected from three hospitals, they showed that diagnosis with the same sensitivity and higher specificity as that of radiologists is possible. Byra et al. [6] applied transfer learning using VGG29 pre-trained with ImageNet [5] to a breast ultrasound image dataset in order to classify benign and malignant breast cancer lesions. They achieved an AUC of 93.6% on their own dataset and an AUC of approximately 89.0% on public datasets. Liu et al. [7] proposed a system that extracts liver membrane features from ultrasound images using a pre-trained CNN model, then classifies liver normality and abnormalities by support-vector machine (SVM) based on the extracted features. These deep learning methods are expected to help radiologists to shorten interpretation times and improve the accuracy of diagnosis.

In addition to ultrasonic images, deep learning is widely applied to radiographic images such as X-ray and Computed Tomography (CT) images. Muresan et al. [8] proposed an approach for automatic tooth detection and disease classification in panoramic X-ray images using deep learning-based image processing. Semantic segmentation and object detection were used to detect tooth regions and label diseases affecting the tooth. Pang et al. [9] proposed a two-step segmentation framework called SpineParseNet for child spine analysis in a volumetric MR image. This model consists of a 3D graph convolutional segmentation network (GCSN) that performs 3D segmentation and a 2D residual U-Net (ResUNet) that performs 2D segmentation. Gu et al. [10] proposed an attention-based CNN (CA-Net) for more accurate and explainable medical image segmentation. Their CA-Net achieved higher accuracy than U-Net in skin lesions, placenta, and fetal brain segmentation. Takeuchi et al. [11] constructed a system for diagnosing esophageal cancer from CT images based on deep learning, and verified its performance. VGG16, which is one of the CNN models used for image recognition, was fine-tuned for classification of the presence or absence of esophageal cancer, and the authors confirmed that esophageal cancer could be detected with high accuracy. Other studies have attempted the detection of landmarks in radiographic images. Payer et al. [12] proposed a system using CNN to predict the position of a landmark in an X-ray image of the hand using heat map regression. Zhong et al. [13] applied landmark regression using a two-stage U-Net to detect anatomical landmarks on cephalometric X-ray images.

Several previous studies have been conducted to automate measurements in ultrasonography using deep learning. Chen et al. [14] proposed a method for the automatic measurement of the width of the fetal lateral ventricle. The lateral ventricle was segmented using a deep convolutional network, and measurement was performed by finding the minimum bounding rectangle of the segmented region. Biswas et al. [15] proposed an automatic measurement method for carotid intima–media thickness. The arterial wall is composed of the intima, media, and adventitia, and the intima–media thickness is the combined thickness of the intima and media. The luminal and media/adventitia regions were segmented using a deep learning method, and the intima–media thickness was obtained from the distance between the boundary surfaces of the regions. Leclerc et al. [16] conducted a study to automatically measure left ventricular volume from echocardiographic images by segmentation using deep learning methods. In these methods, segmentation is performed for measurement; however, creating a mask that serves as training data for segmentation is a time-consuming task. Although research is being conducted to automate measurements in ultrasonography of the heart, carotid artery, and foetation, there have been few studies on abdominal ultrasonography. For example, Jagtap et al. [17] proposed a method to measure the total kidney volume from 3D ultrasound images using CNN. Akkasaligar et al. [18] developed a method for automatic segmentation of renal cysts in ultrasound images using the active contour method and level set segmentation method. However, neither study addressed the prediction of salient landmark positions.

Related studies on deep learning-based analysis of ultrasound images are summarized in the Table 1.

Among the measurement targets of abdominal ultrasonography, renal cysts occur in 20–50% of the population regardless of age [19]. Therefore, the frequency of measurement of renal cysts is high, which leads us to believe that the effects of automating measurement would be high as well.

Saliency map regression is often used to predict the location of landmarks such as salient landmarks; however, previous studies have predicted only a fixed number of landmarks [13]. When assigning salient landmarks to renal cysts, two landmarks are assigned to one renal cyst; because multiple renal cysts may exist in one image, it is necessary to predict the position of a non-constant number of salient landmarks. Therefore, conventional saliency map regression, which can predict only a certain number of landmarks, cannot be used to address this problem.

Table 1. Summary of related studies on deep learning-based analysis of ultrasound images.

Study	Object	Task
Ma et al. [3]	thyroid nodules	detection
Li et al. [4]	thyroid cancer	classification
Byra et al. [6]	breast cancer	classification
Liu et al. [7]	liver membrane	detection & classification
Chen et al. [14]	fetal lateral ventricles	measurement
Biswas et al. [15]	carotid	measurement
Leclerc et al. [16]	left ventricular	measurement
Jagtap et al. [17]	kidney	measurement
Akkasaligar et al. [18]	renal cysts	segmentation
Our study	renal cysts	landmark placement

The following are the main contributions of this study:

- We developed a measurement assistance function for ultrasonic images using deep learning with the aim of supporting the measurement of renal cysts using measurement markers.
- To predict the landmarks for multiple renal cysts within one image, we developed a system in which all renal cysts in the image were detected prior to saliency map regression. Then, we performed saliency map regression to predict the positions of two salient landmarks for each detected renal cyst.
- Because the proposed method only uses the coordinates of the measurement markers when training the models, it is possible to automate the measurement without performing segmentation, thereby avoiding high annotation costs.
- In comparative tests, our method achieved almost the same accuracy as a radiologist. The errors of the measured length and measurement marker coordinates were used as evaluation indices.
- Our results indicate that the proposed method is able to perform measurements at a higher speed than manual measurement and with an accuracy close to that of sonographers.

2. Materials and Methods

In this paper, we propose an automated system for detecting renal cysts from abdominal ultrasonography and assigning a pair of salient landmarks to the detected renal cysts, as shown in Figure 1. The renal cyst measurement task was divided into three steps. First, a YOLOv5 object detection model [20] was trained to detect renal cysts from ultrasound images. Next, the area around each detected renal cyst was extracted from the image, and a heat map expressing the positions of the two measurement markers within that range was predicted using the UNet++ convolutional neural network [21]. Finally, the output heat map was post-processed and the coordinates were corrected to determine the predicted coordinates of the measurement marker. First, we developed a system in which all renal cysts in the image were detected prior to saliency map regression. Then, we performed saliency map regression to predict the positions of two salient landmarks for each detected renal cyst. Thus, two models were required for one for the task of detecting renal cysts and another for saliency map regression to predict the positions of the salient landmarks. The output of the saliency map regression was subjected to post-processing in order to determine the appropriate coordinates of each salient landmark. If the size of the detected renal cyst and measurement result using the predicted salient landmark coordinates were significantly different, the predicted coordinates were corrected. We integrated a renal cyst detection model, a salient landmark position prediction model, and coordinate determination with post-processing and correction to construct an automated system for salient landmark assignment. The renal cyst detection model and the salient landmark position prediction model were trained separately. The performance of this system was compared with that of a radiologist. The system was trained and evaluated using 2664 ultrasound images of renal cysts.

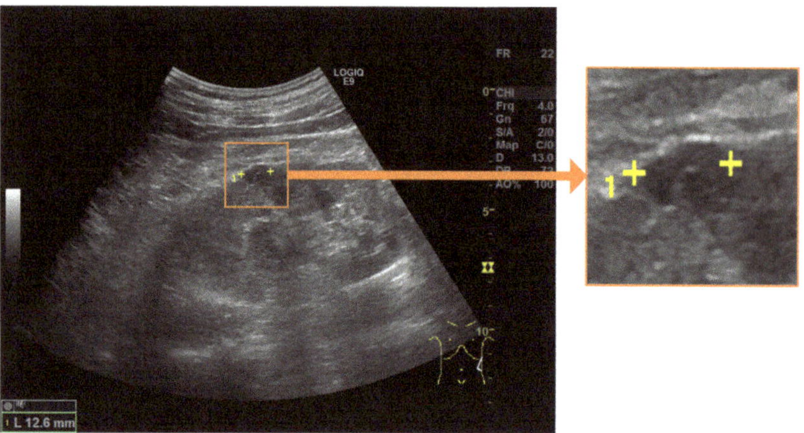

Figure 1. Salient landmarks placed on a renal cyst. A pair of salient landmarks are placed on the longest diameter of the renal cyst.

2.1. Automated System for Assigning Salient Landmarks

Figure 2 shows the processing flow of an automated system that integrates the renal cyst detection model, the salient landmark position prediction model, and coordinate determination by post-processing and correction. First, an ultrasound image was input to the renal cyst detection model and a bounding box surrounding the renal cyst was output. The area surrounded by the output bounding box was extracted from the ultrasound image. Because this process was performed on all bounding boxes output by the renal cyst detection model, a multiple number of bounding boxes and their areas were extracted. Then, the extracted area images were input to the salient landmark position prediction model one by one and a saliency map denoting the position of the salient landmark was output. For each of the obtained saliency maps, post-processing and correction of coordinates were performed as necessary to determine the appropriate coordinates of the salient landmarks. Because salient landmark position prediction was performed for all the bounding boxes output by the renal cyst detection model and because the salient landmark position prediction model predicts the positions of two salient landmarks per bounding box, the number of output salient landmarks was twice the number of detected renal cysts.

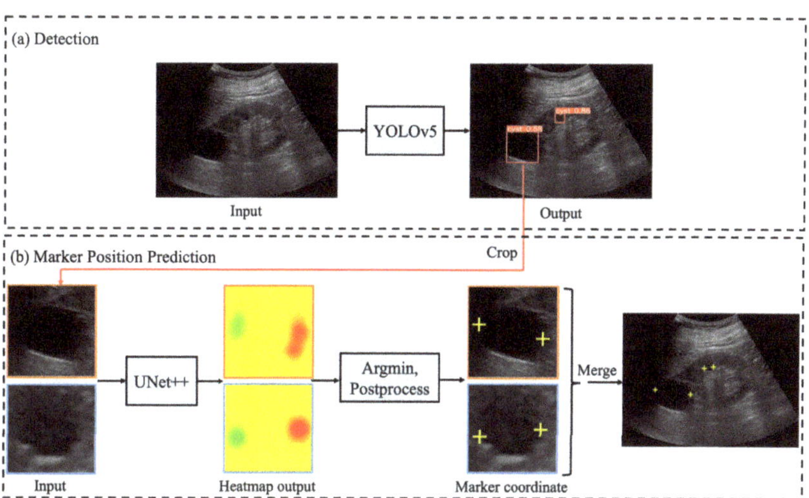

Figure 2. Processing flow of automated system for assigning salient landmarks to renal cysts: (**a**) ultrasound images are input into YOLOv5 [20] to detect renal cysts; (**b**) the area around the detected renal cyst is extracted and input to UNet++ [21] to predict the saliency map (represented by a heatmap) of the salient landmark position; in post-processing, the point with the smallest saliency map value from the output saliency map is selected and used as the appropriate coordinate. If necessary, the coordinates are corrected and the appropriate coordinates determined. Finally, all predicted salient landmarks are plotted on the original image.

2.2. Renal Cyst Detection Model

We constructed a model to detect renal cysts using ultrasound images as input. A renal cyst detection model was trained to predict the bounding box surrounding the renal cyst. The YOLOv5 object detection algorithm was used as the model. YOLOv5 is a model originally proposed by Glenn Jocher in June 2020 [20]; its architecture is shown in Figure 3. Compared with object detection models that require two steps for prediction (i.e., searching for area candidates in which an object appears from an image and identifying its category), YOLO directly predicts the bounding box and its class [22]. Therefore, the calculation speed of YOLO is higher than that of the conventional methods. Moreover, the entire image is used during training, making it possible to consider the surrounding context. Because the detection of renal cysts requires information on whether the background is the kidney, a model that can detect objects based on the surrounding context is suitable. In addition, when the automated system is used for ultrasonic examination, the processing must be faster than the manual placement of salient landmarks by the sonographer. For these reasons, YOLOv5 was selected as a suitable model for this task. The initial parameters of YOLOv5 were pre-trained using the COCO dataset [23], which is a large dataset of RGB images with object bounding boxes and category information. YOLOv5 has multiple models of different sizes, and we used the small (YOLOv5s), medium (YOLOv5m), large (YOLOv5l), and extra-large (YOLOv5x) models for accuracy comparison. The architecture of YOLOv5 consists of three components: BackBone, PANet, and Head. Here, Bottleneck CSP [24] represents the CSP bottleneck architecture proposed by CSPNet, Conv represents the convolutional layer, Upsample represents the upsampling layer, Concat represents the concatenate function, and SPP represents spatial pyramid pooling [25], which is a pooling method that can handle images of various sizes and shapes. First, in the BackBone, namely, CSP Darknet, performs feature extraction twice on multiple scales via Conv and Bottleneck CSP. Second, pooling processing is performed on feature maps with different scales using SPP. This is the backbone of CSP Darknet, which introduces the mechanism proposed by CSPNetinto the Darknet neural network framework in order to reduce the required amount of calculation while maintaining accuracy. Third, the extracted feature map is processed by Neck. PANet is used for Neck; after repeating a series of processing of BottleNeckCSP, Conv, Upsample, and Concat twice, it is processed again by BottleneckCSP. Finally, Conv is performed in Head, and the class, score, position, and size are output as detection results. The loss function of YOLOv5 is the sum of the loss functions of the bounding box regression, confidence, and classification, as indicated in the following equations [26]:

$$LOSS \;=\; L_{GIoU} + L_{conf} + L_{class} \tag{1}$$

$$L_{GIoU} \;=\; \sum_{i=0}^{S^2} \sum_{j=0}^{B} I_{i,j}^{obj}\left[1 - IoU + \frac{A^C - U}{A^C}\right] \tag{2}$$

$$L_{conf} \;=\; -\sum_{i=0}^{S^2}\sum_{j=0}^{B} I_{i,j}^{obj}[\widehat{C}_i^j \log(C_i^j) + (1 - \widehat{C}_i^j)\log(1 - C_i^j)] - \lambda_{nobj}\sum_{i=0}^{S^2}\sum_{j=0}^{B} I_{i,j}^{obj}[\widehat{C}_i^j \log(C_i^j) + (1 - \widehat{C}_i^j)\log(1 - C_i^j)] \tag{3}$$

$$L_{class} \;=\; -\sum_{i=0}^{S^2} I_{i,j}^{nobj} \sum_{c \in classes} [\widehat{P}_i^j \log(P_i^j(c)) + (1 - \widehat{P}_i^j(c))\log(1 - P_i^j(c))] \tag{4}$$

where S^2 is the number of grids, B is the number of bounding boxes in each grid, *obj* means that an object exists in a bounding box, *nobj* means that no object exists in the bounding box, $I_{i,j}^{obj}$ is equal to 1 when an object exists in a bounding box and is otherwise 0, IoU is the Intersection over Union between the predicted bounding box and the real bounding box, A^C is the smallest rectangular box that can completely contain the predicted bounding box and the real bounding box, U is the sum of area of the predicted bounding box and the real bounding box, $\widehat{C}_i^j$ is the prediction confidence of the jth bounding box in the ith grid, C_i^j is the true confidence of the jth bounding box in the ith grid, λ_{nobj} is the confidence weight when no object exists in the bounding box, $\widehat{P}_i^j$ is the probability of predicting the detection object as category c, and $P_i^j(c)$ is the probability of actually being category c.

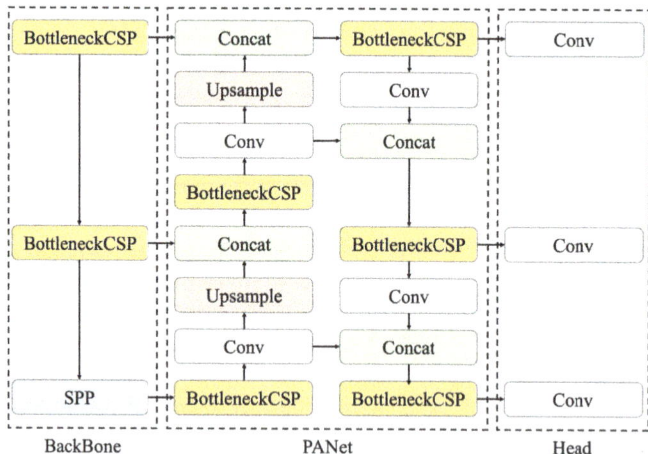

Figure 3. Architecture of YOLOv5, consisting of three components: BackBone, PANet, and Head. BottleNeck CSP refers to CSP Bottleneck, SPP to Spatial Pyramid Pooling, Conv to the Convolutional Layer, and Concat to the Concatenate Function. First, feature extraction is performed on multiple scales using BackBone, then PANet processes the extracted feature map, and finally Head outputs the class, score, position, and size as detection results.

All layers of YOLOv5 were fine-tuned using the renal cyst detection dataset described later in this section. The same single grayscale ultrasound image was input to three channels for RGB in YOLOv5.

2.3. Saliency Map Representing the Location of Salient Landmarks

Our proposed method results in a saliency map predicting and indicating the position of the salient landmarks. Saliency map regression is often used to predict the location of landmarks. In this work, the heatmap is used to represent the saliency map, as shown in Figure 4. Using a Gaussian distribution centered on the position of the salient landmarks, the saliency map value gradually decreases according to the distance from the salient landmark position. Rather than using a uniform gradient, we used the Gaussian distribution to cause the loss function to converge abruptly around the salient landmark position. The saliency map value at the salient landmark position was set to 0, increasing the distance of saliency map value from the salient landmark position. The maximum value was set to 255. The radius of the Gaussian distribution was set to 50. The saliency map of the left landmark used the G channel of the RGB image format, while the saliency map of the right landmark used the R channel. All pixel values of the B channel were set to 0. The left part of Figure 4 shows the positions of the salient landmarks on the ultrasonic image (displayed as yellow crosses), while the right part of Figure 4 shows the corresponding saliency maps; the green part shows the position of the left landmark and the red part shows the position of the right landmark.

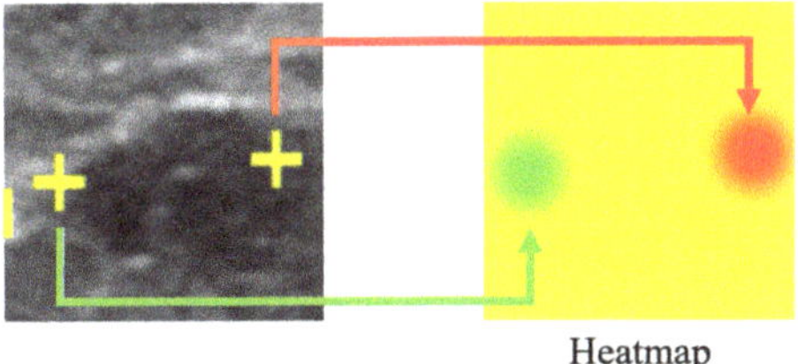

Figure 4. Saliency map showing the location of salient landmarks. The position of the left salient landmark is represented in green and the right one in red.

2.4. Salient Landmark Position Prediction Model

We constructed a salient landmark position prediction model that predicts a saliency map. For the prediction of salient landmark position, we adopted a strategy of predicting the saliency map instead of directly predicting the salient landmark position. In our study, the saliency map is represented by the heatmap. We adopted UNet++ [21] to produce a heatmap as output. UNet++ is an improved version of the U-Net deep convolutional neural network [27], which was developed for segmentation tasks. Using training data consisting of pairs of input images and heatmap outputs representing saliency maps, we trained UNet++ to produce a heatmap instead of segmentation. The salient landmark position prediction dataset (described in a later section) was used for fine-tuning of UNet++ to output a heatmap. U-Net consists of an encoder that extracts features by convolution and downsampling and a decoder that increases the resolution of the feature map by convolution and upsampling, producing segmentation results. A feature of U-Net is a skip connection that directly connects the feature map output in each layer of the encoder to the decoder. UNet++ decodes the feature map outputs at each level of the encoder and then connects them to the decoder by skip connection (Figure 5); this supplements the local features and enables more accurate area detection. Moreover, it reduces the difference in the expression of the encoder/decoder and simplifies the optimization problem [21]. The loss function was the mean square error of the saliency map. DenseNet121 [28] was used for the backbone. The initial parameters of the backbone were pretrained with ImageNet [5], which is a large dataset of RGB images.

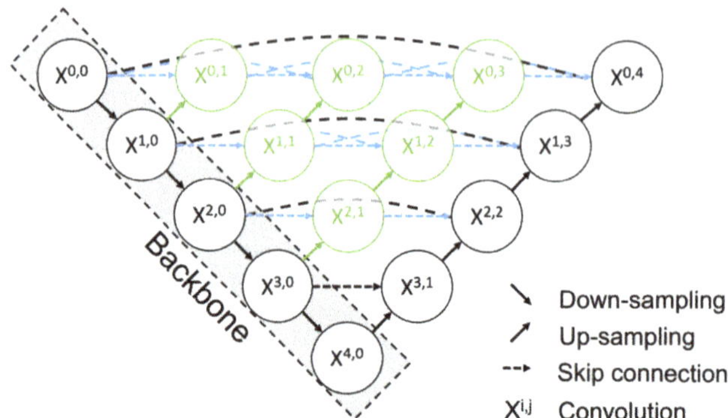

Figure 5. Architecture of UNet++. Each node in the graph represents a convolution block. The down arrow indicates downsampling, the up arrow indicates upsampling, and the dashed arrow indicates the skip connection. Using the skip connection, features with the same resolution from the preceding node are combined. In addition, upsampling combines features from the preceding node with different resolutions. This multi-scale feature aggregation is an advance of UNet++.

Each node in the graph shown in Figure 5 represents a convolution block composed of a Convolution layer, a Batch Normalization layer, and a ReLu layer. This block is stacked in five layers. The down arrow indicates downsampling, the up arrow indicates upsampling, and the dashed arrow indicates the skip connection. Using the skip connection, the features from the preceding node with the same resolution are combined. In addition, upsampling combines features with different resolutions from the preceding node. This multi-scale feature aggregation is one of the improvements available with UNet++. During the fine-tuning process, all layers were trained. The loss function of UNet ++ was as follows:

$$\text{Loss} \;=\; \frac{1}{n}\sum_{i=1}^{n}(\hat{y}_i - y_i)^2 \tag{5}$$

where n is the number of images, y_i is the pixel value of the ith pixel of the correct image, and $\hat{y}_i$ is the pixel value of the ith pixel of the predicted image.

2.5. Post-Processing

Post-processing was performed to determine the appropriate coordinates of the salient landmarks from the salient landmark position image. In the R and G channels of the saliency map showing the position of salient landmarks output by the salient landmark prediction model, the coordinates with the smallest saliency map value were selected and the coordinates were determined as the appropriate coordinates of the two salient landmarks. Note that when multiple coordinates had the same minimum values, we followed the heuristic of selecting the one closest to the top left corner.

2.6. Coordinate Correction

If the size of the detected renal cyst and the distance between the two salient landmarks differed significantly, the predicted coordinates were corrected. Note that the size of the detected renal cyst is defined as the length of the shorter side of the bounding box. Multiple regions with low saliency map values may appear in one channel. If we were to simply select the coordinates in this image with the smallest saliency map value, the coordinates determined from the R channel and G channel might be too close to each other. On the the hand, in the case of a large difference between the distance of the two predicted salient landmarks and the size of the bounding box, it follows that the predicted coordinates must be incorrect. The criteria for determining incorrectness were calculated as follows. Assuming that the predicted coordinates are p_1' and p_2' and the length of the shorter side of the bounding box is l, a correction was made if the following condition (6) was satisfied: there is a difference in the Euclidean distance between the two predicted coordinates (p'_1 and p'_2) and their length (l) that is greater than 5% of the length (l). Note that the double vertical line represents the L2-norm and the single vertical line represents the L1-norm.

$$| \, ||p'_1 - p'_2|| - l \, | \quad > \quad l \times 0.05 \tag{6}$$

The correction method was as follows. First, the coordinates with the lowest saliency map values in each of the R and G channels were selected, then the coordinate with the smaller value between them was selected as the position of the first salient landmark. Second, the coordinates of a point symmetrical to the first salient landmark with respect to the center of the bounding box were selected as the second salient landmark.

Figure 6 shows the coordinates before and after correction. Before correction, the distance between the two salient landmarks, indicated by the light blue crosses, was significantly different from the length of one side of the light blue bounding box; thus, the measurement was considered incorrect. After correction, the distance between the two salient landmarks, indicated by the light blue crosses, was closer to the length of one side of the bounding box. In addition, the measurement was more accurate when compared to the distance between the two true salient landmarks, indicated by the yellow crosses.

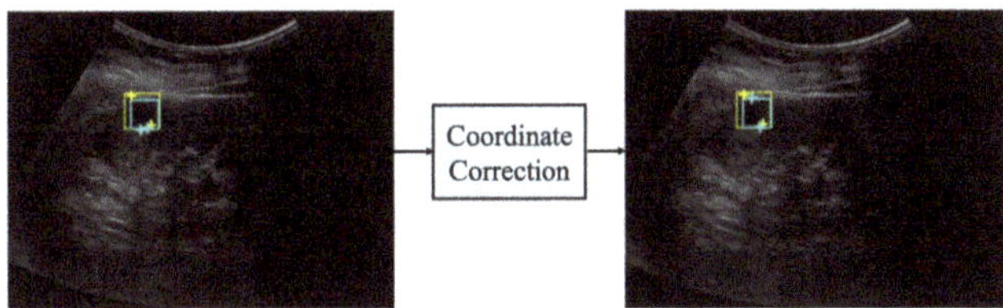

Figure 6. Coordinates before and after coordinate correction. The yellow rectangle is the true bounding box, the light blue rectangle is the bounding box predicted by the renal cyst detection model, the yellow crosses are the true salient landmark coordinates, and the light blue crosses are the salient landmark coordinates determined from the saliency map output by the salient landmark position prediction model. The left side of the figure shows the coordinates before correction and the right side shows the coordinates after correction. After correction, the distance between the two salient landmarks of the prediction is closer to the distance between the two salient landmarks of the true one.

2.7. Evaluation Metrics

We evaluated the accuracy of renal cyst detection and salient landmark coordinate prediction by the automated system. The region of the renal cyst output by the renal cyst detection model was defined as one of following three types: true positive (TP), when the model correctly detected a renal cyst; false positive (FP), when the model identified regions that were not renal cysts as renal cysts; and false negative (FN), when the model failed to detect an existing renal cyst. To establish the criteria for correct detection of a measured renal cyst, a circle with a diameter of a straight line connecting two paired points was drawn for each of the true and predicted salient landmarks. TP was defined as a rate of the intersection over union (IoU) (defined in Equation (7)) of the two circles drawn from the true landmark coordinates and predicted ones that was greater than 0.5. The IoU threshold was determined by reference to a previous study on cyst detection [29].

$$\mathrm{IoU} \quad = \quad \frac{Area\ of\ Intersection}{Area\ of\ Union} \tag{7}$$

Precision (8) and recall (9) were calculated as the detection accuracy.

$$\text{Precision} \quad = \quad \frac{TP}{TP + FP} \tag{8}$$

$$\text{Recall} \quad = \quad \frac{TP}{TP + FN} \tag{9}$$

The position error and diameter length error (DLE) in cyst measurements by both the AI and sonographer were used to evaluate the coordinates of the predicted salient landmarks. The position error (defined in Equation (10)) is defined as the Euclidean distance between the predicted and true coordinates. DLE (defined in Equation (11)) is defined as the absolute value of the difference between the Euclidean distance between the two predicted coordinates and the Euclidean distance between the two true coordinates. If the true coordinates are p_1, p_2 and the predicted coordinates are p'_1, p'_2, then the position error and DLE are defined as follows:

$$\text{Position error} \quad = \quad ||p_1 - p'_1|| + ||p_2 - p'_2|| \tag{10}$$

$$\text{DLE} \quad = \quad ||l - l'|| \tag{11}$$

$$l \quad = \quad ||p_1 - p_2|| \tag{12}$$

$$l' \quad = \quad ||p'_1 - p'_2|| \tag{13}$$

The relationship between the loss function of each model and these evaluation indices is as follows. The loss function of YOLOv5 is the sum of three terms, namely, the loss functions of the bounding box regression, prediction confidence, and classification [26]. The loss function of the bounding box regression is calculated from the IoU of the correct and predicted bounding boxes. Because the salient landmark coordinates are predicted within the bounding box, a smaller loss function of the bounding box regression and more accurate prediction of the bounding box makes for an improvement in the position error and detection accuracy calculated from the bounding box. The loss function of UNet++ is the mean square error. When the output saliency map is closer to the correct answer, the mean square error and position error determined from the output saliency map decrease.

2.8. Performance Comparison of Model and Sonographers

The ground truth coordinates in the test data were set using the annotations of two board-certified radiologists (Sonographers 1 and 4). The annotations of the remaining two radiologists (Sonographers 2 and 3) and the predicted coordinates of the model were compared with the correct coordinates in order to calculate the recall, precision, position error, and diameter length error.

2.9. Post Hoc Evaluation by a Radiologist

In the form of a post hoc evaluation, the predictions of the automated system were manually evaluated by the most experienced radiologist (Sonographer 1). The predictions of salient landmarks by the automated system and predictions of salient landmarks placed by Sonographers 2 and 3 were presented to Sonographer 1 in an anonymous and random order. Sonographer 1 examined the ultrasound image and both predictions, pointed out FPs and FNs, and corrected the coordinates as necessary. The number of FPs and FNs, images with corrected coordinates, salient landmarks, and magnitude of the correction of coordinates were calculated and compared between the automated system and the two radiologists.

2.10. Deep Learning Framework and Computation Time

Python was used as the programming language. In YOLOv5, Torch 1.7.1 version or earlier was used as the framework. The number of training epochs was set to 100, and the weight at the epoch with high mAP (mean Average Precision) was used. SGD was used as the optimizer for training. The batch size was set to 16 and the size of one side of the input image was 256 pixels. In UNet++, TensorFlow GPU version 1.4.0 was used as the framework. The number of training epochs was set to 20, and the weight at the epoch when the loss function was improved was saved. The Adam optimizer was used for training. The hyperparameters, as presented in Table 2, were searched. As a result of this search, the hyperparameters indicated in bold were adopted.

Table 2. The hyperparameter search and its results; the hyperparameters highlighted in bold were adopted.

Parameter	Range of Parameter to Be Searched
CNN architecture	VGG16, ResNet50, **densenet121**
Decode method	**transpose**, upsampling
Number of decoder filters	**(128, 64, 32, 16, 8)**, (256, 128, 64, 32, 16), (512, 256, 128, 64, 32)
Batch size	8 to 32 (**21**)

The computational time required to read the ultrasound image, predict the coordinates of the salient landmarks, plot them, and display the image was measured. This experiment was performed on a computer with an Intel (R) Xeon (R)W-3235 CPU@3.30GH and an NVIDIA Quadro RTX 8000. In addition, the time required for manual assignment of salient landmarks by the radiology specialists was measured for comparison. The methodology source code is available in a public GitHub repository with the following address: https://github.com/henyo245/RenalCystMeasurement, accessed on 6 February 2023.

2.11. Materials

We extracted 170,538 images from 6420 abdominal ultrasound examinations taken by LOGIQE9 or LOGIQS8 GE ultrasonic devices from January 2019 to May 2020 at Keio University Hospital. Of the 6420 examinations, 2134 were identified as "renal cyst" in the report. Among the extracted ultrasound images, 2664 images were selected in which the body marker was located on the kidney and the radiologist determined that renal cysts were measured. Images with no salient landmarks or those determined by the radiologist to not be renal cysts were excluded. The 2664 images were taken from 1444 patients, and therefore contained multiple images of the same patients. All data were annotated by eight radiology technicians and ten radiologists at the clinical site. No double-checking was performed. All data were divided into training and test data at a ratio of 7:3. There was no patient overlap between the training and the test data. Training image data were preprocessed to suit the respective tasks of object detection and salient landmark position prediction. In addition, 100 images were randomly extracted from the test data and used as a dataset in order to compare the performance of the sonographers and the automated system. For the training data, the markers measured at the clinical site were directly used as the true ones. For the test data, the ground truth was regenerated by Sonographers 1 and 4. Sonographer 1 placed the landmarks, Sonographer 4 reviewed the results, and for images with differing opinions, Sonographers 1 and 4 discussed and reassigned the landmarks as ground truth. Patient informed consent for the retrospective datasets was obtained only for this current research work, and has not been confirmed for sharing outside Keio University Hospital.

We created a dataset for training of the renal cyst detection model. The ultrasound images were used as the input data. A bounding box, which is required for object detection training, was created by the following procedure. First, a circle was drawn with its diameter being a straight line connecting the two paired salient landmarks. Next, a square circumscribing this circle was drawn, which was used as a bounding box surrounding the renal cyst. The x and y coordinates, height h, and width w of the center coordinates of the bounding box were saved in a text file and used as the training data.

We created a dataset for use in training the salient landmark position prediction model. The area surrounded by the bounding box for use as the training data of the renal cyst detection model was cropped from the ultrasound image and used as the input image of the salient landmark position prediction model. Then, to ensure that the outline of the renal cyst fit in the image, the cropped area of the bounding box was resized by expanding the area by the length of one side of the bounding box × 0.2 on the top, bottom, left, and right. The cropped images were resized to 256 × 256 pixels and used as the input images. In addition, a saliency map (heatmap) representing the salient landmark position in the area corresponding to the input image was generated and used as training data.

2.12. Ethics

This study was approved by the Ethics Committee of the Keio University School of Medicine (ethical approval code 20170018).

3. Result

3.1. Performance Comparison of Model and Sonographers

Table 3 shows the performance of the automated system on the test data and a performance comparison on the 100 selected images between the automated system and the two radiologists (Sonographers 2 and 3) with the annotation of two specialists (Sonographer 1 and 4) as the ground truth. As a result of the automated system for assigning salient landmarks, the detection accuracy was the highest when YOLOv5m and UNet++ were used and the coordinates were corrected. The precision and recall of the automated system were comparable to Sonographers 2 and 3. The position error and the diameter length error (DLE) of the automated system were comparable or slightly lower than those of the sonographers. No significant differences were found among the YOLO models. Figure 7 shows several examples of annotations by radiologists and the coordinates predicted by the automated system on the ultrasound images.

Table 3. Results of the performance of the automated system in the test data (above) and performance comparison on the 100 selected images (below) between the automated system and the two radiologists (Sonographers 2 and 3) with the annotation of two specialists (Sonographer 1 and 4) as the ground truth. The position error and DLE were calculated only for the true positive predictions of salient landmark positions. * a statistical *t*-test examining the average of IoU values between the "YOLOv5m + UNet++ + Correction" combination method and other combinations, along with the calculated *p*-values.

	Detection Accuracy			Position Error [mm]		DLE [mm]	
	Precision	Recall	*p*-Value * (of *t*-Test for IoU Average)	Mean	Median	Mean	Median
YOLOv5s + UNet++	0.71	0.75	0.07	3.54 ± 2.81	2.54	1.22 ± 1.04	1.02
YOLOv5s + UNet++ + Correction	0.78	0.82	0.07	3.59 ± 2.81	2.63	1.19 ± 1.02	0.93
YOLOv5m + UNet++	0.81	0.81	0.26	3.15 ± 2.48	2.36	1.08 ± 0.83	0.90
YOLOv5m + UNet++ + Correction	0.85	0.86	-	3.22 ± 2.57	2.36	1.09 ± 0.80	0.89
YOLOv5l + UNet++	0.74	0.78	0.07	3.19 ± 2.57	2.51	1.06 ± 1.92	0.90
YOLOv5l + UNet++ + Correction	0.82	0.86	0.18	3.29 ± 2.66	2.60	1.13 ± 1.00	0.88
YOLOv5x + UNet++	0.70	0.73	0.004	3.05 ± 2.72	2.39	1.15 ± 0.87	1.05
YOLOv5x + UNet++ + Correction	0.77	0.81	0.04	3.24 ± 2.73	2.63	1.13 ± 0.89	0.91
	Detection Accuracy		Position Error [mm]		DLE [mm]	
	Precision	Recall	Mean	Median	Mean	Median
Sonographer 2	0.86	0.87	2.56 ± 2.76	1.42	1.21 ± 1.36	0.89
Sonographer 3	0.83	0.84	2.34 ± 2.63	1.53	0.95 ± 1.07	0.63
YOLOv5m + UNet++ + Correction	0.85	0.86	3.22 ± 2.57	2.36	1.09 ± 0.8	0.89

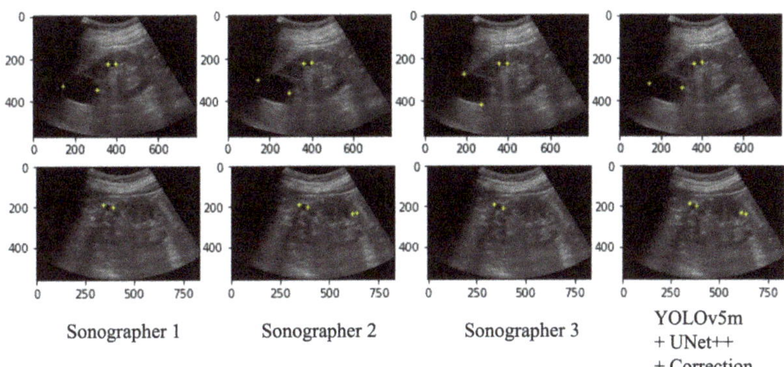

Sonographer 1   Sonographer 2   Sonographer 3   YOLOv5m + UNet++ + Correction

Figure 7. Ultrasound images with salient landmarks placed by sonographers and placed at coordinates predicted by the automated system.

Figure 8 shows the coordinates of the salient landmarks placed by Sonographer 1 and the coordinates predicted by the automation system.

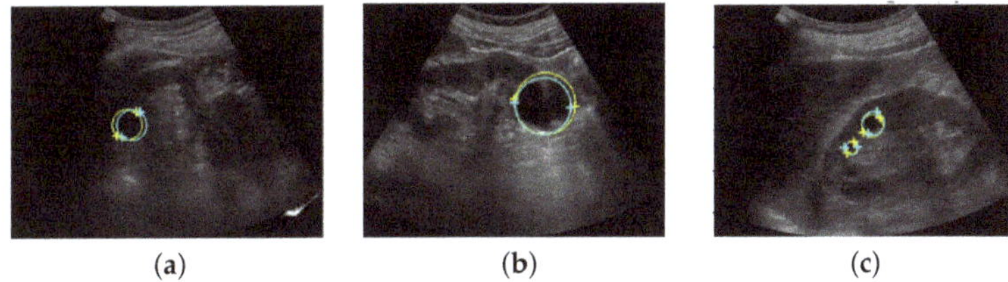

(**a**)   (**b**)   (**c**)

Figure 8. Ultrasound images with salient landmarks placed by sonographers and placed at coordinates predicted by the automated system. The yellow crosses are the coordinates of the salient landmarks placed by Sonographer 1 and the light blue crosses are the coordinates predicted by the automation system. Renal cysts are approximated by a circle with a diameter that is a straight line connecting the two points of salient landmarks. Yellow corresponds to placement by Sonographer 1 and light blue corresponds to prediction by the automated system. (**a**,**b**) show detection of a single renal cyst. (**c**) shows detection of two renal cysts.

3.2. Post Hoc Evaluation by Radiologist

Table 4 presents the results of the post hoc manual evaluation by the most experienced radiologist. The numbers of FPs and FNs produced by the automated system were less than those produced by Sonographer 2 and the same as those produced by Sonographer 3. The number of corrected images and salient landmarks were larger than those produced by Sonographers 2 and 3. The difference between the number of images and the number of salient landmarks is because there were ultrasound images with multiple renal cysts and images in which the coordinates of only one of the pair of salient landmarks were corrected. The magnitude of this modification was the smallest when using the proposed system.

Table 4. Results of post hoc manual evaluation by the most experienced radiologist.

	False Positive [Pair]	False Negative [Pair]	Corrected Coordinates		Position Error [mm]	
			Number of Images [Image]	Number of Landmarks [Point]	Mean	Median
Sonographer 2	3	3	16	18	9.09 ± 5.90	6.80
Sonographer 3	1	0	14	21	8.65 ± 5.40	7.24
YOLOv5m + UNet++ + Correction	1	1	16	22	8.49 ± 8.04	5.47

3.3. Computational Time

The average execution time of the model was 0.45 ± 0.02 s per image. The average time required for measurement by a radiologist was 14.9 ± 4.5 s per image.

4. Discussion

There are a number of limitations to this study. First, this study was a single-center study limited to Japanese patients. In addition, the ultrasound images were taken with a limited number of ultrasonic device models. More ultrasound imaging datasets of renal cysts from multiple institutions are required to build a more accurate system. Moreover, the results may change because of the influence of the amount of noise depending on the sonographer's imaging skills, ghost artifacts (unwanted reflections of ultrasonic waves), and artifacts, such as shadows that darken the back of tissues.

Based on the above, the salient landmark prediction system constructed using deep learning technology has great potential to detect renal cysts faster than radiologists and with comparable accuracy. Further training using larger amounts of data collected from multiple institutions can enable even more accurate detection and measurement of renal cysts. In addition, because the constructed method can be applied to other targets, such as hepatic cysts, we expect artificial intelligence-based measurement support systems for various areas of interest to be developed in the future.

There are a number of issues with the system developed in this study that could represent possibilities for future improvement. Several parameters, including the radius of the Gaussian distribution and the threshold value used for coordinate correction, were determined experimentally; in future work, a more comprehensive and systematic optimization of these parameters is necessary. We simply input the same single grayscale image into three channels for RGB in YOLOv5. Optimizing YOLOv5 to work with only one grayscale channel is another possibility for future work.

5. Conclusions

In this study, we constructed an automated system for assigning salient landmarks to renal cysts using deep learning methods, namely, YOLOv5 and UNet++, with 2664 ultrasound images. Previous studies have relied on segmentation, and have not targeted the abdomen. Here, we developed an automatic measurement method for renal cysts that does not require segmentation. Because the position of the salient landmarks can be predicted with an accuracy close to that of a radiologist in a shorter time, this system is useful for automating the measurement process in ultrasonography.

Author Contributions: M.H., M.J., and Y.S. designed the study and concept. M.H., S.O., and M.J. acquired the data. Y.K., H.H., and Y.S. designed and implemented the automated system. Y.K., M.H., N.T., S.O., H.H., M.J., and Y.S. analyzed and interpreted the data and results. Y.K. and Y.S. wrote the manuscript draft. All authors have read and agreed to the published version of the manuscript.

Funding: This work was supported by a Grant-in-Aid for Scientific Research (A) (KAKENHI) (no. 18H04127) from the JSPS. This work was further supported by GE Healthcare.

Institutional Review Board Statement: This study was approved by the Ethics Committee of the Faculty of Science and Technology of Keio University (protocol code 20170018).

Informed Consent Statement: This study was approved by the institutional review board. Informed consent was obtained from all subjects involved in the study via opt-out method.

Data Availability Statement: Not applicable.

Conflicts of Interest: The authors declare no conflict of interest.

References

1. Sarris, I.; Ioannou, C.; Chamberlain, P.; Ohuma, E.; Roseman, F.; Hoch, L.; Altman, D.G.; Papageorghiou, A.T. Intra- and interobserver variability in fetal ultrasound measurements. *Ultrasound Obstet. Gynecol.* **2012**, *39*, 266–273. [CrossRef] [PubMed]
2. Akkus, Z.; Cai, J.; Boonrod, A.; Zeinoddini, A.; Weston, A.D.; Philbrick, K.A.; Erickson, B.J. A Survey of Deep-Learning Applications in Ultrasound: Artificial Intelligence-Powered Ultrasound for Improving Clinical Workflow. *J. Am. Coll. Radiol.* **2019**, *16*, 1318–1328. [CrossRef]
3. Ma, J.; Wu, F.; Jiang, T.; Zhu, J.; Kong, D. Cascade convolutional neural networks for automatic detection of thyroid nodules in ultrasound images. *Med. Phys.* **2017**, *44*, 1678–1691. [CrossRef]
4. Li, X.; Zhang, S.; Jiang, Q.; Wei, X.; Pan, Y.; Zhao, J.; Xin, X.; Qin, C.; Wang, X.; Li, J.; et al. Diagnosis of thyroid cancer using deep convolutional neural network models applied to sonographic images: A retrospective, multicohort, diagnostic study. *Lancet Oncol.* **2017**, *20*, 193–201. [CrossRef]
5. Deng, J.; Dong, W.; Socher, R.; Li, L.-J.; Li, K.; Fei-Fei, L. Imagenet: A large-scale hierarchical image database. In Proceedings of the IEEE Conference on Computer Vision and Pattern Recognition, Miami, FL, USA, 20–25 June 2009; pp. 248–255.
6. Byra, M.; Galperin, M.; Ojeda-Fournier, H.; Olson, L.; O'Boyle, M.; Comstock, C.; Andre, M. Breast mass classification in sonography with transfer learning using a deep convolutional neural network and color conversion. *Med. Phys.* **2018**, *46*, 746–755. [CrossRef] [PubMed]
7. Liu, X.; Song, J.L.; Wang, S.H.; Chen, Y.Q. Learning to diagnose cirrhosis with liver capsule guided ultrasound image classification. *Sensors* **2017**, *17*, 149. [CrossRef] [PubMed]
8. Muresan, M.P.; Barbura, A.R.; Nedevschi, S. Teeth Detection and Dental Problem Classification in Panoramic X-ray Images using Deep Learning and Image Processing Techniques. In Proceedings of the IEEE 16th International Conference on Intelligent Computer Communication and Processing (ICCP), Cluj-Napoca, Romania, 3–5 September 2020; pp. 457–463.
9. Pang, S.; Pang, C.; Zhao, L.; Chen, Y.; Su, Z.; Zhou, Y.; Huang, M.; Yang, W.; Lu, H.; Feng, Q. SpineParseNet: Spine Parsing for Volumetric MR Image by a Two-Stage Segmentation Framework With Semantic Image Representation. *IEEE Trans. Med. Imaging* **2021**, *40*, 262–273. [CrossRef] [PubMed]
10. Gu, R.; Wang, G.; Song, T.; Huang, R.; Aertsen, M.; Deprest, J.; Ourselin, S.; Vercauteren, T.; Zhang, S. CA-Net: Comprehensive Attention Convolutional Neural Networks for Explainable Medical Image Segmentation. *IEEE Trans. Med. Imaging* **2021**, *40*, 699–711. [CrossRef] [PubMed]
11. Takeuchi, M.; Seto, T.; Hashimoto, M.; Ichihara, N.; Morimoto, Y.; Kawakubo, H.; Suzuki, T.; Jinzaki, M.; Kitagawa, Y.; Miyata, H.; et al. Performance of a deep learning-based identification system for esophageal cancer from CT images. *Esophagus* **2021**, *18*, 612. [CrossRef]
12. Payer, C.; Li, D.; Bischof, H.; Urschler, M. Regressing Heatmaps for Multiple Landmark Localization Using CNNs. *Med. Image Comput. Comput. Assist. Interv.* **2016**, *9901*, 230.
13. Zhong, Z.; Li, J.; Zhang, Z.; Jiao, Z. An attention-guided deep regression model for landmark detection in cephalograms. In Proceedings of the International Conference on Medical Image Computing and Computer-Assisted Intervention, Shenzhen, China, 13–17 October 2019; pp. 540–548.
14. Chen, X.; He, M.; Dan, T.; Wang, N.; Lin, M.; Lin, Z.; Xian, J.; Cai, H.; Xie, H. Automatic measurements of fetal lateral ventricles in 2D ultrasound images using deep learning. *Front. Neurol.* **2020**, *11*, 526. [CrossRef]
15. Biswas, M.; Kuppli, V.; Araki, T.; Edla, D.R.; Godia, E.C.; Saba, L.; Suri, H.S.; Omerzu, T.; Laird, J.; Khanna, N.N.; et al. Deep learning strategy for accurate carotid intima-media thickness measurement: An ultrasound study on Japanese diabetic cohort. *Comput. Biol. Med.* **2018**, *98*, 100–117. [CrossRef] [PubMed]
16. Leclerc, S.; Smistad, E.; Pedrosa, J.; Østvik, A.; Cervenansky, F.; Espinosa, F.; Espeland, T.; Berg, E.A.R.; Jodoin, P.; Grenier, T.; et al. Deep learning for segmentation using an open large-scale dataset in 2D echocardiography. *IEEE Trans. Med. Imaging* **2019**, *38*, 2198–2210. [CrossRef] [PubMed]
17. Jagtap, J.M.; Gregory, A.V.; Homes, H.L.; Wright, D.E.; Edwards, M.E.; Akkus, Z.; Erickson, B.J.; Kline, T.L. Automated measurement of total kidney volume from 3D ultrasound images of patients affected by polycystic kidney disease and comparison to MR measurements. *Abdom. Radiol.* **2022**, *47*, 2408–2419. [CrossRef] [PubMed]
18. Akkasaligar, P.T.; Biradar, S. Automatic Kidney Cysts Segmentation in Digital Ultrasound Images. In *Medical Imaging Methods*; Springer: Berlin/Heidelberg, Germany, 2019; pp. 97–117.
19. Hines, J.J., Jr.; Eacobacci, K.; Goyal, R. The Incidental Renal Mass- Update on Characterization and Management. *Radiol. Clin. N. Am.* **2021**, *59*, 631–646. [CrossRef] [PubMed]
20. YOLOv5 in PyTorch > ONNX > CoreML > TFLite—GitHub. Available online: https://github.com/ultralytics/yolov5 (accessed on 17 January 2022).
21. Zhou, Z.; Siddiquee, M.M.R.; Tajbakhsh, N.; Liang, J. UNet++: Redesigning skip connections to exploit multiscale features in image segmentation. *IEEE Trans. Med. Imaging* **2019**, *39*, 1856–1867. [CrossRef] [PubMed]
22. Redmon, J.; Divvala, S.; Girshick, R.; Farhadi, A. You only look once: Unified, real-time object detection. In Proceedings of the IEEE Conference on Computer Vision and Pattern Recognition, Las Vegas, NV, USA, 27–30 June 2016.
23. Linn, T.Y.; Maire, M.; Belongie, S.; Hays, J.; Perona, P.; Remanan, D.; Dollár, P.; Zitnick, C.L. Microsoft coco: Common objects in context. In Proceedings of the European Conference on Computer Vision, Zurich, Switzerland, 6–12 September 2014.

24. Wang, C.-Y.; Liao, H.Y.M.; Wu, Y.H.; Chen, P.Y.; Hsieh, J.W.; Yeh, I.H. CSPNet: A new backbone that can enhance learning capability of CNN. In Proceedings of the IEEE/CVF Conference on Computer Vision and Pattern Recognition Workshops, Seattle, WA, USA, 14–19 June 2020; pp. 390–391.

25. He, K.; Zhang, X.; Ren, S.; Sun, J. Spatial pyramid pooling in deep convolutional networks for visual recognition. *IEEE Trans. Pattern Anal. Mach. Intell.* **2015**, *37*, 1904–1916. [CrossRef] [PubMed]

26. Song, Q.; Li, S.; Bai, Q.; Yang, J.; Zhang, X.; Li, Z.; Duan, Z. Object Detection Method for Grasping Robot Based on Improved YOLOv5. *Micromachines* **2021**, *12*, 1273. [CrossRef]

27. Ronneberger, O.; Fischer, P.; Brox, T. U-net: Convolutional networks for biomedical image segmentation. In Proceedings of the International Conference on Medical Image Computing and Computer-Assisted Intervention, Munich, Germany, 5–9 October 2015.

28. Huang, G.; Liu, Z.; Maaten, L.; Weinberger, K.Q. Densely connected convolutional networks. In Proceedings of the IEEE Conference on Computer Vision and Pattern Recognition, Honolulu, HI, USA, 21 July 2017.

29. Kwon, O.; Yong, T.H.; Kang, S.R.; Kim, J.E.; Huh, K.H.; Heo, M.S.; Lee, S.S.; Choi, S.C.; Yi, W.J. Automatic diagnosis for cysts and tumors of both jaws on panoramic radiographs using a deep convolution neural network. *Br. Inst. Radiol. Dentomaxillofac. Radiol.* **2020**, *49*, 20200185. [CrossRef] [PubMed]

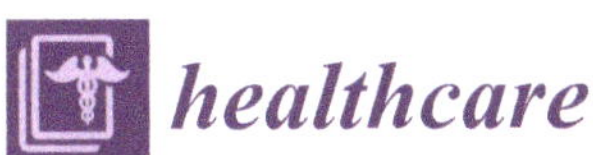

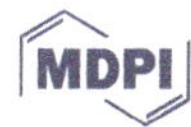

Article

Lung and Infection CT-Scan-Based Segmentation with 3D UNet Architecture and Its Modification

Mohammad Hamid Asnawi [1], Anindya Apriliyanti Pravitasari [1,*], Gumgum Darmawan [1], Triyani Hendrawati [1], Intan Nurma Yulita [2], Jadi Suprijadi [1] and Farid Azhar Lutfi Nugraha [1]

[1] Department of Statistics, Faculty of Mathematics and Natural Sciences, Universitas Padjadjaran, Bandung 45363, Indonesia
[2] Department of Computer Science, Faculty of Mathematics and Natural Sciences, Universitas Padjadjaran, Bandung 45363, Indonesia
* Correspondence: anindya.apriliyanti@unpad.ac.id

Abstract: COVID-19 is the disease that has spread over the world since December 2019. This disease has a negative impact on individuals, governments, and even the global economy, which has caused the WHO to declare COVID-19 as a PHEIC (Public Health Emergency of International Concern). Until now, there has been no medicine that can completely cure COVID-19. Therefore, to prevent the spread and reduce the negative impact of COVID-19, an accurate and fast test is needed. The use of chest radiography imaging technology, such as CXR and CT-scan, plays a significant role in the diagnosis of COVID-19. In this study, CT-scan segmentation will be carried out using the 3D version of the most recommended segmentation algorithm for bio-medical images, namely 3D UNet, and three other architectures from the 3D UNet modifications, namely 3D ResUNet, 3D VGGUNet, and 3D DenseUNet. These four architectures will be used in two cases of segmentation: binary-class segmentation, where each architecture will segment the lung area from a CT scan; and multi-class segmentation, where each architecture will segment the lung and infection area from a CT scan. Before entering the model, the dataset is preprocessed first by applying a minmax scaler to scale the pixel value to a range of zero to one, and the CLAHE method is also applied to eliminate intensity in homogeneity and noise from the data. Of the four models tested in this study, surprisingly, the original 3D UNet produced the most satisfactory results compared to the other three architectures, although it requires more iterations to obtain the maximum results. For the binary-class segmentation case, 3D UNet produced IoU scores, Dice scores, and accuracy of 94.32%, 97.05%, and 99.37%, respectively. For the case of multi-class segmentation, 3D UNet produced IoU scores, Dice scores, and accuracy of 81.58%, 88.61%, and 98.78%, respectively. The use of 3D segmentation architecture will be very helpful for medical personnel because, apart from helping the process of diagnosing someone with COVID-19, they can also find out the severity of the disease through 3D infection projections.

Keywords: COVID-19 CT-scan; 3D image segmentation; 3D UNet; 3D ResUNet; 3D VGGUNet; 3D DenseUNet

Citation: Asnawi, M.H.; Pravitasari, A.A.; Darmawan, G.; Hendrawati, T.; Yulita, I.N.; Suprijadi, J.; Nugraha, F.A.L. Lung and Infection CT-Scan-Based Segmentation with 3D UNet Architecture and Its Modification. *Healthcare* **2023**, *11*, 213. https://doi.org/10.3390/healthcare 11020213

Academic Editor: Mahmudur Rahman

Received: 19 November 2022
Revised: 28 December 2022
Accepted: 4 January 2023
Published: 10 January 2023

1. Introduction

COVID-19 is an infectious respiratory disease caused by SARS-CoV-2 (Severe Acute Respiratory Syndrome Corona Virus 2). This disease has spread over the world since December 2019; it started in one of the cities in China, namely Wuhan, and caused a global pandemic [1,2]. COVID-19 is recognized as a global pandemic because this disease is a highly contagious disease that has caused the WHO (World Health Organization) to declare this COVID-19 disease a PHEIC (Public Health Emergency of International Concern). This is due to the fact that this disease has a significant negative impact on individuals, governments, and even the global economy [3–6]. COVID-19 patients experience symptoms ranging from asymptomatic to symptomatic, including illness, lethargy, fever, cough, loss of smell and taste, and even the potentially fatal ARDS (Acute Respiratory Disease

Syndrome) [7]. COVID-19 mostly affects the lungs, causing lung infection, but it can also induce intestinal infections, resulting in digestive symptoms such as nausea, vomiting, and diarrhea [8].

From 2019 to now, there has still been no medical treatment that has been proven to cure COVID-19 in its entirety [9]. Therefore, one of the most needed precautions to reduce the spread of this COVID-19 virus is accurate and fast testing. The most common COVID-19 disease detection technique used worldwide, and considered the gold standard for testing for COVID-19, is RT-PCR (Reverse Transcription-Polymerase Chain Reaction) [9–11]. In just 4 to 6 h, RT-PCR is able to identify the presence or absence of SARS-CoV-2 RNA from respiratory specimens obtained by nasopharyngeal or oropharyngeal swabs [12]. However, the drawbacks of the RT-PCR test are that this test requires a lot of medical personnel to perform it manually, and each country has a limited stock of RT-PCR test kits. Furthermore, The RT-PCR test has a fairly low sensitivity (range 70 to 90) [13], which causes a high false-negative rate. This is due to many factors, including sample preparation and quality control that is not very mature due to time pressure and the situations around the world that are getting worse [14–16]. In addition to diagnosis using the RT-PCR test, there are also other diagnoses that use chest radiography imaging, namely CXR (Chest X-Ray) and CT-scan (Computed Tomography Scans). Both of these have proven to be more accurate than RT-PCR, but it is necessary for a radiologist to identify and look for radiological signs that show COVID-19 symptoms on the image. Although CXR diagnosis is generally less expensive, faster, and exposes the patient to less radiation than CT-scan [17,18], CT-scan is more recommended for more accurate diagnostic results than CXR.

CT-scan is one of examination tools to diagnose the existence of COVID-19 symptoms trough radiological images [8,19]. The CT-scan is preferable because it can overcome the RT-PCR test's low sensitivity, so that when compared to RT-PCR, CT-scans increase the accuracy and speed of diagnosis [20]. When compared with other chest radiography imaging techniques, specifically CXR, CT-scans are more recommended in the diagnosis of COVID-19 or lung disease in general because CT-scans are not affected by chest tissue, and produce a three-dimensional image output, resulting in better visibility. In addition, one of the significant advantages of CT-scans is their versatility, where CT-scans can diagnose COVID-19 as well as non-covid diseases [16,21,22]. Although CT-scans have proven to be more accurate in diagnosing COVID-19 or lung disease in general, in the diagnostic stage, a radiologist is needed to diagnose and look for radiological signs that show symptoms of COVID-19 on the images. Therefore, it is very necessary to automate the diagnosis of lung disease using CT-scans. In addition to saving time and effort, it is also necessary to avoid errors that occur when performed manually by a radiologist, since the diagnosis depends on the accuracy and experience of the radiologist. Image segmentation is one of the keys in the stage of COVID-19 disease diagnosis automation. With image segmentation, in addition to being useful for knowing the required object segmentation area, it can also be useful for knowing more about the characteristics of a disease from the segmented object area used. Therefore, it is very important to know and find an image segmentation algorithm for medical images, especially CT-Scans, that is effective in helping medical experts diagnose COVID-19 diseases accurately and quickly [23].

With the rapid developments in the field of machine learning, many machine learning algorithms are used for medical image processing needs. One of the deep learning algorithms that is currently the most widely used for medical image processing, or even image processing in general, is the CNN (Convolutional Neural Network) algorithm. CNN has been widely used to diagnose other diseases such as tumors, malaria, cancer, and so on [24–27]. These studies confirm that CNN can also be used to detect the COVID-19 disease. In this study, the 3D UNet architecture and other three 3D UNet modification architectures will be used to segment the lung (binary-class segmentation), and the lung and infection (multi-class segmentation), on CT-scans. Seven models will be compared for each segmentation case (binary and multi-class). The seven models are: pure 3D UNet, 3D ResUNet (ResNet152) without transfer learning, 3D ResUNet (ResNet152) with transfer learning, 3D VGGUNet (VGG19) without transfer learning, 3D VGGUNet (VGG19) without transfer learning, 3D DenseUNet (DenseNet201) with transfer learning, and 3D DenseUNet without transfer learning. The reason for using the 3D UNet architecture and its modification, apart from the fact that the CT-scan data is already in 3D form, is that 3D UNet was chosen so that the image preprocessing and postprocessing processes are simpler. That is different from when we use UNet (2D), with which it is necessary to first separate each slice in the 3D image into one 2D image. Even though the use of the 3D UNet architecture requires larger and more expensive computational resources than UNet (2D), by using 3D UNet, we take advantage of the volume in the image and still consider the image as a single 3D image.

The following are the research's main contributions:

1. To effectively analyze CT-scan images, which are three-dimensional (3D), we have employed 3D deep learning architectures that are capable of analyzing data in a single 3D unit. This approach is distinct from previous research on this problem, where most studies have utilized two-dimensional (2D) architectures that require slicing the 3D image into individual 2D slices. The implementation of 3D architectures can improve the efficiency of CT-scan analysis by eliminating the need for preprocessing before model input and streamlining the post-processing stage through the ability to seamlessly project 3D images.

2. In this research, we have modified the 3D UNet architecture by replacing the encoder with three classification architectures: 3D VGG19, 3D ResNet152, and 3D DenseNet201. This resulted in three distinct image segmentation architectures: 3D VGGUNet, 3D ResUNet, and 3D DenseUNet. To determine which architecture is the most effective, we will compare the performance of these architectures using five evaluation metrics: IoU score, Dice score, accuracy, and F1-score.

3. By using a 3D segmentation architecture on a CT-scan, in addition to being able to help the COVID-19 disease diagnosis process, the 3D output generated from the model can help medical personnel determine the severity of the disease, such as mild, moderate, or severe, through a 3D infection projection that can be easily seen from the output model that generates a file in 3D shape.

The remainder of this paper is structured as follows: In Section 2, several research papers related to the diagnosis of COVID-19 using chest radiography imaging in general and the use of semantic segmentation in CT-scan for COVID-19 diagnosis in particular are discussed. The dataset, data preprocessing, proposed architecture in this study, metrics evaluation, and model setting that were used in this study are explained in Section 3. In Section 4, the result of each proposed architecture is explained and discussed. Finally, Section 5 concludes the paper.

2. Related Works

This section contains works related to our research, including general works on the diagnosis of COVID-19 using chest radiography imaging and the use of semantic segmentation in a specific CT-scan dataset. These works serve as the foundation for our investigation into efficient and effective methods for analyzing CT-scans for COVID-19 diagnosis using image segmentation techniques.

Because of the rapid advancement of technology, several researchers are contributing to the creation of a COVID-19 diagnosis system that uses artificial intelligence with chest radiography imaging media, including CXR and CT-scan. For the use of CXR media, many researchers diagnose COVID-19 using classification methods. In [28], various deep learning architectures, namely ResNet18, ResNet50, SqueezeNet, and DenseNet121, are used for CXR classification, and most of these networks achieve a specificity rate of around 90% and a sensitivity rate of 98%. In [29], COVID-Net was used to classify CXR images into COVID-19, non-COVID, bacterial infection, and normal. Moreover, in [30], high-level features were extracted using various ImageNet pre-trained models, and then all those features were fed into SVM to classify the COVID-19 cases. In addition to using the classification method on CXR, some researchers also use the image segmentation method. For example, in [31], researchers achieve state-of-the-art performance and can provide clinically interpretable saliency maps, which are very useful for COVID-19 diagnosis. In addition, in [32], researchers also applied the image segmentation method on CXR to extend it to cases with extreme abnormalities. CT-scans, in addition to CXR, have been shown in previous studies to be an extremely useful tool for diagnosing COVID-19 [33–35]. Practitioners and doctors use CT abnormalities that correspond to COVID-19. It has been discovered that CT scans show discrete patterns that can be used to identify infected individuals even in the early stages, making automatic CT medical imaging analysis an attractive topic of research among researchers [35]. It has also been discovered that CT diagnosis for COVID-19 anomaly detection can be performed prior to the onset of clinical symptoms [36]. As a result, several research papers have been proposed for the automatic early detection of COVID-19 using the classification and segmentation method infection on CT images [37,38]. Table 1 presents a summary of the method we will use and various previous studies regarding segmentation on CT-scan with the same dataset, namely the COVID-19 CT Lung and Infection Segmentation Dataset [39].

Table 1. A summary of the recently published studies on image segmentation using the same dataset.

Method	Summary
DMDF-Net [40]	DMDF-Net (Dual Multiscale Dilated Fusion Network) is proposed to produce robust segmentation of small lesions in CT images. To achieve superior segmentation performance, this architecture utilizes the power of multiscale deep feature fusion within the encoder and decoder modules in a mutually beneficial manner.
UNet [9]	The UNet architecture is used for precise and fast segmentation of lung and infection areas from CT-scan. CLAHE and cropping were also used in the preprocessing to remove the noise and only use the lung area (region of interest) from each slice.
SSA-Net [41]	SSA-Net (Spatial Self-Attention Network) was created with the aim of automatically identifying areas of infection on CT scans of the lungs. SSA-Net utilizes a self-attention mechanism to broaden the receptive field and improve representation learning by extracting useful contextual information from deeper layers without additional training. In addition, this architecture introduces a spatial convolution layer to accelerate training convergence and strengthen the network.
CHS-Net [42]	CHS-Net (COVID-19 hierarchical segmentation network) is proposed to identify the COVID-19 infected area from CT-scan. In this architecture, two models of RAIU-Net (Residual Attention Inception U-Net) are connected in series, where in the first model a contour map of the lung will be generated and the second model will identify the infected area.
SD-UNet [10]	SD-UNet, this architecture is the modified UNet architecture that combines the SA (Squeeze and Attention) with the Dense ASPP (Dense Atrous Spatial Pyramid Pooling) module. In this architecture, the SA module is used to fully exploit the global context information and strengthen the attention of pixel grouping. The Dense ASPP is used to capture the multi-scale of COVID-19 lessons.
UNet-EfficientB0 [43]	Using EfficientNetB0 as the backbone (encoder) on the UNet architecture
Various 3D UNet (Proposed)	We used the 3D UNet architecture in this study, as well as various types of backbone (encoder) on the 3D UNet architecture using no transfer learning and transfer learning. The backbones being tested in this study are 3D ResNet152, 3D VGG19, and 3D DenseNet201.

Owais et al. [40] introduced DMDF-Net (Dual Multiscale Dilated Fusion Network); this architecture is tailored for precise and fast segmentation of lung and infection areas from CT-scans, and it achieved an IoU score of 67.22%, a Dice similarity coefficient of 75.7%, an average precision of 69.92%, a specificity of 99.79%, a sensitivity of 72.78%, an enhance-alignment of 91.11%, and an MAE of 0.026. The use of CLAHE preprocessing and only cropping the area of interest was carried out by Mahmoudi et al. [9] to improve the image segmentation results when using the UNet architecture, resulting in a Dice score of 98% and 91% for the lung and infection segmentation tasks, respectively. Wang et al. [41] developed a new segmentation architecture, called SSA-Net, with the aim of automatically identifying areas of infection on CT-scans of the lungs. This architecture's main idea is to utilize a self-attention mechanism to broaden the receptive field and improve representation learning by extracting useful contextual information from deeper layers without additional training. Wang et al. [41] conducted experiments using SSA-Net on various datasets, and on dataset [39] obtained an average Dice similarity coefficient of 75.4%. Punn et al. [42] introduced the CHS-Net (COVID-19 hierarchical segmentation network); two RAIU-Net are connected in series in this architecture, and this architecture achieved an accuracy of 96.5%, a precision of 75.6%, a specificity of 96.9%, a recall of 88.5%, a Dice coefficient of 81.6%, and Jaccard similarity of 79.1%. Yin et al. [10] modified the UNet architecture by combining the SA module and the Dense SAPP module so as to create a new architecture called SD-UNet. This architecture achieved the metrics of Jaccard similarity, specificity, accuracy, Dice similarity coefficient, and sensitivity of 77.02% (47.88%), 99.32% (99.07%), 99.06% (98.21%), 86.96% (59.36%), and 89.88% (61.69%), respectively, for the binary-class (multi-class) segmentation. In study conducted by Singh et al. [43], UNet was used again to segment CT-scans. In this study Singh et al. replaced the UNet backbone (encoder) to EfficientNetB0, and it achieved a sensitivity of 84.5%, a specificity of 93.9%, and Dice coefficient of 65%.

Previous research on image segmentation for COVID-19 CT scans has utilized various approaches, many of which utilize convolutional neural networks (CNNs). However, these approaches often rely on 2D architectures, which can lengthen the modeling process, due to the need for data preprocessing to fit the data for 2D architectures and post-processing to project the predicted results into a 3D shape. To address this issue, we propose a solution using 3D CNN architectures in our research. Specifically, we use the 3D version of the well-known UNet architecture for image segmentation, resulting in the 3D UNet architecture. Additionally, we modify the 3D UNet architecture by using three classification architectures, namely VGG 19, ResNet 152, and DenseNet 201, resulting in the 3D VGGUNet, 3D ResUNet, and 3D DenseUNet architectures.

3. Materials and Methods

This section contains our proposed approach and the materials that we will use in this study. We start by describing the dataset that will be used in this study. After that, we will explain what pre-processing stages are applied to the data, the proposed method or architecture that will be used in this study, the metrics evaluation that will be used in the evaluation of our models, and at the end, the model setting for every architecture will be explained, too.

3.1. Dataset

In this study, the lung CT-scan dataset of Ma et al. [39] was used for the CT-scan segmentation modelling (training and testing) process. This dataset consists of 20 CT-scans of COVID-19 patients collected from radiopaedia [44] and the corona-cases initiative (RAIOSS) [45]. In addition to providing CT-scan files, ref. [39] also provides three masks for segmentation purposes, namely 'lung mask', 'infection mask', and 'lung and infection mask'. In the work of Ma et al. [46], it is explained that this dataset was manually annotated by two radiologists and verified by an experienced radiologist. Table 2 presents an overview of the CT-scan dataset used.

In this study, segmentation will be carried out on the "lung mask" and the "lung and infection mask" in each model. Two segmentation cases were carried out to test the strength of each model in the cases of binary-class segmentation (lung mask) and multi-class segmentation (lung and infection mask).

Each CT-scan from the [39] dataset has a different width and height, a depth (slice), and a different level of infection severity. Table 3 shows the more detailed profile of each patient's CT scan used.

Table 2. Three samples (patient 1, patient 2, and patient 20) from the used dataset.

3D Projection of CT-Scan	CT-Scan Slice	Lung Mask	Infection Mask	Lung and Infection Mask

Table 3. Source, infection severity, and size information for each patient's CT-scan.

Patient	Source	Infection Severity	Size (Width × Height × Depth)
Patient 1	RAIOSS	Moderate	512 × 512 × 301
Patient 2	RAIOSS	Mild	512 × 512 × 200
Patient 3	RAIOSS	Severe	512 × 512 × 200
Patient 4	RAIOSS	Mild	512 × 512 × 270
Patient 5	RAIOSS	Mild	512 × 512 × 290
Patient 6	RAIOSS	Moderate	512 × 512 × 213
Patient 7	RAIOSS	Moderate	512 × 512 × 249
Patient 8	RAIOSS	Moderate	512 × 512 × 301
Patient 9	RAIOSS	Moderate	512 × 512 × 256
Patient 10	RAIOSS	Severe	512 × 512 × 301
Patient 11	Radiopaedia	Severe	630 × 630 × 39
Patient 12	Radiopaedia	Severe	630 × 630 × 45
Patient 13	Radiopaedia	Moderate	630 × 630 × 39
Patient 14	Radiopaedia	Moderate	630 × 630 × 418
Patient 15	Radiopaedia	Severe	630 × 401 × 110
Patient 16	Radiopaedia	Moderate	630 × 630 × 66
Patient 17	Radiopaedia	Mild	630 × 630 × 42
Patient 18	Radiopaedia	Mild	630 × 630 × 42
Patient 19	Radiopaedia	Mild	630 × 630 × 45
Patient 20	Radiopaedia	Severe	630 × 630 × 93

3.2. Data Preprocessing

Since we want to use 3D image segmentation architecture, we need to adjust the width, height, and depth of each image to the same size. In this study, we adjusted each CT-scan data to $128 \times 128 \times 128$. The resizing process for each CT-scan data is assisted by ImageJ software, and in the process of resizing the depth of each data, ImageJ applies average upsampling and average downsampling with bilinear interpolation.

Two preprocessing steps will be carried out on the CT-scan image file: scaling the pixel value and applying the CLAHE method. The image scaling process is carried out on each pixel value in the CT-scan into a value with a range of 0 to 1. This scaling stage is carried out using the minmax scaler method.

Furthermore, the CLAHE (Contrast Limited Adaptive Histogram Equalization) method is applied to overcome the contrast problems (noise and intensity inhomogeneity). CLAHE was used to intensify the contrast of the obtained images [47]. This method is a variant of AHE (Adaptive Histogram Equalization). CLAHE's main objective is to determine the mapping for each pixel based on its neighborhood grayscale distribution using a transformation function that reduces contrast amplification in densely packed areas. In [48,49], CLAHE has shown its effectiveness in allocating displayed intensity levels in chest CT-scans. In Table 4, a comparison of the CT-scan slices before CLAHE was applied and after CLAHE was applied is shown.

Table 4. Comparison before and after applying CLAHE preprocessing to CT-scan.

Without CLAHE	CLAHE

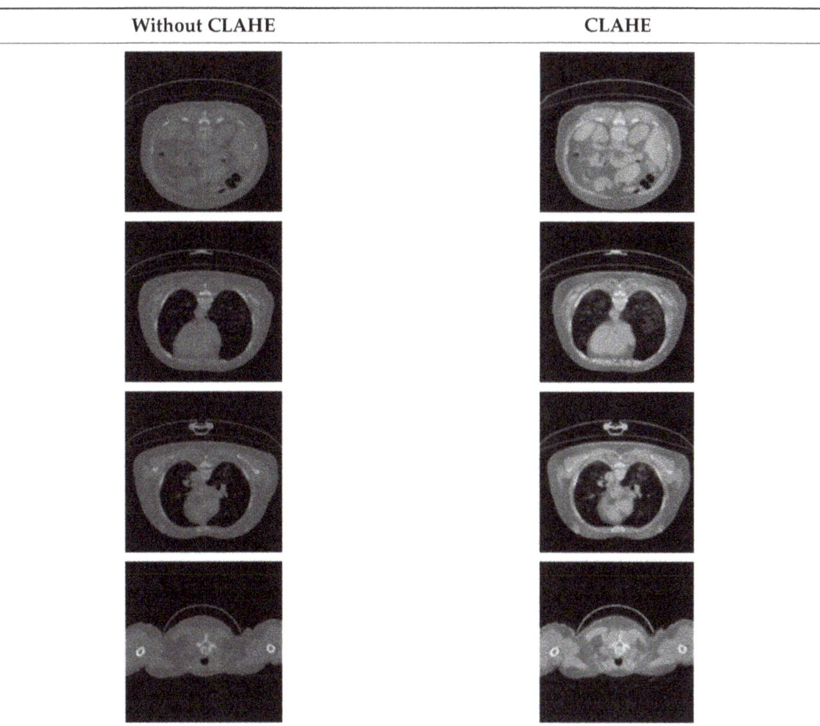

For the case of binary-class segmentation, the lung mask pixels consisting of 0: background, 1: left lung, and 2: right lung are changed to 0: background and 1: lung. The unification of the left lung and right lung masks is not only performed to create a binary-class segmentation case, but it is also performed to facilitate the learning model process because there is no significant difference in the image between the left lung and right lung. The unification of left lung and right lung is also carried out on the lung and infection mask for multi-class segmentation, where, in this multi-class segmentation, the pixel lung and infection mask consist of 0: background, 1: left lung, 2: right lung, and 4: infection is changed to 0: background, 1: warp, and 2: infection.

3.3. Network Architecture

This work proposes four segmentation network architectures, namely 3D UNet [50], 3D ResUNet, 3D VGGUNet, and 3D DenseUNet. Each architecture will be applied in both binary-class CT-scan segmentation (lung segmentation) and multi-class CT-scan segmentation (lung and infection segmentation). For the 3D ResUNet, 3D VGGUNet, and 3D DenseUNet architectures, two experiments will be carried out for each segmentation, using transfer learning and not using transfer learning. From this, a total of seven models will be obtained for each segmentation case.

3D UNet has two main parts, namely the encoder and decoder. The encoder part, also called the contracting part, is in charge of extracting global features from the image. The encoder consists of convolution blocks (consisting of batch normalization, ReLu) and max pooling for downsampling. The decoder part, also known as the expanding path, consists of upconvolution, a concatenation layer with a feature map from the encoder part, and convolutional blocks. To avoid overfitting, a dropout layer is added to each convolutional block. The UNet 3D architecture is shown in Figure 1.

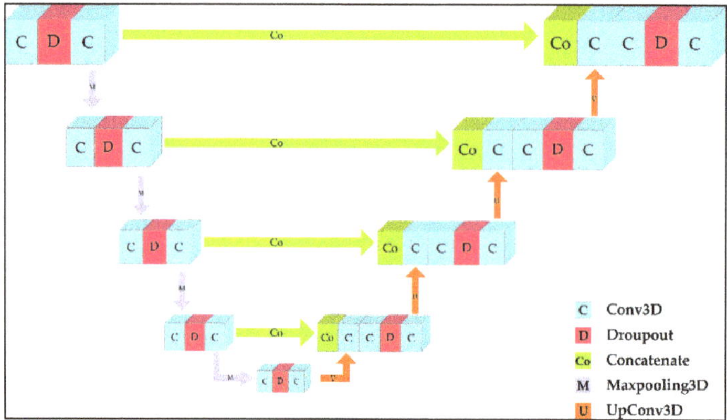

Figure 1. 3D UNet architecture.

The 3D ResUNet, 3D VGGUNet, and 3D DenseUNet architectures are modifications of the 3D UNet architecture. These three architectures replace the encoder portion of 3D UNet with 3D ResNet, 3D VGG, and 3D DenseNet, respectively. 3D ResUNet uses the 3D ResNet152 architecture to replace the encoder part of 3D UNet because the ResNet152 version is the latest version of the 3D ResNet version series available (ResNet18, ResNet34, ResNet50, ResNet152). As with 3D VGGUNet, the latest version of the 3D VGG architecture, namely 3D VGG19, is used as the backbone or encoder of the 3D UNet architecture. The same goes for 3D DenseUNet. DenseNet201's 3D architecture was chosen for the reason of being the most up-to-date version compared to other 3D DenseNet versions (3D DenseNet121, 3D DenseNet169, and 3D DenseNet201). The schematic of these 3 architectures is not much different from the 3D UNet shown in Figure 1. Figure 2 shows the general segmentation process of the 3D VGGUNet, 3D ResUNet, and 3D DenseUNet architectures.

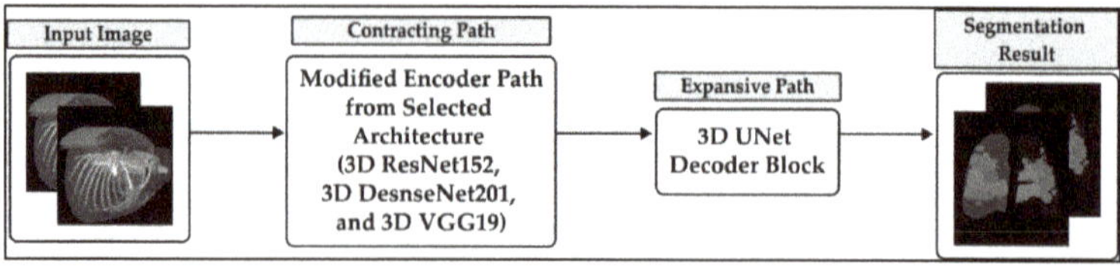

Figure 2. The general segmentation process with scenario of 3D U-Net modified architectures.

The 3D versions of the VGG and ResNet classification architectures were chosen to modify the encoder part of the 3D UNet architecture because these two architectures are some of the most widely used in research, with the ResNet architecture being used in over 142,000 studies and the VGG architecture being used in over 119,000. Apart from being widely used, these two architectures were chosen because both of them have proven to be very good at solving classification problems, as evidenced by their wins in the ImageNet 2014 (VGG) and ImageNet 2015 (ResNet) competitions. The 3D version of the DenseNet architecture was chosen in this study because it is one of the architectures that has recently begun to be widely used, because it has many advantages, such as reducing the vanishing-gradient problem, strengthening feature propagation, encouraging feature reuse, and having parameters that are not too large. This architecture is the development of the most widely used classification architecture, namely ResNet. In the previous study by Alalwan et al. [51], 3D DenseUNet was used to segment liver and tumors from CT-scans, but the DenseNet version of the 3D DenseUNet architecture used in Alalwan et al.'s [51] study is a DenseNet version with a depth of 169. This study will use a deeper version of Densenet, namely DenseNet201. Due to the deep structure of each architecture, visualization will not be possible. Further details on the modified architectures used in this study can be found in Appendix A.

In this study, each modified architecture will be trained using both traditional training and transfer learning approaches. Transfer learning is a machine learning technique in which patterns learned from a pre-trained model are utilized to improve the performance of a model on a new task [52]. This can be particularly useful when working with a small training and testing dataset, as it allows us to leverage the knowledge and experience of the pre-trained model. In this research, we will apply transfer learning to the encoder portion of the architecture, including the 3D VGG19, 3D ResNet152, and 3D DenseNet201. The weights for the transfer learning process will be obtained from models that have been trained on the ImageNet dataset, a large and widely-used dataset for training and evaluating deep learning models. By applying transfer learning and utilizing the knowledge of these pre-trained models, we hope to improve the performance of our modified architectures on the CT-scan image segmentation task.

3.4. Metrics Evaluation

In this study, we use five evaluation metric indices to evaluate the performance of each network: IoU (Intersection Over Union score, also known as the Jaccard Index), DSc (Dice Score, or also known as the F1-score and Sørensen–Dice coefficient), Acc (Accuracy), Pre (Precision), and Rec (Recall). In the case of image segmentation, IoU and Dsc are the most frequently used metrics and are recommended to evaluate the model [53,54]. In general, the Dsc and IoU are used to see the similarity of the results of the segmentation area between the predicted result and the ground truth. The IoU and Dsc formulas are defined as follows:

$$IoU = \frac{|A_1 \cap A_2|}{|A_1 \cup A_2|} \tag{1}$$

$$Dsc = \frac{2|A_1 \cap A_2|}{|A_1| + |A_2|} \tag{2}$$

From Equations (1) and (2), it should be noted that A_1 denotes the ground truth, and A_2 denotes the predicted result by the model.

In addition to using IoU and Dsc, this study also used two classification metrics: accuracy, which measures the ratio of correctly identified predicted pixels to all predicted pixels, and F1 score, which is calculated as the harmonic mean of precision and recall. Precision measures the accuracy of predictions by calculating the ratio of true positive predicted pixels to the total number of positive predictions, and recall measures completeness by calculating the ratio of true positive predicted pixels to the total number of actual positive pixels. The accuracy and F1 score are defined as follows:

$$Acc = \frac{TP + TN}{TP + FP + TN + FN} \qquad (3)$$

$$F1\ score = \frac{2TP}{2TP + FP + FN} \qquad (4)$$

Here, *TP (True Positive)* denotes the number of the lung pixel or infected pixel being correctly identified, *TN (True Negative)* denotes the number of uninfected pixels or non-lung pixels being correctly identified, *FP (False Positive)* represents the number of infected pixels or lung pixels being wrongly identified as the uninfected or non-lung pixels, and *FN (False Negative)* represents the number of the non-lung pixels or the uninfected pixels being wrongly identified as lung or infected pixels.

3.5. Experimental Setting

All models are trained using the ADAM optimizer with a learning rate of 1×10^{-4}. To maximize the learning capabilities of each architecture, we set the maximum epoch to 5000 with an early-stop patience of 250. The loss functions used in the training process are total Dice loss and focal loss. Mixing between focal loss and Dice loss is performed because, after several experiments, the segmentation results using total loss from Dice loss and focal loss are better than using only Dice loss or only using focal loss. The total loss here is obtained by adding up the Dice loss with the focal loss, where each class weight for the Dice loss is set equal. Hold-out validation is used for the process of training and testing models. The data is split by 75% for model training and 25% for model testing. We run all models in this study using Google Colab Pro, with a GPU as a hardware accelerator and high-RAM usage for runtime shape. Figure 3 depicts the modeling scheme used in this study.

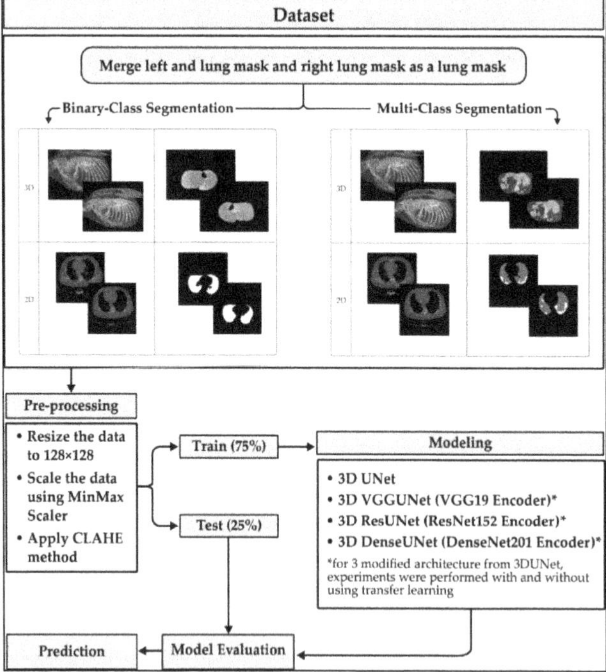

Figure 3. The modeling schemes.

4. Results

In this section, the results of the binary-class and multi-class segmentation experiments on the CT-scan will be shown. As described previously, the case of binary-class segmentation will be applied to segment the lungs from the CT-scan, while the case of multi-class segmentation will be applied to segment the lungs and infection from the CT-scan. We will see the results of the evaluation of metrics from 3D UNet, 3D VGGNet without transfer learning, 3D Res UNet without transfer learning, 3D DenseUNet without transfer learning, 3D VGGUNet with transfer learning, 3D ResUNet with transfer learning, and 3D DenseUNet with transfer learning in each CT-scan segmentation case.

4.1. Lung Segmentation (Binary-Class Segmentation)

For the purpose of comparison, the same hyperparameter values have been set, and the same distribution of training and testing data sets is used for the modeling process in each architecture. Table 5 shows the results of the evaluation metrics for each architecture in lung segmentation.

Table 5. The IoU Score, Dice Score, accuracy, F1-score epoch of learning, and time per epoch results of each architecture for the CT-scan binary-class segmentation.

	Architecture	IoU	DSc	Acc	F1	Epoch [1]	Time
	3D UNet	**0.9432**	**0.9705**	**0.9937**	**0.9707**	1663	±9 s/epoch
Without Transfer Learning	3D VGGUNet	0.9287	0.9624	0.9920	0.9630	230	±24 s/epoch
	3D ResUNet	0.8325	0.9072	0.9793	0.9086	357	±14 s/epoch
	3D DenseUNet	0.9204	0.9580	0.9912	0.9585	93	±13 s/epoch
With Transfer Learning	3D VGGUNet	0.9395	0.9682	0.9934	0.9688	330	±40 s/epoch
	3D ResUNet	0.9183	0.9569	0.9909	0.9574	405	±14 s/epoch
	3D DenseUNet	0.9260	0.9610	0.9919	0.9616	253	±13 s/epoch

[1] The number of epochs is obtained after reducing the total training epochs with a patience value of early stopping. The bolded numbers in the table indicate the highest values compared to other architectures.

Based on the results of the evaluation metrics for each architecture in Table 5, surprisingly, 3D UNet is better than the other six methods. Compared with the 3D VGGUNet architecture with transfer learning, which achieved the second best result on average, 3D UNet improved by 0.37%, 0.23%, 0.03%, and 0,19% in IoU score, Dice score, accuracy, and F1-score, respectively. Although 3D UNet has the best evaluation of metrics compared to other architectures, 3D UNet has the longest maximum learning iteration process of 1663, in contrast to other architectures, which are modifications of 3D UNet, and which have an average maximum learning iteration of 278. Of the seven models that have been tried, 3D DenseUNet obtained first place as the architecture with the fastest learning time, ±4459 s and ±6539 s without transfer learning and using transfer learning, respectively. The 3D UNet architecture stays in the second last position with a learning process time of ±17,217 s, and for the position of the architecture that has the longest training process, it is the 3D VGGUNet, with transfer learning reaching ±23,200 s. The comparison of loss training and testing on the 3D UNet learning process for the lung segmentation is shown in Figure 4. Furthermore, in Table 6, the comparison of ground truth and the prediction results of the 3D UNet model in 2D (slice) and 3D projections for this binary-class segmentation case can be seen.

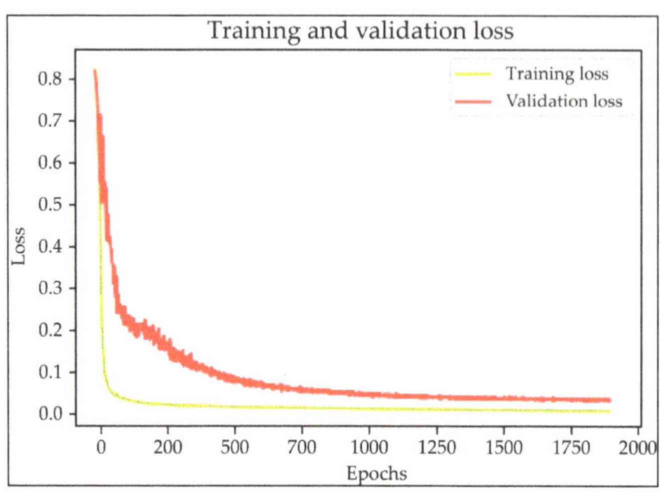

Figure 4. The training and validation loss curve of the 3D UNet architecture CT-scan binary-class segmentation learning process.

Table 6. Comparison between ground truth and prediction results of lung segmentation with 3D UNet architecture.

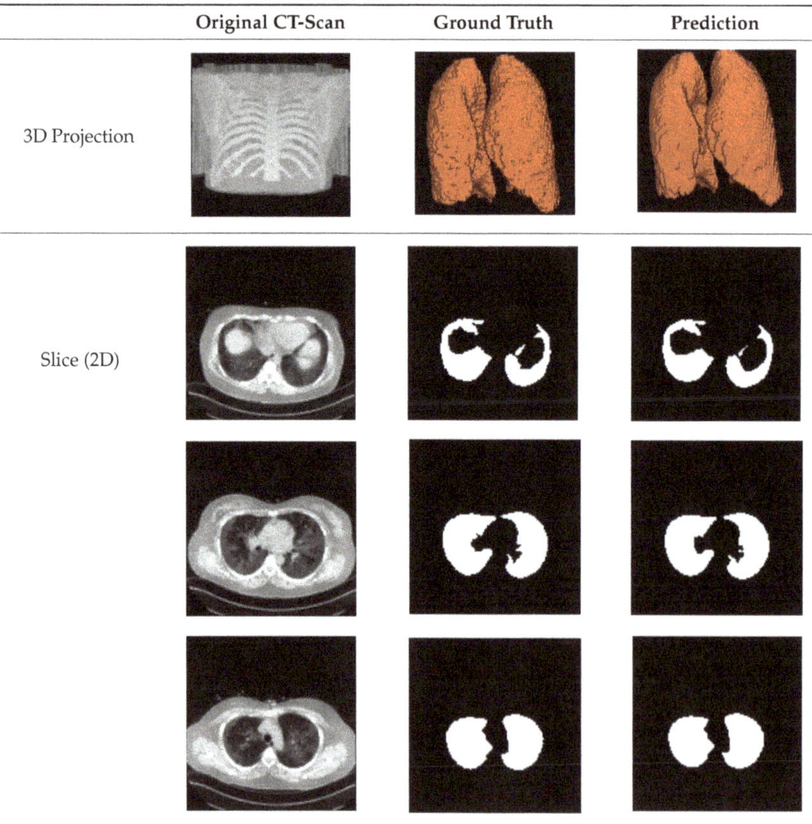

	Original CT-Scan	Ground Truth	Prediction
3D Projection			
Slice (2D)			

4.2. Lung and Infection Segmentation (Multi-Class Segmentation)

Similar to binary-class segmentation, in the case of multi-class segmentation, the same hyperparameter values and training testing data distribution have been established, with the intention of comparing each architecture. Table 7 shows the results of the evaluation metrics for each architecture in lung and infection segmentation.

Table 7. The IoU Score, Dice Score, accuracy, and F1-score, epoch of learning, and time per epoch results of each architecture for the CT-scan multi-class segmentation.

	Architecture	IoU	DSc	Acc	F1	Epoch [1]	Time
	3D UNet	**0.8158**	**0.8861**	**0.9878**	0.9878	1510	±7 s/epoch
Without Transfer Learning	3D VGGUNet	0.7276	0.8049	0.9839	0.9839	146	±24 s/epoch
	3D ResUNet	0.7089	0.7839	0.9833	0.9833	151	±14 s/epoch
	3D DenseUNet	0.7143	0.7916	0.9825	0.9826	104	±13 s/epoch
With Transfer Learning	3D VGGUNet	0.7340	0.8122	0.9840	0.9840	600	±24 s/epoch
	3D ResUNet	0.7381	0.8178	0.9832	0.9832	208	±19 s/epoch
	3D DenseUNet	0.7193	0.7960	0.9835	0.9836	189	±13 s/epoch

[1] The number of epochs is obtained after reducing the total training epochs with a patience value of early stopping. The bolded numbers in the table indicate the highest values compared to other architectures.

Based on the results of the evaluation metrics for each architecture in Table 6, similar to the lung segmentation case, in the lung and infection segmentation case, 3D UNet is better than the other six methods. Compared with the 3D VGGUNet architecture with transfer learning, which achieved the second-best result on average, 3D UNet improved by 8.18%, 7.39%, 0.38% and 0.38% in IoU score, Dice score, accuracy, and F1-score, respectively. Although 3D Unet has the best evaluation of metrics compared to other architectures, 3D UNet has the longest maximum learning iteration process of 1510, in contrast to other architectures, which are modifications of 3D UNet, and which have an average maximum learning iteration of 233. Of the seven models that have been tried, 3D DenseUNet without transfer learning obtained first place as the architecture with the fastest learning time, specifically ±4602 s. The 3D UNet architecture stays in the second to last position with a learning process time of ±12320 s, and in the position of the architecture that has the longest training process is the 3D VGGUNet with transfer learning, reaching ±8702 s. The comparison of loss training and testing on the 3D UNet learning process for the lung and infection segmentation is shown in Figure 5. Furthermore, in Table 8, the comparison of ground truth and the prediction results of the 3D UNet model in 2D (slice) and 3D projections in this multi-class segmentation case can be seen.

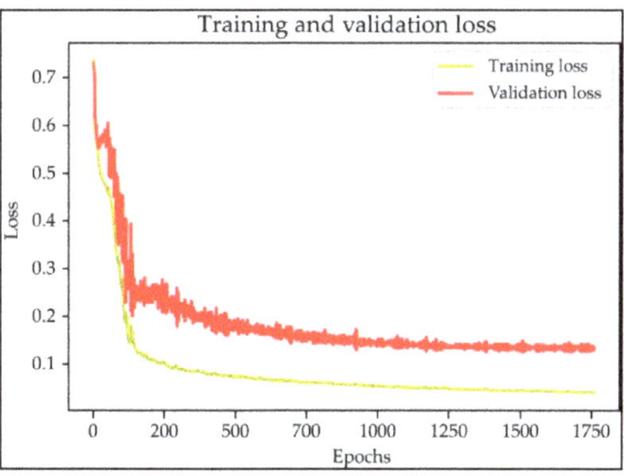

Figure 5. The training and validation loss curve of the 3D UNet architecture CT-scan binary-class segmentation learning process.

Table 8. Comparison between ground truth and prediction results of lung and infection segmentation with 3D UNet architecture.

	Original CT-Scan	Ground Truth	Prediction
3D Projection			
Slice			

4.3. Result Discussion

With the aim of experimenting using the 3D version of the UNet architecture and comparing it with its three modifications, namely 3D VGGUNet, 3D ResUNet, and 3D DenseNet, in the case of binary-class (lung) segmentation and multi-class (lung and infection) segmentation. Surprisingly, the original 3D UNet performs much better in both segmenting the binary-class and the multi-class than the modified 3D UNet. Although, on average, the modified architecture of 3D UNet does not perform as well as the original 3D UNet, the three modified architectures have much faster maximum learning iterations than the original 3D UNet, which is on average below 300 epochs, while for the original 3D UNet it requires more than 1500 epochs to reach the maximum learning iteration. In the case of the modified architectures of 3D UNet, it is also seen that using transfer learning on those three architectures increases the model performance compared to without using transfer learning.

In the case of lung segmentation, which can be seen in Figure 2, the 3D UNet architecture studied the case very well, and there was no indication of overfitting or underfitting in the model. In the case of binary-class segmentation, 3D UNet produces IoU scores, Dice scores, accuracy, and F1-score of 94.32%, 97.05%, 99.37%, and 97.07%, respectively. In this lung segmentation case, if sorted based on the results of the metrics evaluation, it was found that 3D ResUNet became the architecture with the lowest average evaluation metrics, followed by 3D DenseUNet, 3D VGGUNet, and the original 3D UNet, with the best average metrics evaluation from three other architectures.

In the case of multi-class segmentation, as shown in Figure 3, the 3D UNet architecture studies lung and infection segmentation cases quite well. Although not as well as when studying lung segmentation cases, the graph in Figure 3 shows that both lines of training loss and validation loss are close enough that we can assume that the model does not indicate under or over fitting. In the case of lung and infection segmentation, 3D UNet scored 81.58%, 88.61%, 98.78%, and 98.78% for the metrics IoU score, Dice score, accuracy, and F1-score, respectively. Similar to binary-class segmentation, in this multi-class segmentation, 3D UNet gets the best average metrics evaluation, followed by 3D VGGUNet, 3D DenseUNet, and 3D ResUNet, as the architectures with the lowest average metrics evaluation of the other three architectures.

In general, these four architectures obtain acceptable evaluation results for predicting the lung or the lung and infection segmentation because, in addition to preprocessing the data, these four 3D architectures take advantage of the volume/depth of the CT-scan as a single data unit when it is entered into the model in the learning process, in contrast to when using a 2D architecture, which only considers one slice as a single data unit when it is entered into the model in the learning process. It should be noted that in this study, the mask/ground truth from the original data was modified by unifying the left and the right lung. Because of that, the cases used in this study differed from cases used in previous studies, despite the fact that they used the same dataset or same general goal, which is to assist in the process of diagnosing COVID-19 by segmenting images that take advantage of technological advances.

5. Conclusions

In this study, we applied the 3D version as well as three modifications of one of the most used and most recommended architectures for biomedical images, namely 3D UNet, 3D VGGUNet, 3D ResUNet, and 3D DenseUNet, for cases of COVID-19 CT-scan segmentation. All architectures were applied in two cases: binary-class segmentation to segment the lung from CT-scan, and multi-class segmentation to segment the lung and infection from CT-scan. To try and find the best results in the COVID-19 CT-scan segmentation, transfer learning was applied to each of the three modified architectures. The preprocessing operations were also performed on the dataset, namely resizing the height, length, and depth to the same size, with the aim that the data could entered into the 3D architecture, and applying the CLAHE method to the dataset to clarify the data and make it easier for the network to study each case. The experimental result shows that although the 3D UNet has a very large maximum iteration, the 3D UNet has better performance than the other three modified architectures. In the case of lung segmentation, 3D UNet produces very accurate segmentation predictions with an IoU score of 94.32% and a Dice score of 97.05%, and in the case of lung and infection segmentation, 3D UNet also produces a fairly accurate prediction with an IoU score of 81.58% and a Dice score of 88.61%. In general, the 3D UNet architecture gets good results, not only because of the preprocessing that is performed, but also because this architecture utilizes the volume or depth of 3D data. This study proves that UNet's 3D architecture can have a major impact on learning, technological developments, and the diagnosis of COVID-19. However, one of the shortcomings in this study is the limited dataset of COVID-19 labeled CT-scans. This causes insufficient training and testing of data for all models. In the future, this study could be expanded in the following aspects: explore various parameter tunings for each architecture; modify and/or add other blocks to the architecture; and, of course, reapply these architectures to more and larger datasets to obtain better COVID-19 diagnosis performance through CT-scan segmentation.

Author Contributions: M.H.A., A.A.P., G.D., T.H., I.N.Y., J.S. and F.A.L.N. understood and designed the research; M.H.A. analyzed the data and drafted the paper. All authors critically read and revised the draft and approved the final paper. All authors have read and agreed to the published version of the manuscript.

Funding: The authors are grateful to the Universitas Padjadjaran and Directorate for Research and Community Service (DRPM) Ministry of Research, Technology, and Higher Education Indonesia which supports this research under Higher Education Research Grant no. 094/E5/PG.02.00.PT/2022.

Institutional Review Board Statement: Not applicable.

Informed Consent Statement: Not applicable.

Data Availability Statement: Data is available at https://doi.org/10.5281/zenodo.3757476 [39], accessed on 18 November 2022.

Conflicts of Interest: The authors declare no conflict of interest.

Appendix A

Modified Architectures Details

Appendix A gives details structures for each modified architectures used in this study.

Table A1. Details on 3D VGGUNet Architecture.

	Block Type	Block Info	Details on Each Bock/Sub-Block
Encoder part (DenseNet201)	Convolutional Block	1st and 2nd sub-block	Layers: Convolutional 3D + Convolutional 3D + Max Pooling 3D
		3rd–5th sub-block	Layers: Convolutional 3D + Convolutional 3D + Convolutional 3D + Convolutional 3D + Max Pooling 3D
	Convolutional Block	Contains two sub-block	Layers: Convolutional 3D + Batch Normalization + ReLu
Decoder part	Convolutional Block	Contains two sub-blocks	Layers: Up Sampling 3D, Batch Normalization, ReLu, Concatenate, Convultional 3D, Batch Normalization, ReLu
	Output	-	Layers: Convolutional 3D + Softmax/Sigmoid

Table A2. Details on 3D ResUNet Architecture.

	Block Type	Block Info	Details on Each Bock/Sub-Block
	Input Block	-	Layers: Batch Normalization + Zero Padding 3D + Batch Normalization + ReLu + Zero Padding 3D + Max Pooling 3D
	Convolutional Block	1st sub-block	Layers: Convolutional 3D + Batch Normalization + ReLu + Zero Padding 3D + Convolutional 3D + Batch Normalization + ReLu + Convolutional 3D + Convolutional 3D + Concatenate
		2nd and 3rd sub-block	Layers: Convolutional 3D + Batch Normalization + ReLu + Zero Padding 3D + Convolutional 3D + Batch Normalization + ReLu + Convolutional 3D + Concatenate
Encoder part (DenseNet201)	Convolutional Block	1st sub-block	Layers: Convolutional 3D + Batch Normalization + ReLu + Zero Padding 3D + Convolutional 3D + Batch Normalization + ReLu + Convolutional 3D + Convolutional 3D + Concatenate
		2nd–8th sub-block	Layers: Convolutional 3D + Batch Normalization + ReLu + Zero Padding 3D + Convolutional 3D + Batch Normalization + ReLu + Convolutional 3D + Concatenate
	Convolutional Block	1st sub-block	Layers: Convolutional 3D + Batch Normalization + ReLu + Zero Padding 3D + Convolutional 3D + Batch Normalization + ReLu + Convolutional 3D + Convolutional 3D + Concatenate
		2nd–36th sub-block	Layers: Convolutional 3D + Batch Normalization + ReLu + Zero Padding 3D + Convolutional 3D + Batch Normalization + ReLu + Convolutional 3D + Concatenate
	Convolutional Block	1st sub-block	Layers: Convolutional 3D + Batch Normalization + ReLu + Zero Padding 3D + Convolutional 3D + Batch Normalization + ReLu + Convolutional 3D + Convolutional 3D + Concatenate
		2nd and 3rd sub-block	Layers: Convolutional 3D + Batch Normalization + ReLu + Zero Padding 3D + Convolutional 3D + Batch Normalization + ReLu + Convolutional 3D + Concatenate
Decoder part	Convolutional Block	Consists of five sub-blocks	Layers: Batch Normalization + Up Sampling 3D + Concatenate + Convolutional 3D + Batch Normalization + ReLu + Convolutional 3D
	Output	-	Layers: Convolutional 3D + Softmax/Sigmoid

Table A3. Details on 3D DenseUNet Architecture.

	Block Type	Block Info	Details on Each Bock/Sub-Block
	Input Block	-	Layers: Batch Normalization + Convolutional 3D + Batch Normalization + Convolutional 3D + ReLu + Concatenate
	Convolutional Block	Consists of six sub-blocks	Layers: Batch Normalization + ReLu + Convolutional 3D + Batch Normalization + Relu + Convolutional 3D + Concatenate
	Pooling Block	-	Layers: Batch Normalization + ReLu + Convolutional 3D + Average Pooling 3D
Encoder part (DenseNet201)	Convolutional Block	Consists of 12 blocks	Layers: Batch Normalization + ReLu + Convolutional 3D + Batch Normalization + Relu + Convolutional 3D + Concatenate
	Pooling Block	-	Layers: Batch Normalization + ReLu + Convolutional 3D + Average Pooling 3D
	Convolutional Block	Consists of 48 blocks	Layers: Batch Normalization + ReLu + Convolutional 3D + Batch Normalization + Relu + Convolutional 3D + Concatenate
	Pooling Block	-	Layers: Batch Normalization + ReLu + Convolutional 3D + Average Pooling 3D
	Convolutional Block	Consists of 32 blocks	Layers: Batch Normalization + ReLu + Convolutional 3D + Batch Normalization + Relu + Convolutional 3D + Concatenate
Decoder part	Convolutional Block	Consists of five blocks	Layers: Up Sampling 3D + Concatenate + Convolutional 3D + Batch Normalization + ReLu
	Output	-	Layers: Convolutional 3D + Softmax/Sigmoid

References

1. WHO Coronavirus (COVID-19). Available online: https://covid19.who.int (accessed on 12 July 2022).
2. Wang, C.; Horby, P.; Hayden, F.; Gao, G. A novel coronavirus outbreak of global health concern. *Lancet* **2020**, *395*, 470–473. [CrossRef]
3. Wang, W.; Xu, Y.; Gao, R.; Lu, R.; Han, K.; Wu, G.; Tan, W. Detection of SARS-CoV-2 in Different Types of Clinical Specimens. *JAMA* **2020**, *323*, 1843–1844. [CrossRef] [PubMed]
4. WHO Director-General's Opening Remarks at the Media Briefing on COVID-19. Available online: https://www.who.int/director-general/speeches/detail/who-director-general-s-opening-remarks-at-the-media-briefing-on-covid-19---11-march-2020 (accessed on 14 July 2022).
5. Debata, B.; Patnaik, P.; Mishra, A. COVID-19 pandemic! It's impact on people, economy, and environment. *J. Public Aff.* **2020**, *20*, e2372. [CrossRef]
6. Song, L.; Zhou, Y. The COVID-19 Pandemic and Its Impact on the Global Economy: What Does It Take to Turn Crisis into Opportunity? *China World Econ.* **2020**, *28*, 1–25. [CrossRef]
7. Benameur, N.; Mahmoudi, R.; Zaid, S.; Arous, Y.; Hmida, B.; Bedoui, M. SARS-CoV-2 diagnosis using medical imaging techniques and artificial intelligence: A review. *Clin. Imaging* **2021**, *76*, 6–14. [CrossRef] [PubMed]
8. Huang, L.; Han, R.; Ai, T.; Yu, P.; Kang, H.; Tao, Q.; Xia, L. Serial Quantitative Chest CT Assessment of COVID-19: A Deep Learning Approach. *Radiol. Cardiothorac. Imaging* **2020**, *2*, e200075. [CrossRef]
9. Mahmoudi, R.; Benameur, N.; Mabrouk, R.; Mohammed, M.; Garcia-Zapirain, B.; Bedoui, M. A Deep Learning-Based Diagnosis System for COVID-19 Detection and Pneumonia Screening Using CT Imaging. *Appl. Sci.* **2022**, *12*, 4825. [CrossRef]
10. Yin, S.; Deng, H.; Xu, Z.; Zhu, Q.; Cheng, J. SD-UNet: A Novel Segmentation Framework for CT Images of Lung Infections. *Electronics* **2022**, *11*, 130. [CrossRef]
11. Gouda, W.; Almurafeh, M.; Humayun, M.; Jhanjhi, N. Detection of COVID-19 Based on Chest X-rays Using Deep Learning. *Healthcare* **2022**, *10*, 343. [CrossRef]
12. Statement on the Second Meeting of the International Health Regulations (2005). Emergency Committee Regarding the Out-break of Novel Coronavirus (2019-nCoV). Available online: https://www.who.int/news/item/30-01-2020-statement-on-the-second-meeting-of-the-international-health-regulations-(2005)-emergency-committee-regarding-the-outbreak-of-novel-coronavirus-(2019-ncov) (accessed on 14 July 2022).

13. Asai, T. Correction to: COVID-19: Accurate interpretation of diagnostic tests—A statistical point of view. *J. Anesth.* **2021**, *35*, 470. [CrossRef] [PubMed]

14. Tingbo, L.; Yu, L. *Handbook of COVID-19 Prevention and Treatment*; Zhejiang University School of Medicine: Hangzhou, China, 2020.

15. Fang, Y.; Zhang, H.; Xie, J.; Lin, M.; Ying, L.; Pang, P.; Ji, W. Sensitivity of Chest CT for COVID-19: Comparison to RT-PCR. *Radiology* **2020**, *296*, E115–E117. [CrossRef]

16. Ai, T.; Yang, Z.; Hou, H.; Zhan, C.; Chen, C.; Lv, W.; Tao, Q.; Sun, Z.; Xia, L. Correlation of Chest CT and RT-PCR Testing for Coronavirus Disease 2019 (COVID-19) in China: A Report of 1014 Cases. *Radiology* **2020**, *296*, E32–E40. [CrossRef] [PubMed]

17. Gaál, G.; Maga, B.; Lukács, A. Attention u-net based adversarial architectures for chest X-ray lung segmentation. *arXiv* **2020**, arXiv:2003.10304.

18. Narin, A.; Kaya, C.; Pamuk, Z. Automatic detection of coronavirus disease (COVID-19) using X-ray images and deep convolutional neural networks. *Pattern Anal. Appl.* **2021**, *24*, 1207–1220. [CrossRef] [PubMed]

19. Shan, F.; Gao, Y.; Wang, J.; Shi, W.; Shi, N.; Han, M.; Xue, Z.; Shen, D.; Shi, Y. Abnormal lung quantification in chest CT images of COVID-19 patients with deep learning and its application to severity prediction. *Med. Phys.* **2021**, *48*, 1633–1645. [CrossRef]

20. Dong, D.; Tang, Z.; Wang, S.; Hui, H.; Gong, L.; Lu, Y.; Xue, Z.; Liao, H.; Chen, F.; Yang, F.; et al. The Role of Imaging in the Detection and Management of COVID-19: A Review. *IEEE Rev. Biomed. Eng.* **2021**, *14*, 16–29. [CrossRef]

21. Rubin, G.; Ryerson, C.; Haramati, L.; Sverzellati, N.; Kanne, J.; Raoof, S.; Schluger, N.; Volpi, A.; Yim, J.; Martin, I.; et al. The Role of Chest Imaging in Patient Management During the COVID-19 Pandemic. *Chest* **2020**, *158*, 106–116. [CrossRef] [PubMed]

22. Huang, C.; Wang, Y.; Li, X.; Ren, L.; Zhao, J.; Hu, Y.; Zhang, L.; Fan, G.; Xu, J.; Gu, X.; et al. Clinical features of patients infected with 2019 novel coronavirus in Wuhan, China. *Lancet* **2020**, *395*, 497–506. [CrossRef] [PubMed]

23. Patil, D.D.; Deore, S.G. Medical image segmentation: A Review. *Int. J. Comput. Sci. Mob. Comput.* **2013**, *2*, 22–27.

24. Havaei, M.; Davy, A.; Warde-Farley, D.; Biard, A.; Courville, A.; Bengio, Y.; Pal, C.; Jodoin, P.; Larochelle, H. Brain tumor segmentation with Deep Neural Networks. *Med. Image Anal.* **2017**, *35*, 18–31. [CrossRef]

25. Makkapati, V.; Rao, R. Segmentation of malaria parasites in peripheral blood smear images. In Proceedings of the 2009 IEEE International Conference on Acoustics, Speech and Signal Processing, Taipei, Taiwan, 19–24 April 2009.

26. Litjens, G.; Kooi, T.; Bejnordi, B.; Setio, A.; Ciompi, F.; Ghafoorian, M.; van der Laak, J.; van Ginneken, B.; Sánchez, C. A survey on deep learning in medical image analysis. *Med. Image Anal.* **2017**, *42*, 60–88. [CrossRef] [PubMed]

27. Hu, Z.; Tang, J.; Wang, Z.; Zhang, K.; Zhang, L.; Sun, Q. Deep learning for image-based cancer detection and diagnosis − A survey. *Pattern Recognit.* **2018**, *83*, 134–149. [CrossRef]

28. Minaee, S.; Kafieh, R.; Sonka, M.; Yazdani, S.; Jamalipour Soufi, G. Deep-COVID: Predicting COVID-19 from chest X-ray images using deep transfer learning. *Med. Image Anal.* **2020**, *65*, 101794. [CrossRef] [PubMed]

29. Wang, L.; Lin, Z.; Wong, A. COVID-Net: A tailored deep convolutional neural network design for detection of COVID-19 cases from chest X-ray images. *Sci. Rep.* **2020**, *10*, 19549. [CrossRef] [PubMed]

30. Sethy, P.; Behera, S.; Ratha, P.; Biswas, P. Detection of coronavirus Disease (COVID-19) based on Deep Features and Support Vector Machine. *Int. J. Math. Eng. Manag. Sci.* **2020**, *5*, 643–651. [CrossRef]

31. Oh, Y.; Park, S.; Ye, J. Deep Learning COVID-19 Features on CXR Using Limited Training Data Sets. *IEEE Trans. Med. Imaging* **2020**, *39*, 2688–2700. [CrossRef]

32. Selvan, R.; B. Dam, E.; S. Detlefsen, N.; Rischel, S.; Sheng, K.; Nielsen, M.; Pai, A. Lung Segmentation from Chest X-rays using Variational Data Imputation. *arXiv* **2020**, arXiv:2005.10052.

33. Li, Y.; Xia, L. Coronavirus Disease 2019 (COVID-19): Role of Chest CT in Diagnosis and Management. *Am. J. Roentgenol.* **2020**, *214*, 1280–1286. [CrossRef] [PubMed]

34. Ding, X.; Xu, J.; Zhou, J.; Long, Q. Chest CT findings of COVID-19 pneumonia by duration of symptoms. *Eur. J. Radiol.* **2020**, *127*, 109009. [CrossRef]

35. Meng, H.; Xiong, R.; He, R.; Lin, W.; Hao, B.; Zhang, L.; Lu, Z.; Shen, X.; Fan, T.; Jiang, W. CT imaging and clinical course of asymptomatic cases with COVID-19 pneumonia at admission in Wuhan, China. *J. Infect.* **2020**, *81*, e33–e39. [CrossRef]

36. Kenny, J. An Illustrated Guide to the Chest CT in COVID-19. Available online: https://pulmccm.org/uncategorized/an-illustrated-guide-to-the-chest-ct-in-covid-19/ (accessed on 20 July 2022).

37. Shi, F.; Wang, J.; Shi, J.; Wu, Z.; Wang, Q.; Tang, Z.; He, K.; Shi, Y.; Shen, D. Review of Artificial Intelligence Techniques in Imaging Data Acquisition, Segmentation, and Diagnosis for COVID-19. *IEEE Rev. Biomed. Eng.* **2021**, *14*, 4–15. [CrossRef] [PubMed]

38. Shoeibi, A.; Khodatars, M.; Alizadehsani, R.; Ghassemi, N.; Jafari, M.; Moridian, P.; Khadem, A.; Sadeghi, D.; Hussain, S.; Zare, A. Automated Detection and Forecasting of COVID-19 using Deep Learning Techniques: A Review. *arXiv* **2022**, arXiv:2007.10785.

39. Ma, J.; Ge, C.; Wang, Y.; An, X.; Gao, J.; Yu, Z. COVID-19 CT Lung and Infection Segmentation Dataset. *OpenAIRE* **2020**. [CrossRef]

40. Owais, M.; Baek, N.; Park, K. DMDF-Net: Dual multiscale dilated fusion network for accurate segmentation of lesions related to COVID-19 in lung radiographic scans. *Expert Syst. Appl.* **2022**, *202*, 117360. [CrossRef]

41. Wang, X.; Yuan, Y.; Guo, D.; Huang, X.; Cui, Y.; Xia, M.; Wang, Z.; Bai, C.; Chen, S. SSA-Net: Spatial self-attention network for COVID-19 pneumonia infection segmentation with semi-supervised few-shot learning. *Med. Image Anal.* **2022**, *79*, 102459. [CrossRef] [PubMed]

42. Punn, N.; Agarwal, S. CHS-Net: A Deep Learning Approach for Hierarchical Segmentation of COVID-19 via CT Images. *Neural Process. Lett.* **2022**, *54*, 3771–3792. [CrossRef]

43. Singh, A.; Kaur, A.; Dhillon, A.; Ahuja, S.; Vohra, H. Software system to predict the infection in COVID-19 patients using deep learning and web of things. *Softw. Pract. Exp.* **2021**, *52*, 868–886. [CrossRef]
44. Radiopaedia Pty Ltd. ACN 133 562 722. Available online: https://radiopaedia.org/ (accessed on 23 July 2022).
45. RAIOSS.com. Coronacases. Available online: https://coronacases.org/ (accessed on 23 July 2022).
46. Ma, J.; Wang, Y.; An, X.; Ge, C.; Yu, Z.; Chen, J.; Zhu, Q.; Dong, G.; He, J.; He, Z.; et al. Towards Data-Efficient Learning: A Benchmark for COVID-19 CT Lung and Infection Segmentation. *arXiv* **2020**, arXiv:arXiv:2004.12537. [CrossRef]
47. Pizer, S.M.; Amburn, E.P.; Austin, J.D.; Cromartie, R.; Geselowitz, A.; Greer, T.; ter Haar Romeny, B.; Zimmerman, J.B.; Zuiderveld, K. Adaptive histogram equalization and its variations. *Comput. Vis. Graph. Image Process.* **1987**, *39*, 355–368. [CrossRef]
48. Zimmerman, J.; Pizer, S.; Staab, E.; Perry, J.; McCartney, W.; Brenton, B. An evaluation of the effectiveness of adaptive histogram equalization for contrast enhancement. *IEEE Trans. Med. Imaging* **1988**, *7*, 304–312. [CrossRef]
49. Pizer, S.; Johnston, R.; Ericksen, J.; Yankaskas, B.; Muller, K. Contrast-limited adaptive histogram equalization: Speed and effectiveness. In Proceedings of the First Conference on Visualization in Biomedical Computing, Atlanta, GA, USA, 22–25 May 1990; pp. 337–345.
50. Çiçek, Ö.; Abdulkadir, A.; S. Lienkamp, S.; Brox, T.; Ronneberger, O. 3D U-Net: Learning Dense Volumetric Segmentation from Sparse Annotation. *arXiv* **2022**, arXiv:arXiv:1606.06650.
51. Alalwan, N.; Abozeid, A.; ElHabshy, A.; Alzahrani, A. Efficient 3D Deep Learning Model for Medical Image Semantic Segmentation. *Alex. Eng. J.* **2021**, *60*, 1231–1239. [CrossRef]
52. Pravitasari, A.A.; Iriawan, N.; Almuhayar, M.; Azmi, T.; Irhamah, I.; Fithriasari, K.; Purnami, S.W.; Ferriastuti, W. UNET-VGG16 with transfer learning for MRI-based brain tumor segmentation. *TELKOMNIKA (Telecommunication Computing Electronics and Control)* **2020**, *18*, 1310–1318. [CrossRef]
53. Ronneberger, O.; Fischer, P.; Brox, T. U-Net: Convolutional Networks for Biomedical Image Segmentation. *Lect. Notes Comput. Sci.* **2015**, *9351*, 234–241.
54. Kamnitsas, K.; Ledig, C.; Newcombe, V.; Simpson, J.; Kane, A.; Menon, D.; Rueckert, D.; Glocker, B. Efficient multi-scale 3D CNN with fully connected CRF for accurate brain lesion segmentation. *Med. Image Anal.* **2017**, *36*, 61–78. [CrossRef] [PubMed]

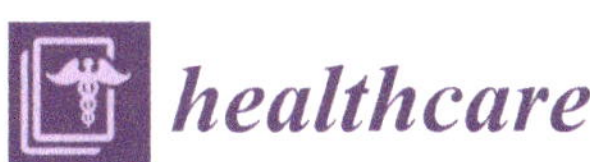

Article

Artificial-Intelligence-Based Decision Making for Oral Potentially Malignant Disorder Diagnosis in Internet of Medical Things Environment

Rana Alabdan [1], Abdulrahman Alruban [2], Anwer Mustafa Hilal [3,*] and Abdelwahed Motwakel [4]

[1] Department of Information Systems, College of Computer and Information Science, Majmaah University, Majmaah 11952, Saudi Arabia
[2] Department of Information Technology, College of Computer and Information Sciences, Majmaah University, Majmaah 11952, Saudi Arabia
[3] Department of Computer and Self Development, Preparatory Year Deanship, Prince Sattam bin Abdulaziz University, AlKharj 16278, Saudi Arabia
[4] Department of Information Systems, College of Business Administration in Hawtat bani Tamim, Prince Sattam bin Abdulaziz University, AlKharj 16278, Saudi Arabia
* Correspondence: a.hilal@psau.edu.sa

Abstract: Oral cancer is considered one of the most common cancer types in several counties. Earlier-stage identification is essential for better prognosis, treatment, and survival. To enhance precision medicine, Internet of Medical Things (IoMT) and deep learning (DL) models can be developed for automated oral cancer classification to improve detection rate and decrease cancer-specific mortality. This article focuses on the design of an optimal Inception-Deep Convolution Neural Network for Oral Potentially Malignant Disorder Detection (OIDCNN-OPMDD) technique in the IoMT environment. The presented OIDCNN-OPMDD technique mainly concentrates on identifying and classifying oral cancer by using an IoMT device-based data collection process. In this study, the feature extraction and classification process are performed using the IDCNN model, which integrates the Inception module with DCNN. To enhance the classification performance of the IDCNN model, the moth flame optimization (MFO) technique can be employed. The experimental results of the OIDCNN-OPMDD technique are investigated, and the results are inspected under specific measures. The experimental outcome pointed out the enhanced performance of the OIDCNN-OPMDD model over other DL models.

Keywords: Internet of Medical Things; oral cancer; biomedical imaging; artificial intelligence; Inception model; hybrid deep learning

Citation: Alabdan, R.; Alruban, A.; Hilal, A.M.; Motwakel, A. Artificial-Intelligence-Based Decision Making for Oral Potentially Malignant Disorder Diagnosis in Internet of Medical Things Environment. *Healthcare* **2023**, *11*, 113. https://doi.org/10.3390/healthcare11010113

Academic Editor: Mahmudur Rahman

Received: 11 December 2022
Revised: 25 December 2022
Accepted: 26 December 2022
Published: 30 December 2022

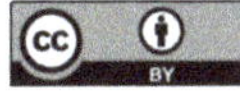

1. Introduction

The Internet of Medical Things (IoMT) is an extended version of the Internet of Things (IoT), which encompasses several interlinked devices that can be employed for timely support to patients and the healthcare sector [1]. Oral squamous cell carcinoma (OSCC) is a common cancer, and its existing rate seems to be increasing worldwide. Usually, the preferred therapy, primary cornerstone therapy, is a surgical treatment for OSCC [2,3]. In addition, considering the aggressive nature of OSCC, and most patients were identified with advanced locoregionally diseases, multimodality therapy and concomitant chemora-diotherapy can be imperative [4–6]. Instead of the above-stated treatment possibilities, the higher occurrence rate and the suboptimal treatment result form an important concern to date. The initial analysis is very important for better treatment, survival, and prognosis [7]. At the same time, a late diagnosis will hamper the quest for precision medicine in spite of the new developments in understanding the molecular system of tumors [8]. Hence, the deep machine learning (ML) method was touted to improve initial identification and decrease cancer-specific morbidity and mortality. Automatic image analysis can assist clinicians and pathologists in the initial level of OSCC and makes informed decisions regarding cancer management [9].

The dependability of automatic decisions is higher for real clinical applications [10]. Even with the promising performance, conventional deep learning (DL)-related classification lacks doctors' capability to quantify decision uncertainty [11]. Without uncertainty measurements, physicians could not depend on decisions from DL-related automated systems in practical clinical routines. Irrespective of the robustness of a DL technique, tough diagnostic cases were unavoidable and might result in serious consequences for patients when the method is not referred for more analysis [12]. Previous methods have yet to learn that model how much confidence an individual output has. In this study, the author devises a DL oral cancer image classification structure that quantifies the output uncertainty of the methods and recommends that problematic cases with higher uncertainty values are mentioned for more analyses. This DL technique has uncertainty predictions and is compiled to assist and accelerate conventional medical workflows, not replace them [13,14]. DL techniques are frequently considered a 'black-box'; however, the techniques are highly trustable and reliable by offering uncertain data and possibly rising overall performance [15]. In such a case, the automatic classifier is a tireless front-line clinician who requires no rest, presenting diagnoses when confident and denoting tough cases to experienced experts when uncertain.

The author in [16] applied and evaluated the efficiency of six deep convolution neural network (DCNN) methods, including the TL approach, for directly identifying precancerous tongue lesions using small data of medically annotated images to identify earlier signs of OCC. DCNN method could differentiate between pre-cancerous tongue lesions and benign and distinguish five classes of tongue lesions, viz., geographic tongue, hairy tongue, fissured tongue, oral hairy leukoplakia, and strawberry tongue, with higher classifier performance. In [17], the authors developed an image classification model using the Inception-ResNet-V2 model. The authors also generated an automatic heat map to emphasize the region of the images probably to be included in the decision-making process.

Rajan et al. [18] developed a novel methodology that exploits an adapted vesselness measurement and DCNN to recognize oral cancer areas in IoT-related smart healthcare schemes. The strong vesselness filter system manages noise when preserving smaller structures. In contrast, the CNN framework significantly increases classifier performance by deblurring region of interest (ROI), which is focused on combining multi-dimension data from the feature vector selecting stage. The marked feature vector point is derived from every interconnected module in the region and applied as input to train the CNN. The author in [19] discovered the prospective application of deep learning and computer vision methods in oral cancer in the scope of images and examined the prospect of an automatic scheme for potentially recognizing oral malignant disorder having two phase channels.

Bhandari et al. [20] intend to raise the detection and classifying performances of oral tumors in a decreased processing duration. The presented method has a CNN with an adapted loss function for minimizing the fault in classifying and forecasting oral cancers by decreasing the over-fitting dataset and supporting a multiclass classifier. The presented method was tested on data samples from various data sets with four classes of oral cancers. Chan et al. [21] present a new DCNN compiled with texture mapping to identify cancerous areas and automatically mark the ROI in one method. The presented DCNN method has two collaborative branches: the lower branch performs semantic segmentation and ROI marking, whereas the upper one performs oral cancer detection. The network method will extract the tumorous regions with the upper branch and the lower one making the tumorous regions very accurate. A sliding window can be implemented for computing the texture images' standard deviation values.

This article focuses on designing an optimal Inception-Deep Convolution Neural Network for Oral Potentially Malignant Disorder Detection (OIDCNN-OPMDD) technique. The presented OIDCNN-OPMDD technique mainly concentrates on identifying and classifying oral cancer. In this study, the feature extraction and classification process are performed using the IDCNN model, which integrates the Inception module with DCNN. To enhance the classification performance of the IDCNN model, the moth flame optimization (MFO) technique can be employed. The experimental results of the OIDCNN-OPMDD technique are investigated, and the results are inspected under various measures.

2. Methods

In this article, a new OIDCNN-OPMDD technique was projected to identify and classify oral cancer in the IoMT environment. In this study, the feature extraction and classification process can be executed by using the IDCNN model, which integrates the Inception module with DCNN. To enhance the classification performance of the IDCNN method, the MFO algorithm is utilized in this study. Figure 1 depicts the overall process of the OIDCNN-OPMDD approach.

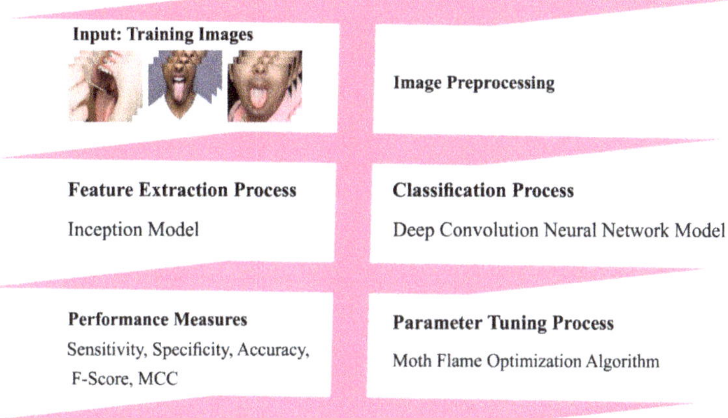

Figure 1. Working outline of OIDCNN-OPMDD approach.

2.1. Pre-Processing

Firstly, this work implemented several preprocessing levels to normalize the input images. At first, the images were resized to an even size by bi-cubic interpolation on 4×4 neighborhood pixels. The image was resized by padlocking the sustaining quality and aspect ratio. Generally, the retinal image is yellow and has a dark background. The input image overlaps with the background image and gets eliminated to decrease noise. Matching the black contextual of the input image results in darkness as prolonged into the image details. So, pre-processing was agreed upon for eliminating the black background by fixing the pixel values for non-zero and zero to the bright zone. Then, the application of threshold, the abstraction of the green channel, was applied. The green channel will conserve extra retinal data, except red or blue. The performance of CLAHE, which is contrast-limited adaptive histogram equalization, arrived to enhance smaller areas and the retinal image quality. Then, the weighted Gaussian blur was used to increase image structure and reduce noise. The σ standard deviation and Gaussian function in 2D (x, y) are mathematically articulated in Equation (1).

$$G(x,y) = \frac{1}{2\pi\sigma^2}\epsilon^{\frac{x^2+y^2}{2\sigma^2}}$$

(1)

2.2. Oral Cancer Recognition Module

In order to detect and classify oral cancer, the IDCNN model was utilized in this work. In this research, a DCNN mechanism with pre-trained Inception-v3 was developed [22]. The presented method is based on DTL, which aims at identifying the oral tumor from the input datasets. To extract features from the datasets, this study used pre-trained Inception-v3 architecture, and the classification model used DCNN. TL is a DL technique that exploits the module trained for the particular task as a primary point for model training for a related task. Typically, it is simpler and much quicker for network fine tuning with TL when compared to training a network from scratch. In this work, a DTL method-based Inception-v3 was carried out. The suggested method was applied for extracting features through its learned weight on the ImageNet datasets and CNN.

- Inception-v3 based DCNN method is deliberated to retrain; this technique comprises convolution, AvgPool, concat layer, maxpool, full connection layer, softmax function, and dropout.
- Average Pooling. It is a 2*D* function with a pooling size of (8×8) that reduces the computational complexity and the variance of the dataset. This layer enables the outcomes to flow toward the following layer.
- Convolution. A $299 \times 299 \times 3$ input size is utilized through convolutional operation, and this layer produces the feature map by convoluting the input dataset.
- Maxpool. It is a 2D *max* pooling operation, decreasing the dataset's variance and computation difficulty.
- Classified Result features like edges and average pooling are utilized to feature extraction.
- Concatenation. This layer is used for concatenating the different input blobs into an individual blob of output. It takes a tensor as the input, from which a similar kind of shape expect concatenation axes and return the output of individual tensor when concatenating every input.
- It is regarded as the normalization technique for minimizing the over-fitting in the ANN by overwhelming complex coadaptation from the trained dataset. Now, the dropout scale is regarded as 0.4, and robust model to execute averaging with the NN method. Furthermore, dropout represents the units' hidden and visible sides in the NN model.
- Fully Connected. This is utilized for connecting each neuron from one layer to others that operate according to the traditional MLP-NN model.
- Softmax. This is utilized as the output function that operates correspondingly towards the *max* layer once it is a parameter to train through gradient descent. The exponential function causes an increment in the likelihood of the previous layer and correspondingly compares with other values; each output summation is equivalent to one.

Generally, a 2D plane forms different independent neurons, and the DCNN is composed of different layers with many 2D feature mapping plane models. There exist 4 rimary segments of the DCNN. The initial one is the local perception that the global image does not need to be deduced through all the neurons in a neural network, and global and local data are attained by gathering local datasets. The second one is the convolution method. The convolution functionality is used to extract image features, and the convolutional kernels decrease the overall variables. The next one is weight sharing. This implies that the parameter of the related convolutional kernel was exploited for the whole image. Due to distinct locations in the image, the weight in the convolutional kernel would not be altered. Furthermore, convolutional operation weight sharing would considerably decrease the parameter of the convolutional kernels. The last one is the pooling layer, which is usually fixed in the CNN behindhand convolutional layer, employed to decrease the feature dimension of the efficiency of the preceding convolutional layer instantaneously to preserve data of the satisfactory crucial image.

To estimate the dot product of weight and the value in the input, a filter that is an array of weights was utilized in a convolution layer that slides over the input from a preceding layer. The procedure of backpropagation of error finds out such weights. Afterwards, an activation function that integrates component-wise non-linearity generates a feature map using every entry signifying a single neuron output from a small local area of the input. Then, the feature map is utilized for training a NN model.

As a filter is regarded, once the number of filters is high, it can extract additional feature maps and improve the model performance. Therefore, the relative imprints of 32-32-64, 32-32-32, 64-64-64, and 64-64-128 filters are employed to select the proper filter on the condition that computation resource and DCNN network performance were regraded on keeping the different influencing unchanged factors and distinct hierarchical architectures. Therefore, 64-64-64 was selected as the convolutional filter, which considers the performance, and each corresponding field size is 5×5.

For Inception-v3, the likelihood of each label $k \in \{1, \ldots, K\}$ for all the training instances is estimated as follows

$$Q(k|z) = \frac{\exp (y_k)}{\sum_i^k \exp (y_i)},\tag{2}$$

In Equation (2), y signifies the non-normalized log probability. The distribution of ground truth over label $p(k|z)$ was normalized; therefore, $\sum_k p(k|z) = 1$. For these systems, the loss was given using cross-entropy:

$$C = \sum_{k=1}^{K} \log (q(k))p(k).\tag{3}$$

For logits yk, the cross-entropy loss can be distinguishable, and thus it is employed in in-depth module gradient training, whose gradient has the simplest form of $\partial C/\partial y_k = q(k) - p(k)$, bounds between -1 and 1. Generally, this implies that the log probability of accurate labels can be increased after the cross-entropy is minimalized. Therefore, it produces some over-fitting problems. Inception-v3 regarded the distribution on labels with smooth variable $\in$ independent of trained instances (k), from which the label distribution $p(k|z) = Z_{k,z}$ was interchanged using

$$p'^{(k|z)} = (1 - \epsilon)\partial_{k,z} + \epsilon v(k),\tag{4}$$

that is a combination of the original $p(k|z)$ distribution with $1 - \epsilon$ weights and the $v(k)$ fixed distribution with ϵ weight.

For a uniform distribution $v(k) = 1/K$, label smoothing normalization is employed so that it turns out to be

$$p'^{(k|z)} = (1 - \varepsilon)\delta_{k,z} + \frac{\varepsilon}{K}.\tag{5}$$

Consecutively, this is inferred as cross-entropy in the following

$$H(p',q) = -\sum_{k=1}^{K} \log (q(k))p'^{(k)} = (1 - \epsilon)H(p',q) + \epsilon H(v,q).\tag{6}$$

Different activation features exist in the activation layer, namely softmax, sigmoid, and ReLU. The process is to integrate non-linear factors to improve the model condition; subsequently, it should be non-linear, and it is formulated by using Equation (7)

$$f(x) = \frac{1}{1 + e^{-x}}.\tag{7}$$

The activation function of ReLU can be formulated in the following:

$$f(x) = \begin{cases} 0, & x \leq 0, \\ x, & x > 0. \end{cases}\tag{8}$$

The activation function of the *softmax* layer can be formulated in Equation (9):

$$f(x_j) = \frac{e^{x_j}}{\sum e^{x_i}}.\tag{9}$$

From the equation, $f(x)$ indicates the activation function, and x denotes the activation function input. This is a non-linear function such as sigmoid or ReLU that can be employed for the element of convolution named activation function. If more than one pooling layer has been used for the feature map produced through the convolution layer, the computation perplexity of CNN can be decreased.

2.3. Hyperparameter Tuning Model

To enhance the classification performance of the IDCNN method, the MFO algorithm is utilized. MFO is an MH technique that mimics the behavior of moths in nature [23]. The major stages of MFO are defined below:

$$MFO = (R, V, T),\qquad(10)$$

In Equation (10), R is used for randomly initializing the population of moths; the fitness value, V, determines the major function that moves the moth around the search space, and T shows a flag of the stopping condition.

In the major function (V), the moth location is upgraded using flames as follows:

$$\vec{A} = S(\vec{A}_i, F_j),\qquad(11)$$

In Equation (11), S denotes the spiral function, A_i shows the i-th moths, and F_j indicates the j-th flames and expresses in the following:

$$S(\vec{A}_i, \vec{F}_j) = \vec{D}_i \cdot e^{bl} \cdot \cos(2\pi l) + \vec{F}_j,\qquad(12)$$

$$\vec{D} = |\vec{F}_j - \vec{A}_i|,\qquad(13)$$

In Equation (12), b shows a constant to define the logarithmic spiral curve, and $l \in [-1, 1]$ is randomly produced. Define the distance of i-th moths to j-th flames.

The optimal solution exploitation degrades owing to the changing of moth location w.r.t N_{pop} different locations in the problem. To resolve these issues there exists a method used to resolve these problems by offering more than one flame (Fno) as follows:

$$Fno = round\left(N - iter_c \times \frac{N_{pop} - 1}{iter_{max}}\right),\qquad(14)$$

Equation (14) $iter_c$ indicates the iterative number, N_{pop} describes the maximal flame number, and $iter_{max}$ specifies the stopping condition (the maximal iteration count). Algorithm 1 illustrates the key procedure of the MFO approach.

Algorithm 1 Pseudocode of MFO Algorithm

1: Generate early population of moths (A);
2: Compute the value of the fitness function of A;
3: while not T do
4:       Compute the number of flames based on Equation (14):
5:       FA = the value of fitness function of (A);
6:       if Loop == 1 then
7:           = $sort(A)$;
8:           = $sort(FA)$;
9:     else
10:        $F = sort(A_{c-1}, A_c)$;
11:      = $sort(A_{c-1}, A_c)$;
12:     end if
13:     for $i = 1 : n$ do
14:     for $j = 1 : n2$ do
15:        Upgrade b and t
16:        Calculate D
17:        Upgrade $A(i, j)$ by Equation (12)
18:       end for
19:       end for
20: end while
21: $y_j = A$
22: Output: Optimum flames

---

3. Results and Discussion

The oral cancer classification results of the OIDCNN-OPMDD method are investigated utilizing the oral cancer dataset from the Kaggle repository [24]. Table 1 showcases the details of the dataset. A few sample images are depicted in Figure 2. The dataset holds 131 samples with two classes. The proposed model is simulated using Python 3.6.5 tool on PC i5-8600 k, GeForce 1050 Ti 4 GB, 16 GB RAM, 250 GB SSD, and 1 TB HDD. The parameter settings are learning rate: 0.01, dropout: 0.5, batch size: 5, epoch count: 50, and activation: ReLU.

Table 1. Dataset details.

Class	No. of Samples
Cancer	87
Non-Cancer	44
Total Number of Samples	131

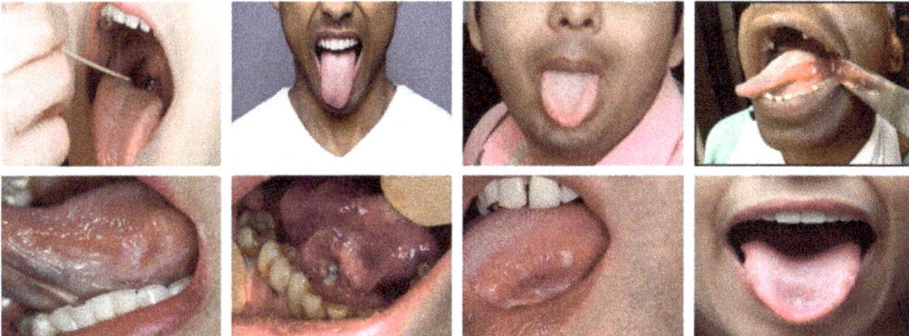

Figure 2. Sample images.

Figure 3 illustrates the confusion matrices generated by the OIDCNN-OPMDD model. With 80% of TR data, the OIDCNN-OPMDD method categorized 66 cases into cancer and 33 into non-cancer classes. In parallel, with 20% of TS data, the OIDCNN-OPMDD algorithm categorized 18 cases into the cancer class and 8 into the non-cancer class. At the same time, with 70% of TR data, the OIDCNN-OPMDD technique categorized 62 instances into the cancer class and 24 instances into the non-cancer class. In addition, with 30% of TS data, the OIDCNN-OPMDD approach categorized 22 instances into the cancer class and 17 into the non-cancer class.

Table 2 and Figure 4 provide the oral cancer classification results of the OIDCNN-OPMDD model on 80% of TR data. The OIDCNN-OPMDD model identified cancer class instances with $accu_y$, $sens_y$, $spec_y$, F_{score}, and MCC of 95.19%, 97.06%, 91.67%, 96.35%, and 89.33%, respectively. In addition, the OIDCNN-OPMDD model categorized non-cancer class instances with $accu_y$, $sens_y$, $spec_y$, F_{score}, and MCC of 95.19%, 91.67%, 97.06%, 92.96%, and 89.33%, respectively. In addition, the OIDCNN-OPMDD model attained average $accu_y$, $sens_y$, $spec_y$, F_{score}, and MCC of 95.19%, 94.36%, 94.36%, 94.65%, and 89.33%, correspondingly.

Table 3 and Figure 5 offer the oral cancer classification outcomes of the OIDCNN-OPMDD algorithm on 20% of TS data. The OIDCNN-OPMDD approach identified cancer class instances with $accu_y$, $sens_y$, $spec_y$, F_{score}, and MCC of 96.30%, 94.74%, 100%, 97.30%, and 91.77%, correspondingly. Moreover, the OIDCNN-OPMDD method categorized non-cancer class instances with $accu_y$, $sens_y$, $spec_y$, F_{score}, and MCC of 96.30%, 100%, 94.74%, 94.12%, and 91.77%, respectively. Further, the OIDCNN-OPMDD approach gained average $accu_y$, $sens_y$, $spec_y$, F_{score}, and MCC of 96.30%, 97.37%, 97.37%, 95.71%, and 91.77%, correspondingly.

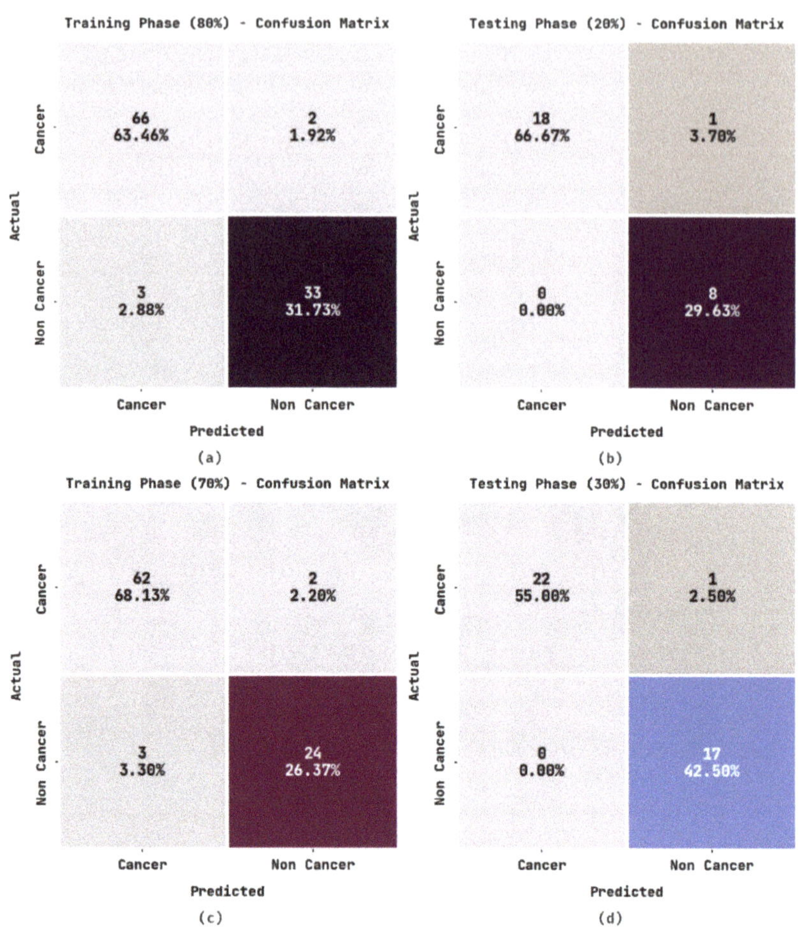

Figure 3. Confusion matrices of OIDCNN-OPMDD approach: (**a**) 80% of TR data, (**b**) 20% of TS data, (**c**) 70% of TR data, and (**d**) 30% of TS data.

Table 2. Result analysis of OIDCNN-OPMDD approach with distinct class labels under 80% of TR data.

	Training Phase (80%)				
Labels	**Accuracy**	**Sensitivity**	**Specificity**	**F-Score**	**MCC**
Cancer	95.19	97.06	91.67	96.35	89.33
Non-Cancer	95.19	91.67	97.06	92.96	89.33
Average	95.19	94.36	94.36	94.65	89.33

Table 4 and Figure 6 present the oral cancer classification results of the OIDCNN-OPMDD method on 70% of TR data. The OIDCNN-OPMDD approach identified cancer class instances with $accu_y$, $sens_y$, $spec_y$, F_{score}, and MCC of 94.51%, 96.88%, 88.89%, 96.12%, and 86.72% correspondingly. Likewise, the OIDCNN-OPMDD technique categorized non-cancer class instances with $accu_y$, $sens_y$, $spec_y$, F_{score}, and MCC of 94.51%, 88.89%, 96.88%, 90.57%, and 86.72% correspondingly. Moreover, the OIDCNN-OPMDD approach acquired average $accu_y$, $sens_y$, $spec_y$, F_{score}, and MCC of 94.51%, 92.88%, 92.88%, 93.35%, and 86.72%, correspondingly.

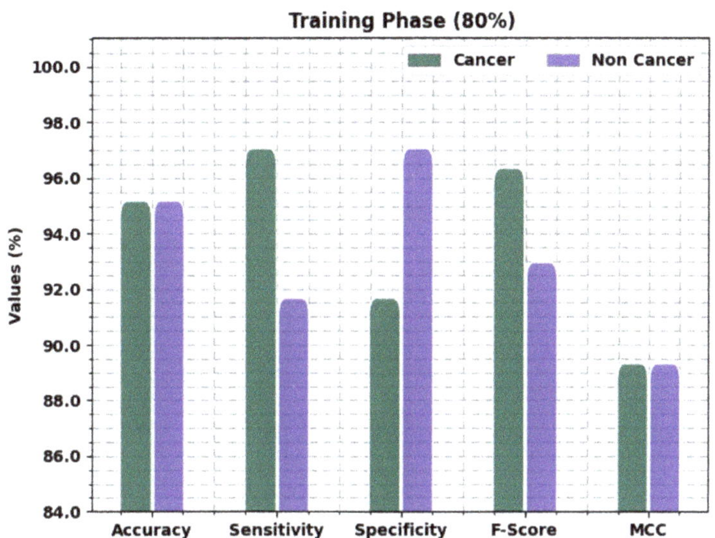

Figure 4. Result analysis of OIDCNN-OPMDD approach under 80% of TR data.

Table 3. Result analysis of OIDCNN-OPMDD approach with distinct class labels under 20% of TS data.

Testing Phase (20%)					
Labels	Accuracy	Sensitivity	Specificity	F-Score	MCC
Cancer	96.30	94.74	100.00	97.30	91.77
Non-Cancer	96.30	100.00	94.74	94.12	91.77
Average	96.30	97.37	97.37	95.71	91.77

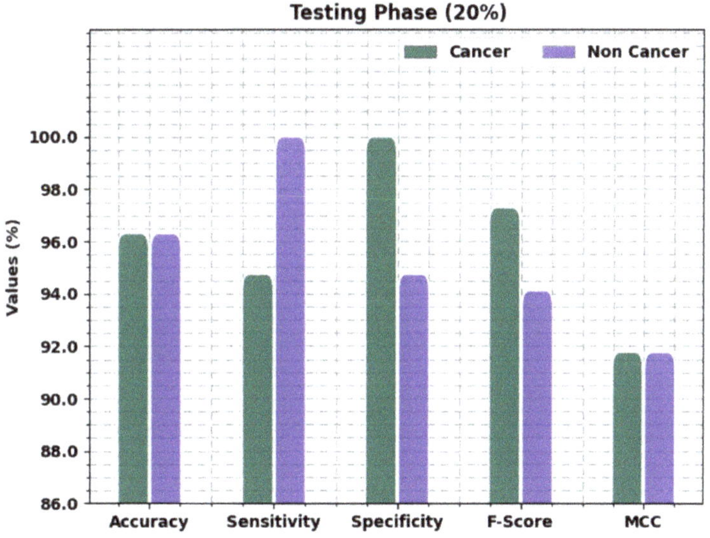

Figure 5. Result analysis of OIDCNN-OPMDD approach under 20% of TS data.

Table 4. Result analysis of OIDCNN-OPMDD approach with distinct class labels under 70% of TR data.

Training Phase (70%)					
Labels	Accuracy	Sensitivity	Specificity	F-Score	MCC
Cancer	94.51	96.88	88.89	96.12	86.72
Non-Cancer	94.51	88.89	96.88	90.57	86.72
Average	94.51	92.88	92.88	93.35	86.72

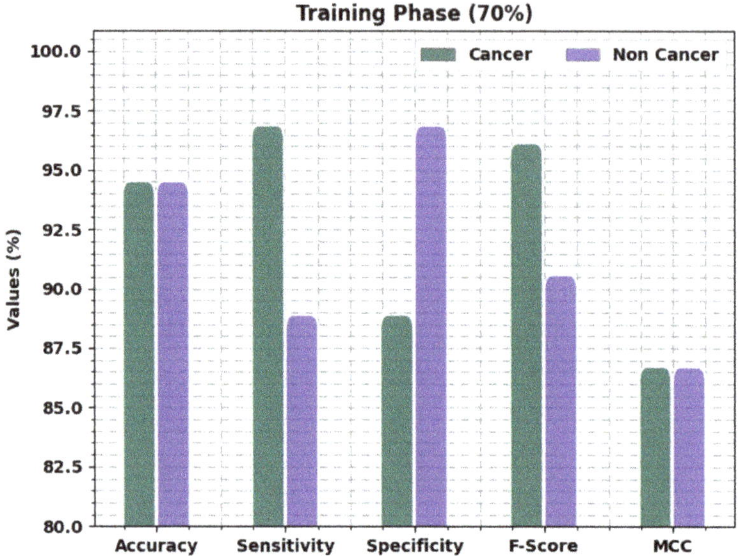

Figure 6. Result analysis of OIDCNN-OPMDD approach under 70% of TR data.

Table 5 and Figure 7 present the oral cancer classification results of the OIDCNN-OPMDD approach on 30% of TS data. The OIDCNN-OPMDD technique identified cancer class instances with $accu_y$, $sens_y$, $spec_y$, F_{score}, and MCC of 97.50%, 95.65%, 100%, 97.78%, and 95.05% correspondingly. Further, the OIDCNN-OPMDD approach categorized non-cancer class instances with $accu_y$, $sens_y$, $spec_y$, F_{score}, and MCC of 97.50%, 100%, 95.65%, 97.14%, and 95.05% correspondingly. Along with that, the OIDCNN-OPMDD algorithm gained average $accu_y$, $sens_y$, $spec_y$, F_{score}, and MCC of 97.50%, 97.83%, 97.83%, 97.46%, and 95.05% correspondingly.

Table 5. Result analysis of OIDCNN-OPMDD approach with distinct class labels under 30% of TS data.

Testing Phase (30%)					
Labels	Accuracy	Sensitivity	Specificity	F-Score	MCC
Cancer	97.50	95.65	100.00	97.78	95.05
Non-Cancer	97.50	100.00	95.65	97.14	95.05
Average	97.50	97.83	97.83	97.46	95.05

The training accuracy (TRA) and validation accuracy (VLA) acquired by the OIDCNN-OPMDD approach on the test dataset is displayed in Figure 8. The experimental result inferred that the OIDCNN-OPMDD approach had achieved maximal values of TRA and VLA. The VLA is greater than TRA.

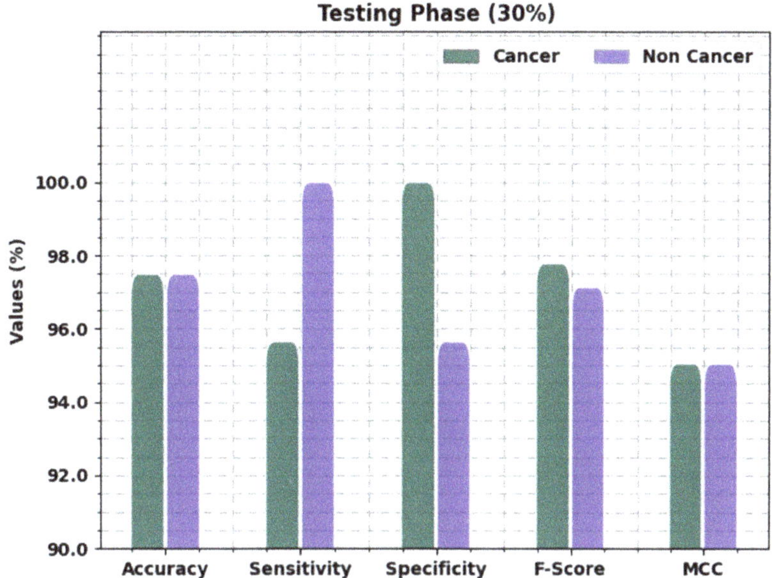

Figure 7. Result analysis of OIDCNN-OPMDD approach under 30% of TS data.

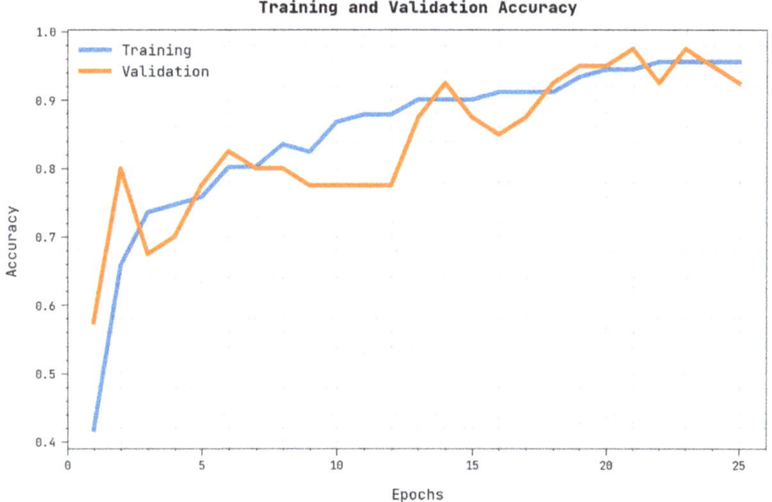

Figure 8. TRA and VLA analysis of OIDCNN-OPMDD approach.

The training loss (TRL) and validation loss (VLL) obtained by the OIDCNN-OPMDD technique on the test dataset are exhibited in Figure 9. The experimental result implied the OIDCNN-OPMDD method had established minimal values of TRL and VLL. Particularly, the VLL is lesser than TRL.

A clear precision–recall examination of the OIDCNN-OPMDD algorithm on the test dataset is shown in Figure 10. The figure denoted the OIDCNN-OPMDD approach has enhanced values of precision–recall values under all classes.

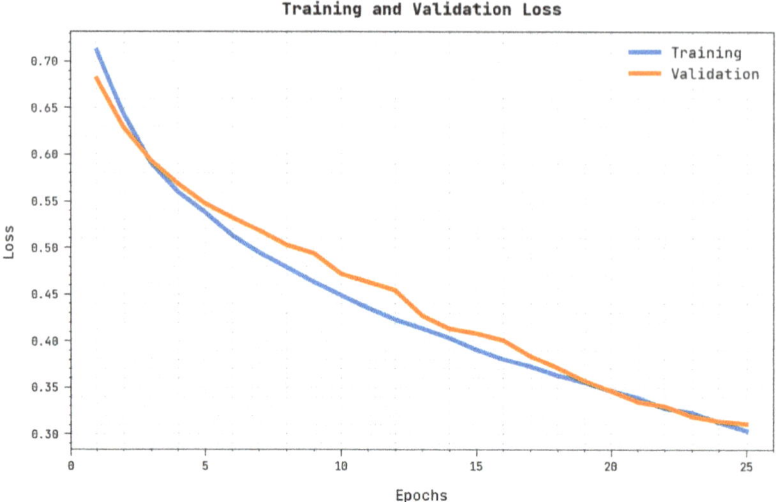

Figure 9. TRL and VLL analysis of OIDCNN-OPMDD approach.

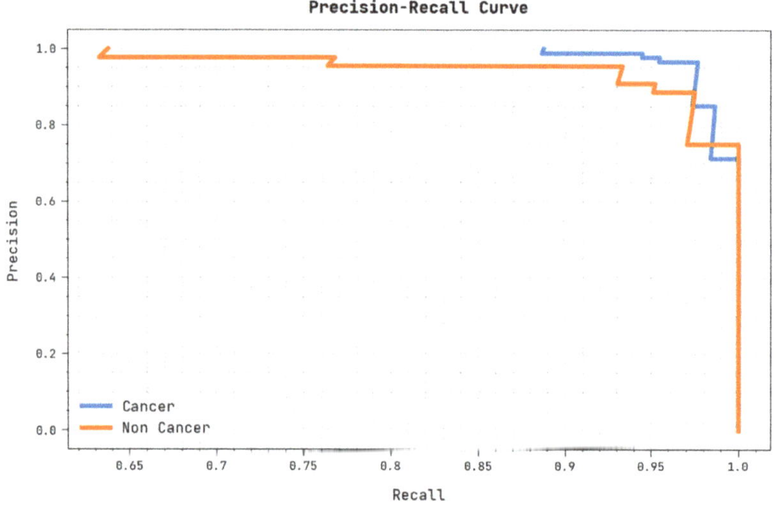

Figure 10. Precision–recall analysis of OIDCNN-OPMDD approach.

A brief ROC inquiry of the OIDCNN-OPMDD technique on the test dataset is displayed in Figure 11. The outcomes denoted by the OIDCNN-OPMDD method have shown their ability to categorize distinct classes on the test dataset.

Table 6 depicts detailed comparative oral classification outcomes of the OIDCNN-OPMDD model with recent DL models [10,19]. Figure 12 offers a comparative study of the OIDCNN-OPMDD model with existing models in terms of $accu_y$. These results indicated the ineffectual outcome of the Inception-v4 model with a minimal $accu_y$ of 85.14%, whereas the DBN model reported a slightly improved $accu_y$ of 86.36%. In addition, the DenseNet-161 method reached reasonable outcomes with an $accu_y$ of 90.06%. Next, the CNN model resulted in considerable performance with an $accu_y$ of 94.14%. However, the OIDCNN-OPMDD model outperformed the other ones with an increased $accu_y$ of 97.50%.

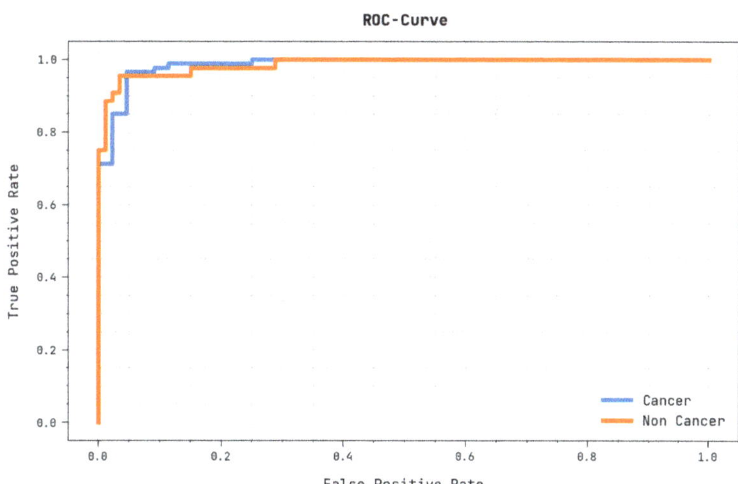

Figure 11. ROC analysis of OIDCNN-OPMDD approach.

Table 6. Comparative analysis of OIDCNN-OPMDD approach with existing algorithms [10,19].

Methods	Accuracy	Sensitivity	Specificity	F-Score
OIDCNN-OPMDD	97.50	97.83	97.83	97.46
DBN	86.36	84.12	91.15	85.74
CNN	94.14	93.93	96.89	95.39
Inception-v4	85.14	86.68	89.42	87.24
DenseNet-161	90.06	88.21	85.59	86.22

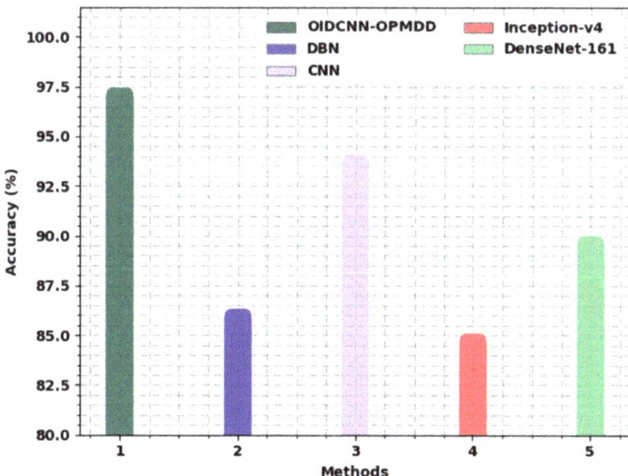

Figure 12. $accu_y$ analysis of the OIDCNN-OPMDD approach with existing algorithms.

Figure 13 portrays a comparative analysis of the OIDCNN-OPMDD algorithm with existing models in terms of $sens_y$. These results represented the ineffectual outcome of the Inception-v4 approach with a minimal $sens_y$ of 86.68%, whereas the DBN method reported a slightly improved $sens_y$ of 84.12%. In addition, the DenseNet-161 algorithm reached reasonable outcomes with a $sens_y$ of 88.21%. Then, the CNN technique resulted in notable performance with a $sens_y$ of 93.93%. However, the OIDCNN-OPMDD approach outperformed the others with an increased $sens_y$ of 97.83%.

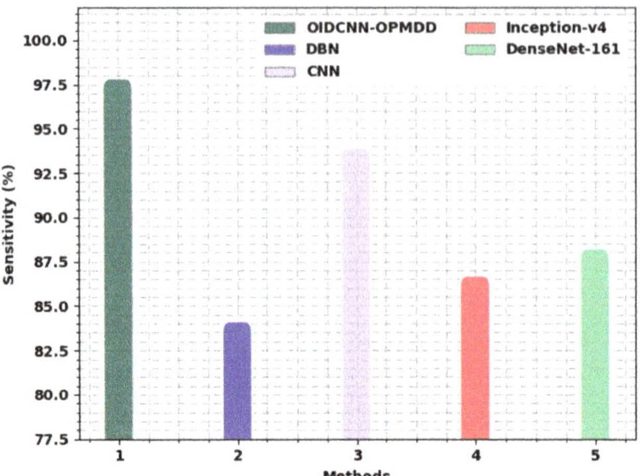

Figure 13. *Sens$_y$* analysis of the OIDCNN-OPMDD approach with existing algorithms.

Figure 14 displays the detailed study of the OIDCNN-OPMDD approach with existing algorithms in terms of *spec$_y$*. These results implicit the ineffectual outcome of the Inception-v4 technique with a minimal *spec$_y$* of 89.42%, whereas the DBN approach managed to report a slightly improved *spec$_y$* of 91.15%. In addition, the DenseNet-161 methodology reached reasonable outcomes with a *spec$_y$* of 85.59%. Then, the CNN algorithm resulted in notable performance with a *spec$_y$* of 96.89%. However, the OIDCNN-OPMDD methodology outperformed the others with an increased *spec$_y$* of 97.83%.

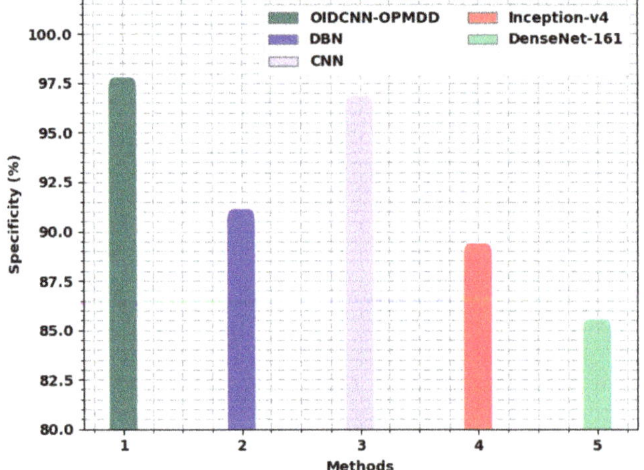

Figure 14. *Spec$_y$* analysis of OIDCNN-OPMDD approach with existing algorithms.

Figure 15 exemplifies the comprehensive inception of the OIDCNN-OPMDD algorithm with existing models in terms of *F$_{score}$*. These results denoted the ineffectual outcome of the Inception-v4 technique with a minimal *F$_{score}$* of 87.24%, whereas the DBN approach managed to report a slightly improved *F$_{score}$* of 85.74%. Moreover, the DenseNet-161 methodology reached reasonable outcomes with a *F$_{score}$* of 86.22%. Next, the CNN technique resulted in notable performance with a *F$_{score}$* of 95.39%. However, the OIDCNN-OPMDD approach outperformed the other ones with an increased *F$_{score}$* of 97.46%.

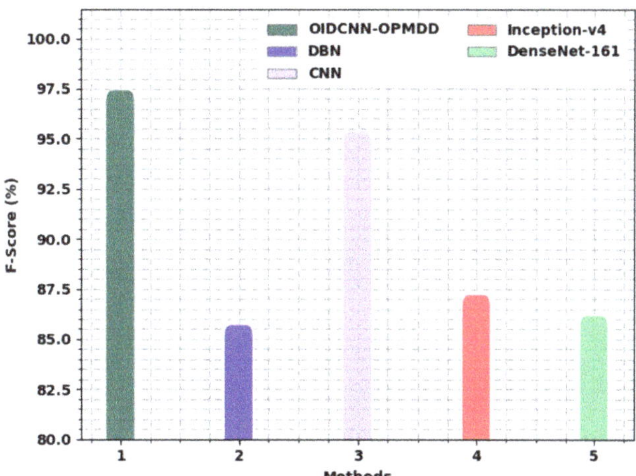

Figure 15. F_{score} analysis of OIDCNN-OPMDD approach with existing algorithms.

Thus, the OIDCNN-OPMDD model is found to be a productive solution for oral cancer detection. The enhanced performance of the proposed model is due to the optimal hyperparameter tuning using the MFO algorithm.

4. Conclusions

In this article, a novel OIDCNN-OPMDD approach was devised for the identification and classification of oral cancer. In this study, the feature extraction and classification process are performed using the IDCNN model, which integrates the Inception module with DCNN. To enhance the classification performance of the IDCNN method, the MFO algorithm is utilized in this study. The experimental results of the OIDCNN-OPMDD technique were investigated, and the outcomes were scrutinized under specific measures. The experimental outcome pointed out the enhanced performance of the OIDCNN-OPMDD model over other DL models. Thus, the OIDCNN-OPMDD model can be utilized for automated oral cancer recognition and classification process. In the future, the deep instance segmentation process can be combined with the OIDCNN-OPMDD model to boost the overall classification outcomes.

Author Contributions: Conceptualization, R.A. and A.A.; methodology, A.M.H.; software, A.M.; validation, R.A., A.A. and A.M.H.; formal analysis, A.M.; investigation, A.A.; resources, R.A.; data curation, A.M.; writing—original draft preparation, R.A., A.A. and A.M.H.; writing—review and editing, A.M.H. and A.A.; visualization, A.M.; supervision, R.A.; project administration, A.M.H.; funding acquisition, R.A. All authors have read and agreed to the published version of the manuscript.

Funding: The authors extend their appreciation to the deputyship for research and innovation, ministry education in Saudi Arabia for funding this research work through the project number (IFP-2022-25).

Institutional Review Board Statement: This article does not contain any studies with human participants performed by any of the authors.

Informed Consent Statement: Not applicable.

Data Availability Statement: Data sharing is not applicable to this article as no datasets were generated during the current study.

Conflicts of Interest: The authors declare that they have no conflict of interest. The manuscript was written through contributions of all authors. All authors have given approval for the final version of the manuscript.

References

1. Kim, Y.; Kang, J.W.; Kang, J.; Kwon, E.J.; Ha, M.; Kim, Y.K.; Lee, H.; Rhee, J.K.; Kim, Y.H. Novel deep learning-based survival prediction for oral cancer by analyzing tumor-infiltrating lymphocyte profiles through CIBERSORT. *Oncoimmunology* **2021**, *10*, 1904573. [CrossRef] [PubMed]
2. Song, B.; Sunny, S.; Uthoff, R.D.; Patrick, S.; Suresh, A.; Kolur, T.; Keerthi, G.; Anbarani, A.; Wilder-Smith, P.; Kuriakose, M.A.; et al. Automatic classification of dual-modalilty, smartphone-based oral dysplasia and malignancy images using deep learning. *Biomed. Opt. Express* **2018**, *9*, 5318–5329. [CrossRef] [PubMed]
3. Chu, C.; Lee, N.; Ho, J.; Choi, S.; Thomson, P. Deep learning for clinical image analyses in oral squamous cell carcinoma: A review. *JAMA Otolaryngol. Head Neck Surg.* **2021**, *147*, 893–900. [CrossRef] [PubMed]
4. Alabi, R.O.; Almangush, A.; Elmusrati, M.; Leivo, I.; Mäkitie, A. Measuring the usability and quality of explanations of a machine learning web-based tool for Oral Tongue Cancer Prognostication. *Int. J. Environ. Res. Public Health* **2022**, *19*, 8366. [CrossRef]
5. Saraswat, N.; Pillay, R.; Prabhu, N.; Everett, B.; George, A. Perceptions and practices of general practitioners towards oral cancer and emerging risk factors among Indian immigrants in Australia: A qualitative study. *Int. J. Environ. Res. Public Health* **2021**, *18*, 11111. [CrossRef]
6. Adeoye, J.; Choi, S.W.; Thomson, P. Bayesian disease mapping and The 'high-risk' oral cancer population in Hong Kong. *J. Oral Pathol. Med.* **2020**, *49*, 907–913. [CrossRef]
7. Calado, G.; Behl, I.; Daniel, A.; Byrne, H.J.; Lyng, F.M. Raman spectroscopic analysis of Saliva for the diagnosis of oral cancer: A systematic review. *Transl. Biophotonics* **2019**, *1*, e201900001. [CrossRef]
8. Ariji, Y.; Fukuda, M.; Kise, Y.; Nozawa, M.; Yanashita, Y.; Fujita, H.; Katsumata, A.; Ariji, E. Contrast-enhanced computed tomography image assessment of cervical lymph node metastasis in patients with oral cancer by using a deep learning system of artificial intelligence. *Oral Surg. Oral Med. Oral Pathol. Oral Radiol.* **2019**, *127*, 458–463. [CrossRef]
9. Azimi, S.; Ghorbani, Z.; Tennant, M.; Kruger, E.; Safiaghdam, H.; Rafieian, N. Population survey of knowledge about oral cancer and related factors in the capital of Iran. *J. Cancer Educ.* **2017**, *34*, 116–123. [CrossRef]
10. Jeyaraj, P.; Nadar, E.S. Computer-assisted medical image classification for early diagnosis of oral cancer employing deep learning algorithm. *J. Cancer Res. Clin. Oncol.* **2019**, *145*, 829–837. [CrossRef]
11. Rahman, A.U.; Alqahtani, A.; Aldhafferi, N.; Nasir, M.U.; Khan, M.F.; Khan, M.A.; Mosavi, A. Histopathologic Oral Cancer Prediction Using Oral Squamous Cell Carcinoma Biopsy Empowered with Transfer Learning. *Sensors* **2022**, *22*, 3833. [CrossRef]
12. Figueroa, K.C.; Song, B.; Sunny, S.; Li, S.; Gurushanth, K.; Mendonca, P.; Mukhia, N.; Patrick, S.; Gurudath, S.; Raghavan, S.; et al. Interpretable deep learning approach for oral cancer classification using guided attention inference network. *J. Biomed. Opt.* **2022**, *27*, 015001. [CrossRef]
13. Jubair, F.; Al-karadsheh, O.; Malamos, D.; Al Mahdi, S.; Saad, Y.; Hassona, Y. A novel lightweight deep convolutional neural network for early detection of oral cancer. *Oral Dis.* **2022**, *28*, 1123–1130. [CrossRef]
14. Song, B.; Sunny, S.; Li, S.; Gurushanth, K.; Mendonca, P.; Mukhia, N.; Patrick, S.; Gurudath, S.; Raghavan, S.; Tsusennaro, I.; et al. Bayesian deep learning for reliable oral cancer image classification. *Biomed. Opt. Express* **2021**, *12*, 6422–6430. [CrossRef]
15. Song, B.; Li, S.; Sunny, S.; Gurushanth, K.; Mendonca, P.; Mukhia, N.; Patrick, S.; Gurudath, S.; Raghavan, S.; Tsusennaro, I.; et al. Classification of imbalanced oral cancer image data from high-risk population. *J. Biomed. Opt.* **2021**, *26*, 105001. [CrossRef]
16. Shamim, M.Z.; Syed, S.; Shiblee, M.; Usman, M.; Ali, S.J.; Hussein, H.S.; Farrag, M. Automated detection of oral pre-cancerous tongue lesions using deep learning for early diagnosis of oral cavity cancer. *Comput. J.* **2022**, *65*, 91–104. [CrossRef]
17. Camalan, S.; Mahmood, H.; Binol, H.; Araújo, A.L.; Santos-Silva, A.R.; Vargas, P.A.; Lopes, M.A.; Khurram, S.A.; Gurcan, M.N. Convolutional neural network-based clinical predictors of oral dysplasia: Class activation map analysis of deep learning results. *Cancers* **2021**, *13*, 1291. [CrossRef]
18. Rajan, J.P.; Rajan, S.E.; Martis, R.J.; Panigrahi, B.K. Fog computing employed computer aided cancer classification system using deep neural network in internet of things based healthcare system. *J. Med. Syst.* **2020**, *44*, 34. [CrossRef]
19. Tanriver, G.; Tekkesin, M.S.; Ergen, O. Automated detection and classification of oral lesions using deep learning to detect oral potentially malignant disorders. *Cancers* **2021**, *13*, 2766. [CrossRef]
20. Bhandari, B.; Alsadoon, A.; Prasad, P.; Abdullah, S.; Haddad, S. Deep learning neural network for texture feature extraction in oral cancer: Enhanced loss function. *Multimed. Tools Appl.* **2020**, *79*, 27867–27890. [CrossRef]
21. Chan, C.H.; Huang, T.T.; Chen, C.Y.; Lee, C.C.; Chan, M.Y.; Chung, P.C. Texture-map-based branch-collaborative network for oral cancer detection. *IEEE Trans. Biomed. Circuits Syst.* **2019**, *13*, 766–780. [CrossRef]
22. Mirzabagherian, H.; Sardari, M.A.; Menhaj, M.B.; Suratgar, A.A. Classification of Raw Spinal Cord Injury EEG Data Based on the Temporal-Spatial Inception Deep Convolutional Neural Network. In Proceedings of the 9th RSI International Conference on Robotics and Mechatronics (ICRoM), Prague, Czech Republic, 20–22 April 2021; pp. 43–50. [CrossRef]
23. Shehab, M.; Abualigah, L.; Al Hamad, H.; Alabool, H.; Alshinwan, M.; Khasawneh, A.M. Moth–flame optimization algorithm: Variants and applications. *Neural Comput. Appl.* **2020**, *32*, 9859–9884. [CrossRef]
24. Available online: https://www.kaggle.com/datasets/shivam17299/oral-cancer-lips-and-tongue-images (accessed on 12 September 2022).

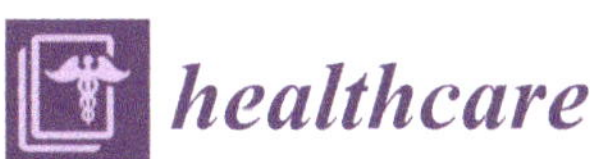

Article

Equilibrium Optimization Algorithm with Ensemble Learning Based Cervical Precancerous Lesion Classification Model

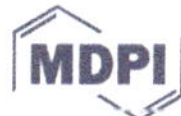

Rasha A. Mansouri [1] and **Mahmoud Ragab** [2,3,*]

1 Department of Biochemistry, Faculty of Sciences, King Abdulaziz University, Jeddah 21589, Saudi Arabia
2 Information Technology Department, Faculty of Computing and Information Technology, King Abdulaziz University, Jeddah 21589, Saudi Arabia
3 Department of Mathematics, Faculty of Science, Al-Azhar University, Naser City, Cairo 11884, Egypt
* Correspondence: mragab@kau.edu.sa

Abstract: Recently, artificial intelligence (AI) with deep learning (DL) and machine learning (ML) has been extensively used to automate labor-intensive and time-consuming work and to help in prognosis and diagnosis. AI's role in biomedical and biological imaging is an emerging field of research and reveals future trends. Cervical cell (CCL) classification is crucial in screening cervical cancer (CC) at an earlier stage. Unlike the traditional classification method, which depends on hand-engineered or crafted features, convolution neural network (CNN) usually categorizes CCLs through learned features. Moreover, the latent correlation of images might be disregarded in CNN feature learning and thereby influence the representative capability of the CNN feature. This study develops an equilibrium optimizer with ensemble learning-based cervical precancerous lesion classification on colposcopy images (EOEL-PCLCCI) technique. The presented EOEL-PCLCCI technique mainly focuses on identifying and classifying cervical cancer on colposcopy images. In the presented EOEL-PCLCCI technique, the DenseNet-264 architecture is used for the feature extractor, and the EO algorithm is applied as a hyperparameter optimizer. An ensemble of weighted voting classifications, namely long short-term memory (LSTM) and gated recurrent unit (GRU), is used for the classification process. A widespread simulation analysis is performed on a benchmark dataset to depict the superior performance of the EOEL-PCLCCI approach, and the results demonstrated the betterment of the EOEL-PCLCCI algorithm over other DL models.

Keywords: medical imaging; healthcare; decision making; cervical cancer; ensemble learning

Citation: A. Mansouri, R.; Ragab, M. Equilibrium Optimization Algorithm with Ensemble Learning Based Cervical Precancerous Lesion Classification Model. *Healthcare* **2023**, *11*, 55. https://doi.org/10.3390/healthcare11010055

Academic Editor: Mahmudur Rahman

Received: 11 November 2022
Revised: 17 December 2022
Accepted: 21 December 2022
Published: 25 December 2022

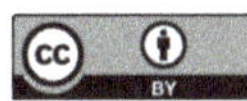

1. Introduction

Cervical cancer (CC) ranks as the fourth most common cancer in females. As per the statistical report by WHO, approximately 604,000 new cases occurred worldwide in 2020, particularly 6.5% of cancer cases in females [1]. Although the initial treatment rate of CC is high, lack of symptoms and signs hinders the initial diagnoses. An effective screening program may prevent CC deaths and decrease the persistence and incidence of the disease. The statistical reports stated that over 311,000 CC deaths occurred annually [2]. Because of amateur healthcare staff and inadequate screening funds, CC screening facilities seem to be very scarce in developing nations [3]. Thus, employing effective and automated screening techniques is essential to reduce the cost of initial detection of CC. CC screening follows the following workflow: colposcopy, HPV test, biopsy, and PAP smear test or cytology.

Numerous tools reinforce the task, which make it inexpensive, practical, and very effective [4]. The PAP smear image screening can be used for the treatment of CC; however, it needs several microscopic analyses to find non-cancer and cancer patients, and even if it takes more time and necessitates skilled professionals, there comes a chance of missing the positive case with the use of the traditional screening technique [5]. The HPV testing and PAP smear are expensive medications and offer less sensitivity. In contrast, colposcopy treatment can be broadly employed in developing nations. Colposcopy screening is employed to address the limitations of HPV testing and PAP smear images [6]. The cervical and other cancers are probably treated at the initial level. However, the lack of symptoms at this phase will hinder the initial diagnosis. CC deaths are evaded by effective screening methods and result in impermanence and lowered sickness [7]. CC screening facilities are very sparse in middle-and-low-income countries due to a lack of educated and experienced healthcare professionals and inadequate funding to fund screening mechanisms.

Some of the important advancements of deep learning (DL) in various applications are battery health monitoring, natural language processing (NLP), forecasting, and computer vision (CV) [8]. Medical image processing, which includes registration, classification, segmentation, and identification, had a significant role in diagnosing disease. Medical images of blood smears, MRI, ultrasound, and CT constitute the major part of the image data processed [9]. The multilayer neural network perception system of DL has more extracted features in images and was anticipated to overcome the challenges plaguing standard CAD systems. Still, the DL methods have to be reinforced with a wide range of datasets, particularly for positive cases [10]. Several ensemble learning and transfer learning (TL) methods were used to solve this problem [11–13].

This study develops an equilibrium optimizer with ensemble learning-based cervical precancerous lesion classification on colposcopy images (EOEL-PCLCCI) technique. The presented EOEL-PCLCCI technique mainly focuses on identifying and classifying cervical cancer on colposcopy images. In the presented EOEL-PCLCCI technique, the DenseNet-264 architecture is used for the feature extractor. Since the trial and error method for hyperparameter tuning is tedious and erroneous, metaheuristic algorithms can be applied. Therefore, in this work, we employ the EO algorithm for the parameter selection of the DenseNet model. An ensemble of weighted voting classifiers, namely long short-term memory (LSTM) and gated recurrent unit (GRU), is used for the classification process. A widespread simulation analysis is performed on a benchmark dataset to depict the enhanced performance of the EOEL-PCLCCI algorithm.

2. Related Works

Khamparia et al. [14] developed a new Internet of Health Things (IoHT)-based DL algorithm for classifying and recognizing CC in pap smear images with a TL model. Then, CNN was fused with outdated ML approaches. In this work, feature extraction from cervical images can be carried out by pre-trained CNN modules such as ResNet50, InceptionV3, VGG19, and SqueezeNet and are fed into flattened and dense layers for the classification of normal and abnormal CCLs. Shi et al. [15] recommend a classification of CCLs based GCN model. The study aims at exploring the possible relations of CCL images for enhancing the accuracy of classification. The CNN feature of each CCL image was clustered initially, and the inherent relationship of images can be exposed earlier through the clustering. A graph model has been constructed to capture the fundamental correlation among the clusters further.

Allehaibi et al. [16] propose a CCL segmentation with mask regional CNN (Mask R-CNN) and categorizes by a small VGG-like Net. ResNet10 uses prior knowledge and spatial information as the backbone of Mask R-CNN. Chen et al. [17] developed a TL-based snapshot ensemble (TLSE) technique by incorporating them in a unified and coordinated manner. SE technique offers ensemble advantages within a single model training method, whereas TL emphasizes the smaller sampling problems in CCL classification. Archana and Panicker [18] advise a new methodology for the multiclass classification of CCLs with less computing power, optimum feature extraction, and minimal parameters. The application of ConvNet with the TL method validates substantial diagnoses of cancer cells.

Dong et al. [19] proposed a cell classification technique which combines artificial and Inceptionv3 features that considerably enhance the performance of CCL detection. Furthermore, the study inherits the stronger learning capability from TL to address the under-fitting problems and perform effectual DL training with a less quantity of medicinal datasets and accomplishes precise and effective CCL image classification based on Herlev data. Li et al. [20] introduced an L-PCNN which incorporates a global context dataset and attention module for categorizing CCLs. The cell image was transferred to the improved ResNet50 model for extracting DL features. For extracting deep features, every convolutional block presents an attention module for guiding the network to emphasize the cell region. Next, the network includes a pyramid pooling layer and an LSTM for aggregating image features in distinct areas.

3. The Proposed Model

In this study, we introduced an automated cervical cancer classification model, the EOEL-PCLCCI technique, on colposcopy images. The EOEL-PCLCCI technique uses a DenseNet-264 feature extractor, EO hyperparameter optimizer, and weighted voting classifier. Figure 1 illustrates the working process of the EOEL-PCLCCI system.

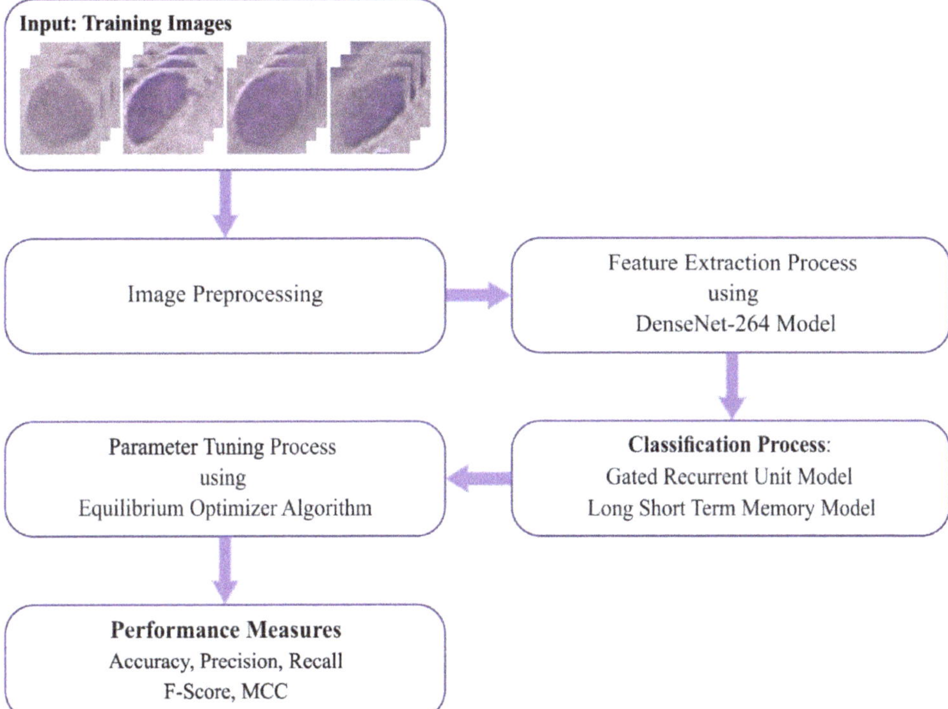

Figure 1. Working process of EOEL-PCLCCI system.

3.1. Feature Extraction

In the presented EOEL-PCLCCI technique, the DenseNet-264 architecture is used for the feature extraction. In the typical CNN, every layer is gradually interconnected, making the network difficult to go deeper and wider. Meanwhile, it has a gradient exploding or vanishing problem [21]. Consequently, DenseNet analyzes the module by successively concatenating all the feature maps instead of outputting feature maps from every prior layer in the following:

$$x_l = H_l(x_{l-1}) \tag{1}$$

$$x_l = H_l(x_{l-1}) + x_{l-1} \tag{2}$$

$$x_l = H_l([x_0, x_1, x_2, \dots, x_{l-1}]) \tag{3}$$

H indicates the nonlinear function from the expression, and l characterizes the layer index. x_l symbolizes the feature of l-th layers. DenseNet concurs all the feature maps from previous layers, indicating that all the feature maps are propagated toward the last layer and interconnected toward the new feature maps. The recently designed DenseNet has certain benefits, namely feature reutilization and reduction in gradient exploding or vanishing problems. Once the size of feature maps continuously changes, the concatenation function becomes impossible to be implemented. Among the dense blocks, transition layers exist: convolution, pooling, and BN operations. Meanwhile, each layer receives feature maps from all the previous layers. Note that k feature maps are constructed for each H_l operation. Meanwhile, there exist five layers, and we obtain $k_0 + 4k$ feature maps. k_0 symbolizes the number of feature maps from prior layers.

However, there exists a huge quantity of inputs, and bottleneck layers are introduced for the DenseNet, viz., implemented using the 1×1 convolution layer beforehand 3×3 convolution layers that are beneficial to save the computational cost and decrease the feature map. Subsequently, considering the model compactness, a transition layer is applied to reduce the feature maps: consider m feature maps are constructed using DenseBlock and assume the compression factors $\theta\epsilon(0,1)$. If $\theta = 1$, the quantity of feature maps remains unchanged. The DenseNet module encompasses transition layers, input layers, Dense Blocks, and global average pooling (GAP). The transition layer comprises the BN layer, $1 \times 12 \times 2$ convolution, and average pooling layers with a stride of 2.

To adjust the hyperparameters associated with the DenseNet-264 model, the EO algorithm is exploited in this work. The fundamental idea of single objective EO has been established based on the dynamic mass balance [22]. This characteristic can maintain the balance between exploitation and detection and the ability to retain flexibility among individual solutions. In the initialization, EO uses a certain group, while each particle explains the vector of focus that has solutions to the problem.

$$Y_j^{initial} = lb + rand_j(ub - lb), \; j = 0, 1, 2, 3, \ldots, n \tag{4}$$

$Y_j^{initial}$ denotes the vector focus on jth particles, ub and lb represent the upper and lower boundaries of each parameter, $rand_j$ indicates the arbitrary integer within $[0, 1]$, and n shows the number of particles. Hence, it assigns an equilibrium candidate to the optimal four particles from the population. In the exploitation and exploration methods, these five equilibrium candidate assists EO. The initial four candidates seek optimal exploration. However, the 5th candidate with average values seeks alteration from exploitation.

$$\vec{C}_{eq,pool} = \left\{ \vec{C}_{eq(1)}, \vec{C}_{eq(2)}, \vec{C}_{eq(3)}, \vec{C}_{eq(4)}, \vec{C}_{eq(ave)} \right\} \tag{5}$$

The upgrade of concentration enables EO to balance exploitation and exploration equally:

$$\vec{F} = e^{-\vec{\lambda}(t-t_0)} \tag{6}$$

Equation (6) $\vec{\lambda}$ indicates the arbitrary integer within $[0, 1]$, and t reduces as the iteration amount enhances.

$$t = \left(1 - \frac{It}{Max\_it}\right)^{\left(a_2 \frac{It}{Max\_it}\right)} \tag{7}$$

It and *Max_it* denote existing and maximal iteration counts, and a_2 shows the constant control of the ability for exploiting. Another parameter, a_1, has been employed to enhance exploration and exploitation:

$$t = \frac{1}{\vec{\lambda}} \ln\left(-a_1 \, \text{sign}\left(\vec{r} - 0.5 \right) \left[1 - e^{-\vec{\lambda} t} \right] \right) + t \tag{8}$$

The generation rate is denoted as G rises exploitation:

$$\vec{G} = \vec{G}_0 e^{-\vec{l}(t - t_0)} \tag{9}$$

Equation (9) $\vec{l}$ denotes the arbitrary number within $[0, 1]$, and the initial generation rate represented by $\vec{G}_0$:

$$\vec{G}_0 = \vec{GCP}\left(\vec{C}_{eq} - \vec{\lambda}\vec{C} \right) \tag{10}$$

$$\vec{GCP} = \begin{cases} 0.5 r_1, r_2 \geq GP \\ 0, r_2 < GP \end{cases} \tag{11}$$

From the expression, the arbitrary integers are denoted by r_1 and r_2 and vary between zero and one. The vector $\vec{GCP}$ represents the variable which controls the generation rate executed for the upgrading phase.

$$\vec{C} = \vec{C} + \left(\vec{C} - \vec{C}_{eq} \right) \cdot \vec{F} + \frac{\vec{C}}{\vec{\lambda} V}\left(1 - \vec{F} \right) \tag{12}$$

The value of V corresponds to 1.

3.2. Weighted Voting-Based Ensemble Classification

An ensemble of weighted voting classifiers, GRU and LSTM, is used for the classification process. The DL algorithm is incorporated, and the maximal result is preferred by the weighted voting method [23]. Considering the D base classification and amount of classes as n for voting, the predictive class c_k of weighted voting for every instance, k, can be defined by:

$$c_k = \text{argmax}_j \sum_{i=1}^{D} \left(\Delta_{ji} \times w_i \right) \tag{13}$$

The expression Δ_{ji} indicates the binary variable. As soon as the i-th base classification classifies the k instances into j-th classes, then $\Delta_{ji} = 1$, or else, $\Delta_{ji} = 0$. w_i shows the weight of i-th base classifications:

$$Acc = \frac{\sum_k \{1 | c_k \text{ is the true class of instance } k\}}{\text{Size of test instances}} \times 100\%. \tag{14}$$

3.2.1. GRU Model

GRU is an LSTM network which inherits the advantages of RNN: it learns features automatically and effectively models long dependency datasets. It is utilized for short-term traffic prediction. Intuitively, input and forget gates are integrated as a reset gate in GRU, which determines how to incorporate the novel input dataset in the previous time. Another gate in GRU is an update gate; it determines the information stored from the previous time to the existing time. Therefore, GRU is one gate lower than LSTM. This makes the

GRU network have faster training speed and lesser variables and needs lesser datasets for efficiently generalizing the system:

$$z_n = \sigma f(W_z \cdot [h_{n-1}, \, x_n]) \tag{15}$$

$$r_n = \sigma f(W_r \cdot [h_{n-1}, \, x_n]) \tag{16}$$

$$\overline{h}_n = \tanh\,(W \cdot [r * h_{n-1}, \, x_n]) \tag{17}$$

$$h_n = (1 - z_n) * h_{n-1} + z_n * \overline{h} \tag{18}$$

Equations (15) and (16) illustrate how r_n, z_n reset, and update gates are evaluated. W_z is the weight of z_n, 0 denotes the sigmoid function, W_r characterizes the weight of r_n. A larger value of z_n denotes that data were retained through the present cell r_n and proposes that when the value corresponds to 0, the dataset from the prior cell is eliminated. Equations (17) and (18) demonstrate the estimation of h_n and $\overline{h}$ final and pending output of GRU-NN. W characterizes the weight of z_n, h_{n-1} denotes the output from the preceding cell, and $\tan h$ denotes the hyperbolic tangent function. $\overline{h}_n$ can be obtained by multiplying h_{n-1} of the prior cell using r_n and x_n, multiplying by W and $\tan h$. h_n denotes the amount of two vectors.

3.2.2. LSTM Model

The RNN approach was widely employed for predicting and analyzing time sequence datasets. RNN often undergoes the gradient vanishing problem. Hence, it is hard to remember the previous dataset, namely the long dependence problem. To overcome these problems, the LSTM is introduced and applies a gate-controlling method for altering data flow and systematically determines the count of received datasets that are regathered from each time step. Figure 2 represents the architecture of LSTM.

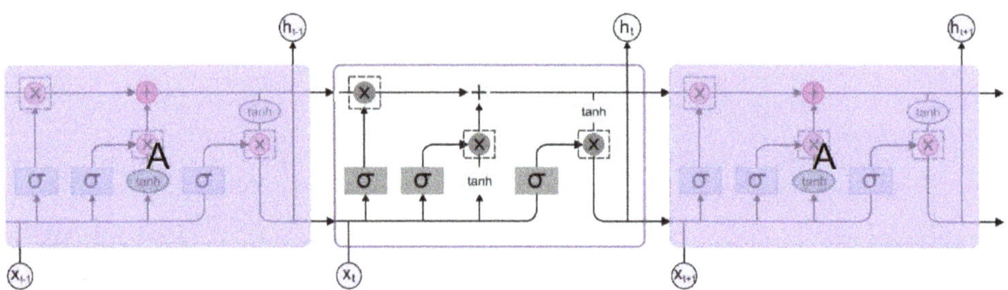

Figure 2. The architecture of LSTM.

The architecture of the LSTM unit is encompassed by storing unit and three control gates (forget, input, and output gates). x_z and h_z correspond to the input and hidden state of time z. f_z, i_z, and o_z determine the forgetting, input, and output gates. $\overrightarrow{C}_z$ indicates the candidate dataset to the input.

$$f_z = \sigma f\left(W_f \cdot [h_{z-1}, \, x_z] + b_f\right) \tag{19}$$

$$i_z = \sigma(W_i \cdot [h_{z-1}, \, x_z] + b_i) \tag{20}$$

$$o_z = \sigma(W_o \cdot [h_{z-1}, \, x_z] + b_o) \tag{21}$$

$$\widetilde{C} = \tanh\,(W_C \cdot [h_{z-1}, \, x_z] + b_C) \tag{22}$$

$$C_z = f_z \cdot C_{z-1} + i_t \cdot \widetilde{C} \tag{23}$$

$$h_z = o_z \cdot \tanh\,(C_z) \tag{24}$$

W_f, W_i, W_o, and W_c b_f, b_i, b_o, and b_c correspondingly denote the weight matrices and bias vector of forget, input, output, and update state. x^z represents the time sequence dataset of the existing time interval z, and h_{z-1} denotes the resultant memory unit from the previous time interval $z - 1$.

4. Results and Discussion

The proposed method is simulated using a Python tool. The experimental results of the EOEL-PCLCCI model are tested using the Herlev database [21]. Figure 3 demonstrates some sample images. The proposed model is simulated using Python 3.6.5 tool on PC i5-8600k, GeForce 1050Ti 4 GB, 16 GB RAM, 250 GB SSD, and 1 TB HDD. The parameter settings are learning rate: 0.01, dropout: 0.5, batch size: 5, epoch count: 50, and activation: ReLU.

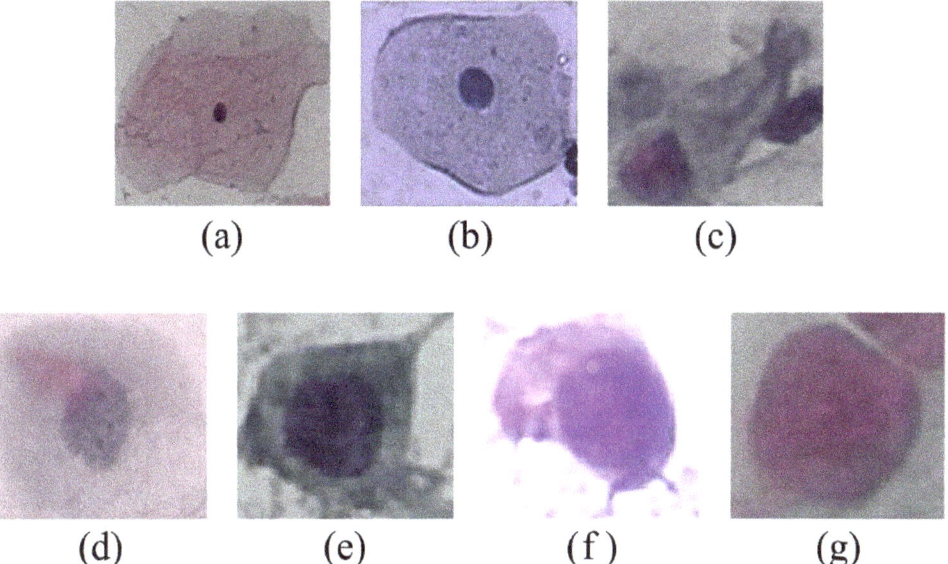

Figure 3. Sample images. (**a**) Superficial squamous (SSE), (**b**) intermediate squamous (ISE), (**c**) columnar (CE), (**d**) mild dysplasia (MS-NKD), (**e**) moderate dysplasia (MOS-NKD), (**f**) severe dysplasia (SS-NKD), (**g**) carcinoma in situ (SCCSI).

In Figure 4, the confusion matrices of the EOEL-PCLCCI model on cervical cancer classification performance are provided. The figure implied that the EOEL-PCLCCI model detected all cervical cancer classes.

Table 1 and Figure 5 demonstrate the overall cervical cancer classification results of the EOEL-PCLCCI technique on entire datasets. The experimental value indicates that the EOEL-PCLCCI method has recognized all different class labels. It is observed that the EOEL-PCLCCI approach has reached an average $accu_y$ of 98.94%, $prec_n$ of 96%, $reca_l$ of 95.61%, F_{score} of 95.80%, and MCC of 95.18%.

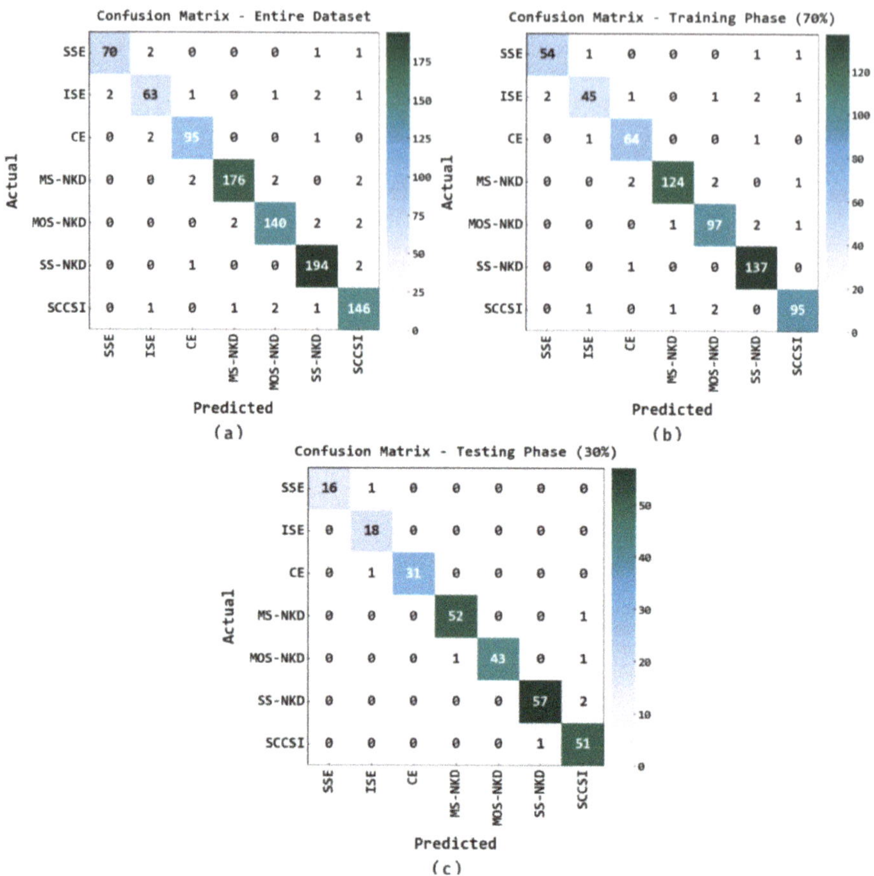

Figure 4. Confusion matrices of EOEL-PCLCCI system on cervical cancer classification; (**a**) entire database, (**b**) 70% of TR database, and (**c**) 30% of TS database.

Table 1. CC outcome of EOEL-PCLCCI system with various classes under entire database.

	Entire Dataset				
Labels	$Accu_y$	$Prec_n$	$Reca_l$	F_{score}	**MCC**
SSE	99.35	97.22	94.59	95.89	95.55
ISE	98.69	92.65	90.00	91.30	90.61
CE	99.24	95.96	96.94	96.45	96.02
MS-NKD	99.02	98.32	96.70	97.51	96.90
MOS-NKD	98.80	96.55	95.89	96.22	95.51
SS-NKD	98.91	96.52	98.48	97.49	96.80
SCCSI	98.58	94.81	96.69	95.74	94.90
Average	98.94	96.00	95.61	95.80	95.18

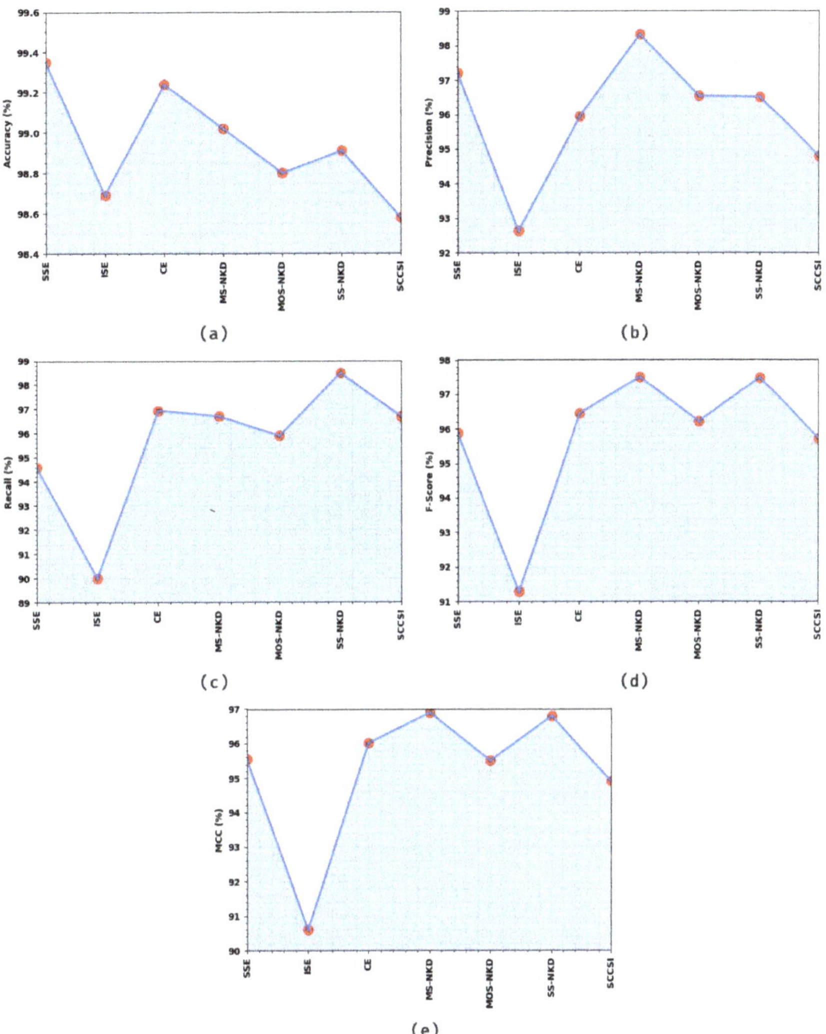

Figure 5. Result analysis of the EOEL-PCLCCI system on the entire database in terms of different measures (**a**) $Accu_y$, (**b**) $Prec_n$, (**c**) $Reca_l$, (**d**) F_{score}, and (**e**) MCC.

Table 2 and Figure 6 illustrate the overall cervical cancer classification results of the EOEL-PCLCCI technique on the TR database. The simulation values exhibited that the EOEL-PCLCCI approach recognized all different class labels. The EOEL-PCLCCI algorithm has attained an average $accu_y$ of 98.84%, $prec_n$ of 95.65%, $reca_l$ of 95.09%, F_{score} of 95.34%, and MCC of 94.68%.

Table 3 and Figure 7 show the overall cervical cancer classification results of the EOEL-PCLCCI approach on the TS database. The simulation values designated that the EOEL-PCLCCI approach has recognized all different class labels. The EOEL-PCLCCI technique has gained an average $accu_y$ of 99.17%, $prec_n$ of 97.02%, $reca_l$ of 97.05%, F_{score} of 96.96%, and MCC of 96.51%.

Table 2. CC outcome of EOEL-PCLCCI system with various classes under TR database.

	Training Phase (70%)				
Labels	$Accu_y$	$Prec_n$	$Reca_l$	F_{score}	MCC
SSE	99.22	96.43	94.74	95.58	95.15
ISE	98.44	93.75	86.54	90.00	89.24
CE	99.07	94.12	96.97	95.52	95.01
MS-NKD	98.91	98.41	96.12	97.25	96.59
MOS-NKD	98.60	95.10	96.04	95.57	94.74
SS-NKD	98.91	95.80	99.28	97.51	96.84
SCCSI	98.75	95.96	95.96	95.96	95.22
Average	98.84	95.65	95.09	95.34	94.68

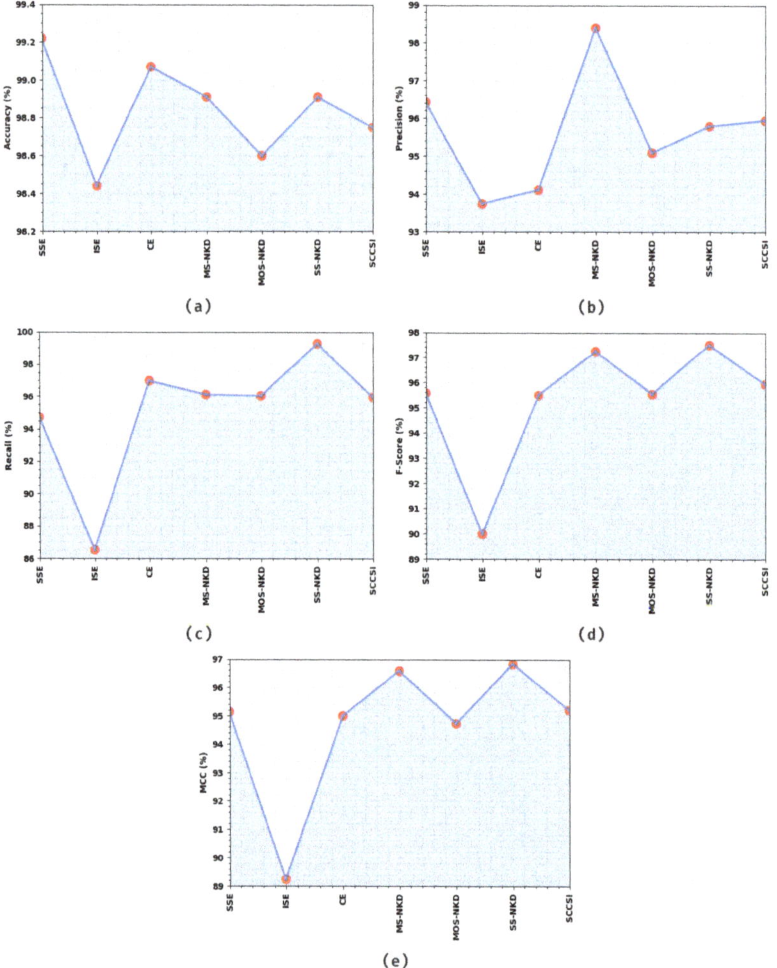

Figure 6. Result analysis of EOEL-PCLCCI system on 70% of TR database in terms of different measures (**a**) $Accu_y$, (**b**) $Prec_n$, (**c**) $Reca_l$, (**d**) F_{score}, and (**e**) MCC.

Table 3. CC outcome of EOEL-PCLCCI system with various classes under TS database.

	Testing Phase (30%)				
Labels	$Accu_y$	$Prec_n$	$Reca_l$	F_{score}	**MCC**
SSE	99.64	100.00	94.12	96.97	96.83
ISE	99.28	90.00	100.00	94.74	94.50
CE	99.64	100.00	96.88	98.41	98.22
MS-NKD	99.28	98.11	98.11	98.11	97.66
MOS-NKD	99.28	100.00	95.56	97.73	97.33
SS-NKD	98.91	98.28	96.61	97.44	96.75
SCCSI	98.19	92.73	98.08	95.33	94.26
Average	99.17	97.02	97.05	96.96	96.51

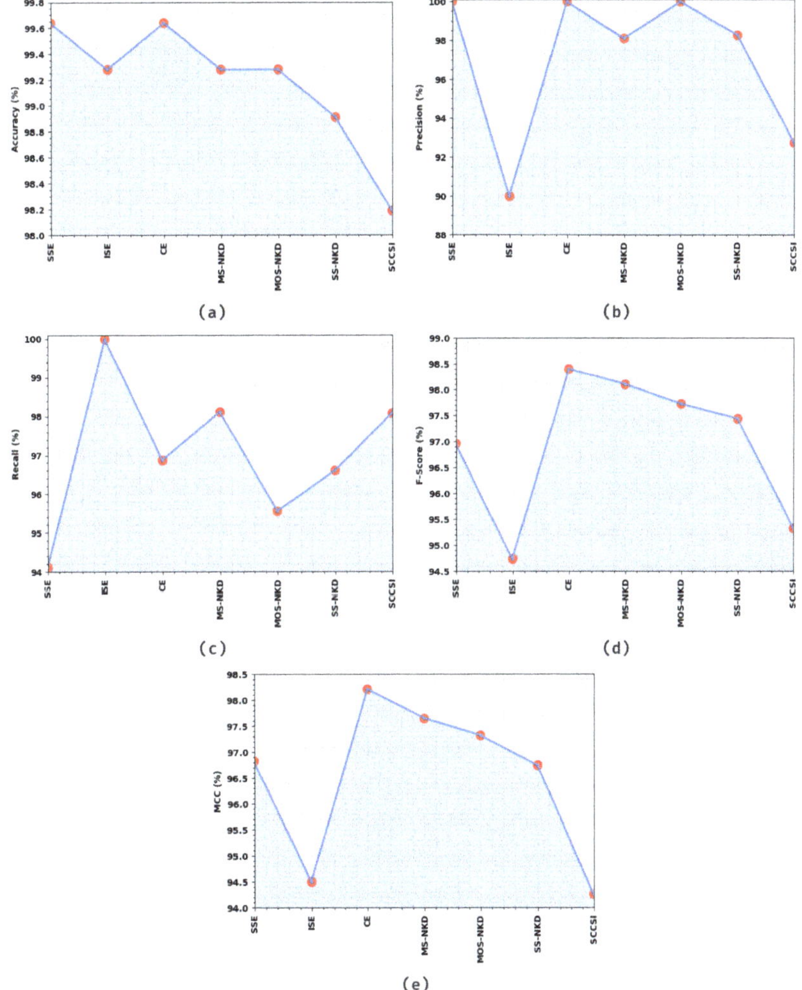

Figure 7. Result analysis of EOEL-PCLCCI system on 30% of TS database in terms of different measures (**a**) $Accu_y$, (**b**) $Prec_n$, (**c**) $Reca_l$, (**d**) F_{score}, and (**e**) MCC.

The TACC and VACC of the EOEL-PCLCCI method are investigated on CC performance in Figure 8. The figure implied that the EOEL-PCLCCI methodology has exhibited improved performance with increased values of TACC and VACC. It is noted that the EOEL-PCLCCI approach has reached maximum TACC outcomes.

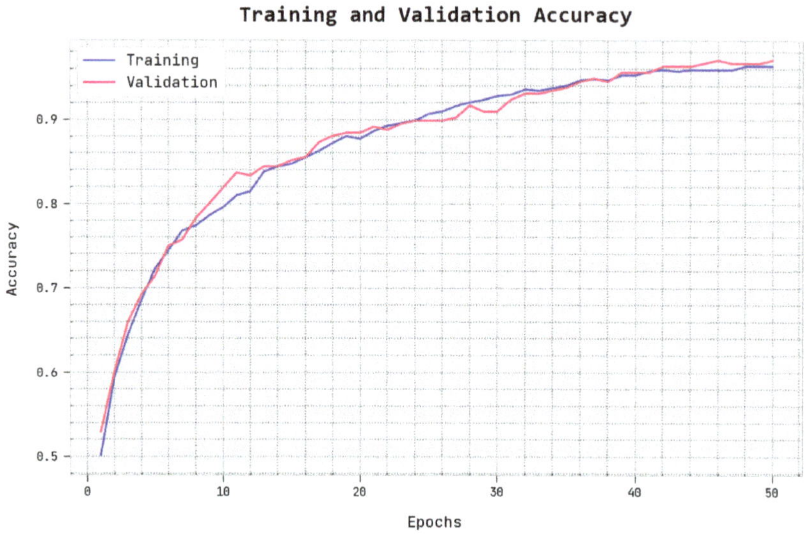

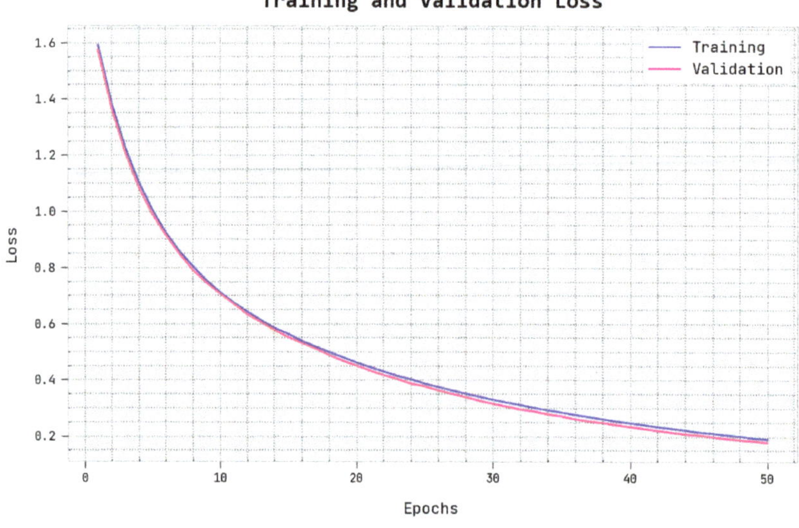

Figure 8. TACC and VACC analysis of EOEL-PCLCCI system.

The TLS and VLS of the EOEL-PCLCCI method are tested on CC performance in Figure 9. The figure designated the EOEL-PCLCCI approach has revealed better performance with minimal values of TLS and VLS. It is noted the EOEL-PCLCCI approach has resulted in reduced VLS outcomes.

Figure 9. TLS and VLS analysis of EOEL-PCLCCI system.

A clear precision-recall inspection of the EOEL-PCLCCI system under test database is shown in Figure 10. The precision-recall curve shows the tradeoff between precision and recall for different threshold. A high area under the curve represents both high recall and high precision, where high precision relates to a low false positive rate, and high recall relates to a low false negative rate. The figure shows the EOEL-PCLCCI method has resulted in superior values of precision-recall value in all the class labels.

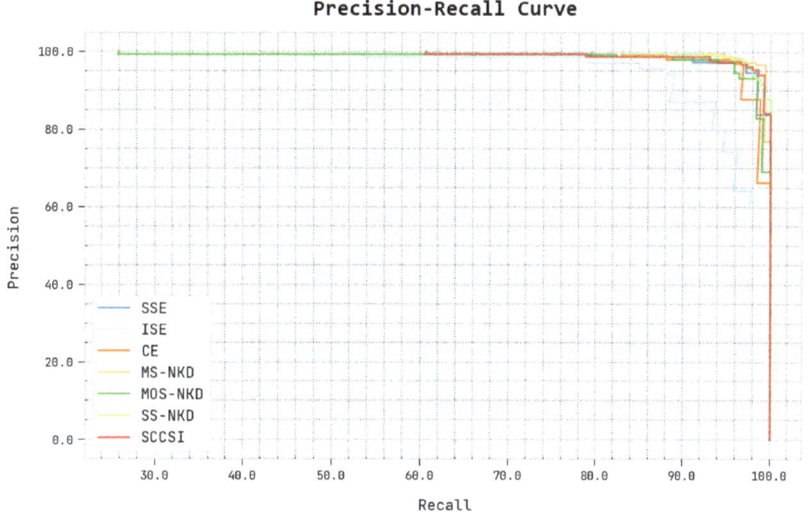

Figure 10. Precision-recall analysis of EOEL-PCLCCI system.

The detailed ROC analysis of the EOEL-PCLCCI system under the test database is shown in Figure 11. ROC curves summarize the trade-off between the true positive rate and false positive rate for a predictive model using different probability thresholds. The outcomes exhibited by the EOEL-PCLCCI methodology has signified its ability to categorize distinct classes in test database.

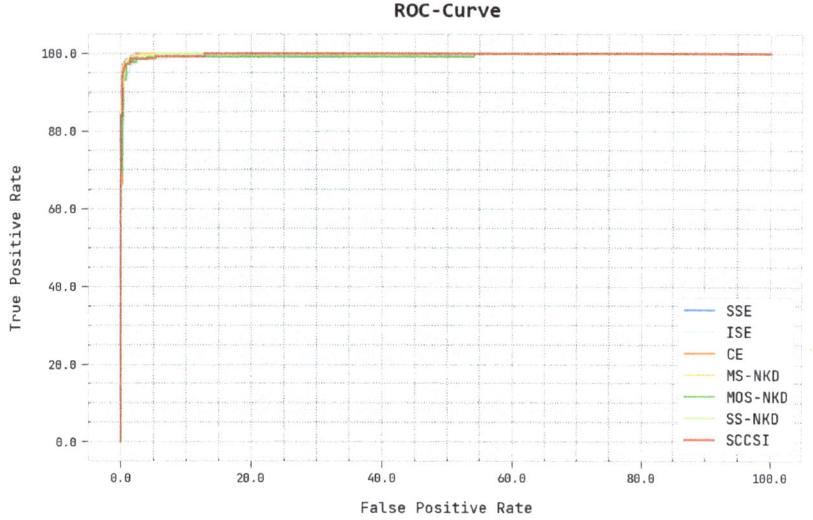

Figure 11. ROC curve analysis of EOEL-PCLCCI system.

The experimental results of the EOEL-PCLCCI model are compared with other DL models in Table 4 and Figure 12 [24,25]. The result implies that the ShuffleNet and ShuffleNet_SE models have shown lower performance, whereas the ResNet34 and DenseNet121 models have reported moderately improved performance.

Table 4. Comparative analysis of EOEL-PCLCCI algorithm with recent approaches.

Methods	$Accu_y$	$Prec_n$	$Reca_l$	F_{score}
EOEL-PCLCCI	99.17	97.02	97.05	96.96
GCN	96.28	92.41	95.38	92.79
Mor-27	94.34	87.55	96.36	86.57
ResNet-101	91.58	88.70	96.75	90.73
ResNet34	83.47	85.59	80.94	83.08
DenseNet121	86.40	86.45	84.42	85.46
ShuffleNet	79.78	79.97	78.66	79.78
ShuffleNet_SE	80.90	81.79	81.04	81.22

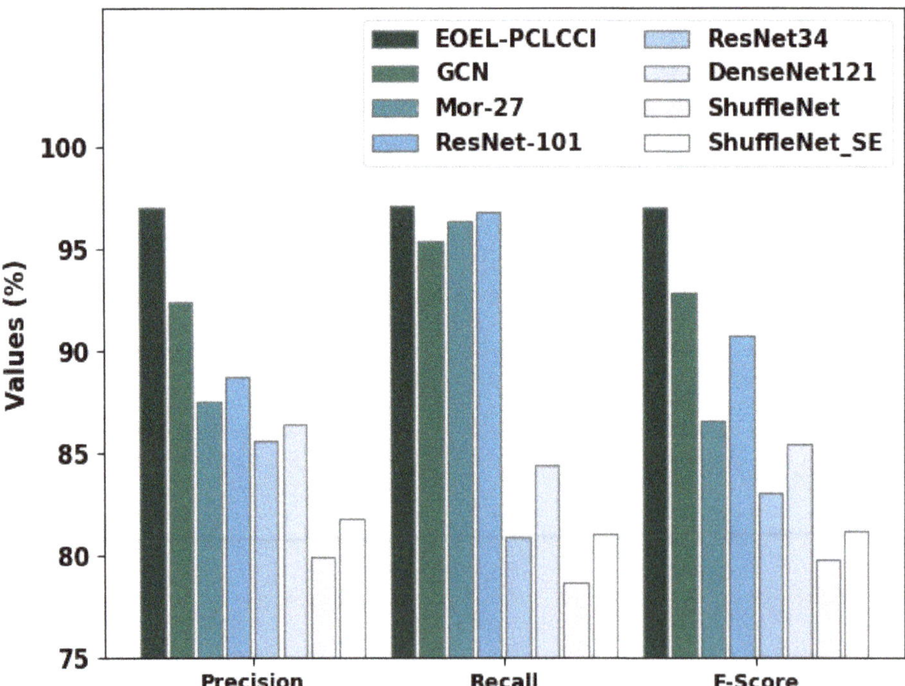

Figure 12. Comparative analysis of EOEL-PCLCCI algorithm with recent approaches.

In contrast, the Mor-27 and ResNet-101 models have tried to obtain reasonable outcomes. Although the GCN model has shown near-optimal performance, the EOEL-PCLCCI model has shown enhanced results with $accu_y$ of 99.17%, $prec_n$ of 97.02%, $reca_l$ of 97.05%, and F_{score} of 96.96%. Therefore, the EOEL-PCLCCI model has shown superior results over other models.

5. Conclusions

In this study, we have introduced an automated cervical cancer classification method, named EOEL-PCLCCI algorithm on colposcopy images. In the presented EOEL-PCLCCI technique, the DenseNet-264 architecture is used for feature extraction and EO algorithm is applied as a hyperparameter optimizer. For classification process, an ensemble of weighted voting classifiers namely GRU and LSTM is used. A widespread simulation analysis is performed on benchmark dataset to depict the superior performance of the EOEL-PCLCCI technique, and the results demonstrate the superiority of the EOEL-PCLCCI algorithm over other DL models with maximum accuracy of 99.17%. Thus, the EOEL-PCLCCI approach can be used for cervical cancer classification effectively. In the future, the performance of EOEL-PCLCCI technique needs to be enhanced by deep instance segmentation.

Author Contributions: Conceptualization, R.A.M.; Methodology, R.A.M.; Software, M.R.; Formal analysis, R.A.M.; Investigation, R.A.M.; Resources, M.R.; Data curation, R.A.M.; Writing—original draft, R.A.M.; Writing—review & editing, M.R.; Supervision, M.R.; Funding acquisition, M.R. All authors have read and agreed to the published version of the manuscript.

Funding: This project was financed by the Deanship of Scientific Research (DSR) at King Abdul-Aziz University (KAU), Jeddah, Saudi Arabia, under grant no. (G: 246-247-1443). The authors, therefore, thank DSR for technical and financial support.

Institutional Review Board Statement: Not applicable.

Informed Consent Statement: This article does not contain any studies with human participants performed by authors.

Data Availability Statement: Data sharing does not apply to this article as no datasets were generated during the current study.

Conflicts of Interest: The authors declare that they have no conflict of interest. The manuscript was written through the contributions of all authors. All authors have approved the final version of the manuscript.

References

1. Kuko, M.; Pourhomayoun, M. Single and clustered cervical cell classification with the ensemble and deep learning methods. *Inf. Syst. Front.* **2020**, *22*, 1039–1051. [CrossRef]
2. Zhao, S.; He, Y.; Qin, J.; Wang, Z. A Semi-supervised Deep Learning Method for Cervical Cell Classification. *Anal. Cell. Pathol.* **2022**, *2022*, 4376178. [CrossRef] [PubMed]
3. Nirmal Jith, O.U.; Harinarayanan, K.K.; Gautam, S.; Bhavsar, A.; Sao, A.K. DeepCerv: Deep Neural Network for Segmentation Free Robust Cervical Cell Classification. In *Computational Pathology and Ophthalmic Medical Image Analysis*; Springer: Cham, Switzerland, 2018; pp. 86–94.
4. Sompawong, N.; Mopan, J.; Pooprasert, P.; Himakhun, W.; Suwannarurk, K.; Ngamvirojcharoen, J.; Vachiramon, T.; Tantibundhit, C. Automated Pap Smear Cervical Cancer Screening Using Deep Learning. In Proceedings of the 2019 41st Annual International Conference of the IEEE Engineering in Medicine and Biology Society (EMBC), Berlin, Germany, 23–27 July 2019; IEEE: Piscataway, NJ, USA, 2019; pp. 7044–7048.
5. Chen, W.; Gao, L.; Li, X.; Shen, W. Lightweight convolutional neural network with knowledge distillation for cervical cells classification. *Biomed. Signal Process. Control.* **2022**, *71*, 103177. [CrossRef]
6. Rahaman, M.M.; Li, C.; Yao, Y.; Kulwa, F.; Wu, X.; Li, X.; Wang, Q. DeepCervix: A deep learning-based framework for the classification of cervical cells using hybrid deep feature fusion techniques. *Comput. Biol. Med.* **2021**, *136*, 104649. [CrossRef]
7. Zhang, C.; Jia, D.; Li, Z.; Wu, N. Auxiliary classification of cervical cells based on multi-domain hybrid deep learning framework. *Biomed. Signal Process. Control.* **2022**, *77*, 103739. [CrossRef]
8. Lin, H.; Hu, Y.; Chen, S.; Yao, J.; Zhang, L. Fine-grained classification of cervical cells using morphological and appearance based convolutional neural networks. *IEEE Access* **2019**, *7*, 71541–71549. [CrossRef]
9. Tripathi, A.; Arora, A.; Bhan, A. Classification of Cervical Cancer Using Deep Learning Algorithm. In Proceedings of the 2021 5th International Conference on Intelligent Computing and Control Systems (ICICCS), Madurai, India, 6–8 May 2021; IEEE: Piscataway, NJ, USA, 2021; pp. 1210–1218.
10. Rahaman, M.M.; Li, C.; Wu, X.; Yao, Y.; Hu, Z.; Jiang, T.; Li, X.; Qi, S. A survey for cervical cytopathology image analysis using deep learning. *IEEE Access* **2020**, *8*, 61687–61710. [CrossRef]
11. Ragab, M.; Albukhari, A.; Alyami, J.; Mansour, R.F. Ensemble deep-learning-enabled clinical decision support system for breast cancer diagnosis and classification on ultrasound images. *Biology* **2022**, *11*, 439. [CrossRef] [PubMed]

12. Alsuhibany, S.A.; Abdel-Khalek, S.; Algarni, A.; Fayomi, A.; Gupta, D.; Kumar, V.; Mansour, R.F. Ensemble of Deep Learning Based Clinical Decision Support System for Chronic Kidney Disease Diagnosis in Medical Internet of Things Environment. *Comput. Intell. Neurosci.* **2021**, *2021*, 4931450. [CrossRef] [PubMed]

13. Ragab, M.; Alshehri, S.; Alhakamy, N.A.; Mansour, R.F.; Koundal, D. Multiclass Classification of Chest X-ray Images for the Prediction of COVID-19 Using Capsule Network. *Comput. Intell. Neurosci.* **2022**, *2022*, 6185013. [CrossRef] [PubMed]

14. Khamparia, A.; Gupta, D.; de Albuquerque, V.H.C.; Sangaiah, A.K.; Jhaveri, R.H. Internet of health things-driven deep learning system for detection and classification of cervical cells using transfer learning. *J. Supercomput.* **2020**, *76*, 8590–8608. [CrossRef]

15. Shi, J.; Wang, R.; Zheng, Y.; Jiang, Z.; Zhang, H.; Yu, L. Cervical cell classification with graph convolutional network. *Comput. Methods Programs Biomed.* **2021**, *198*, 105807. [CrossRef] [PubMed]

16. Allehaibi, K.H.S.; Nugroho, L.E.; Lazuardi, L.; Prabuwono, A.S.; Mantoro, T. Segmentation and classification of cervical cells using deep learning. *IEEE Access* **2019**, *7*, 116925–116941.

17. Chen, W.; Li, X.; Gao, L.; Shen, W. Improving computer-aided cervical cells classification using transfer learning based snapshot ensemble. *Appl. Sci.* **2020**, *10*, 7292. [CrossRef]

18. Archana, M.C.P.; Panicker, J.V. Deep Convolutional Neural Networks for Multiclass Cervical Cell Classification. In Proceedings of the 2022 International Conference on Wireless Communications Signal Processing and Networking (WiSPNET), Chennai, India, 24–26 March 2022; IEEE: Piscataway, NJ, USA, 2022; pp. 376–380.

19. Dong, N.; Zhao, L.; Wu, C.H.; Chang, J.F. Inception v3 based cervical cell classification combined with artificially extracted features. *Appl. Soft Comput.* **2020**, *93*, 106311. [CrossRef]

20. Li, J.; Dou, Q.; Yang, H.; Liu, J.; Fu, L.; Zhang, Y.; Zheng, L.; Zhang, D. Cervical cell multi-classification algorithm using global context information and attention mechanism. *Tissue Cell* **2022**, *74*, 101677. [CrossRef] [PubMed]

21. Zheng, K.; Zha, Z.J.; Cao, Y.; Chen, X.; Wu, F. La-Net: Layout-Aware Dense Network for Monocular Depth Estimation. In Proceedings of the 26th ACM international conference on Multimedia, Seoul, Republic of Korea, 22–26 October 2018; pp. 1381–1388.

22. Gupta, S.; Deep, K.; Mirjalili, S. An efficient equilibrium optimizer with mutation strategy for numerical optimization. *Appl. Soft Comput.* **2020**, *96*, 106542. [CrossRef]

23. Alzubi, O.A.; Qiqieh, I.; Alzubi, J.A. Fusion of deep learning based cyberattack detection and classification model for intelligent systems. *Clust. Comput.* **2022**, 1–12. [CrossRef]

24. Available online: http://mde-lab.aegean.gr/index.php/downloads (accessed on 10 November 2022).

25. Fang, S.; Yang, J.; Wang, M.; Liu, C.; Liu, S. An Improved Image Classification Method for Cervical Precancerous Lesions Based on ShuffleNet. *Comput. Intell. Neurosci.* **2022**, *2022*, 9675628. [CrossRef] [PubMed]

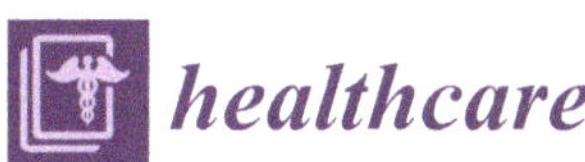

Article

Melanoma Detection Using Deep Learning-Based Classifications

Ghadah Alwakid [1,*], **Walaa Gouda** [2], **Mamoona Humayun** [3] **and Najm Us Sama** [4]

[1] Department of Computer Science, College of Computer and Information Sciences, Jouf University, Sakaka 72341, Al Jouf, Saudi Arabia

[2] Department of Computer Engineering and Networks, College of Computer and Information Sciences, Jouf University, Sakaka 72341, Al Jouf, Saudi Arabia

[3] Department of Information Systems, College of Computer and Information Sciences, Jouf University, Sakaka 72341, Al Jouf, Saudi Arabia

[4] Faculty of Computer Science and Information Technology, Universiti Malaysia Sarawak, Kota Samarahan 94300, Sarawak, Malaysia

* Correspondence: gnalwakid@ju.edu.sa

Abstract: One of the most prevalent cancers worldwide is skin cancer, and it is becoming more common as the population ages. As a general rule, the earlier skin cancer can be diagnosed, the better. As a result of the success of deep learning (DL) algorithms in other industries, there has been a substantial increase in automated diagnosis systems in healthcare. This work proposes DL as a method for extracting a lesion zone with precision. First, the image is enhanced using Enhanced Super-Resolution Generative Adversarial Networks (ESRGAN) to improve the image's quality. Then, segmentation is used to segment Regions of Interest (ROI) from the full image. We employed data augmentation to rectify the data disparity. The image is then analyzed with a convolutional neural network (CNN) and a modified version of Resnet-50 to classify skin lesions. This analysis utilized an unequal sample of seven kinds of skin cancer from the HAM10000 dataset. With an accuracy of 0.86, a precision of 0.84, a recall of 0.86, and an F-score of 0.86, the proposed CNN-based Model outperformed the earlier study's results by a significant margin. The study culminates with an improved automated method for diagnosing skin cancer that benefits medical professionals and patients.

Keywords: deep learning; machine learning; convolutional neural network; HAM10000; skin lesion; ESRGAN

Citation: Alwakid, G.; Gouda, W.; Humayun, M.; Sama, N.U. Melanoma Detection Using Deep Learning-Based Classifications. *Healthcare* **2022**, *10*, 2481. https://doi.org/10.3390/healthcare10122481

Academic Editor: Mahmudur Rahman

Received: 14 November 2022
Accepted: 5 December 2022
Published: 8 December 2022

Publisher's Note: MDPI stays neutral with regard to jurisdictional claims in published maps and institutional affiliations.

1. Introduction

Cells that proliferate and divide uncontrollably are referred to as "cancer"; they can quickly spread and invade nearby tissues if left untreated. Any sort of cancer, not just skin cancer, has the most significant probability of developing into a malignant tumor [1,2]. Melanoma (mel), Basal-cell carcinoma (BCC), nonmelanoma skin cancer (NMSC), and squamous-cell carcinoma (SCC) are the most common forms of skin cancer. It should be noted that some kinds of skin cancer, such as actinic keratosis (akiec), Kaposi sarcoma (KS), and sun keratosis (SK) are scarce [3]. Skin cancer of all varieties is increasing, as illustrated in Figure 1.

Malignant and non-malignant skin cancers are the most common [1,5]. The presence of cancerous lesions exacerbates cancer morbidity and healthcare expenses. Consequently, scientists have focused their efforts on creating algorithms that are both highly precise and flexible when it comes to spotting early signs of cancer in the skin. Malignant melanocyte cells proliferate, invade, and disseminate rapidly; therefore, early detection is critical [6]. Dermoscopy and epiluminescence microscopy (ELM) are frequently used by specialists to identify if a skin lesion is benign or cancerous.

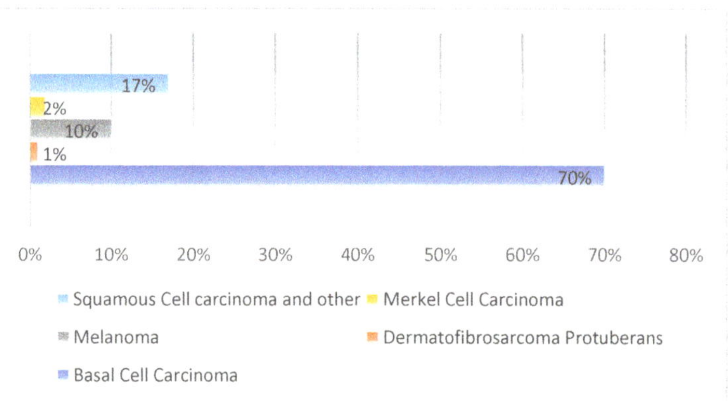

Figure 1. According to Reference [4], a number of different types of skin cancer are widespread.

A magnifying lens and light in dermatology are used to see medical patterns better such as hues, veils, pigmented nets, globs, and ramifications [7,8].. Visually impaired people can see the morphological structures that are otherwise hidden. These include the ABCD (Asymmetrical form, Border anomaly, Color discrepancy, Diameter, and Evolution) [9], 7-point checklist [10], and pattern analysis [11]. Non-professional dermoscopic images have a predictive value of 75% to 80% for Melanoma, but the interpretation takes time and is highly subjective, depending on the experience of the dermatologist [12]. Computer-Aided Diagnosis (CAD) approaches have made it easier to overcome these difficulties [8,12]. CAD of malignancies made a giant leap forward thanks to Deep Learning (DL)-based Artificial Intelligence (AI) [13,14]. In rural areas, dermatologists and labs are in poor supply; therefore, using DL approaches to classify skin lesions could help automate skin cancer screening and early detection [15,16]. To classify images in the past, dermoscopic images strongly depended on the extraction of handcrafted characteristics [17,18]. Throughout these promising scientific advances, the actual deployment of DCNN-based dermoscopic pictures has yielded amazing results. Still, future development of diagnosis accuracy is hampered by various obstacles, such as inadequate training data and imbalanced datasets, especially for rare and comparable lesion types. Regardless of the restrictions of the dataset, it is vital to maximize the performance of DCNNs for the correct Classification of skin lesions [14,19].

Models such as CNN, and modified Resnet50, are used in this research. We found that the invented CNN model beats existing DCNNs in classification accuracy while testing their performance on the HAM10000 dataset. To select the best network for diverse medical imaging datasets, it may be necessary to conduct multiple experiments. Accordingly, the paper's primary contributions can be summarized in this way:

1. We used an enhanced generative adversarial network with super-high resolution (ESRGAN) with 10,000 training photos to produce high-quality images for the Human Against Machine dataset (HAM10000 dataset [20]) to enhance the visibility of the images. ERSGAN improves the accuracy of Classification.
2. Segmentation is performed for each image in the dataset to specify ROI to facilitate the learning process.
3. We used Augmentation to ensure that the HAM10000 dataset had an even distribution of data.
4. The feasibility of the suggested system is determined by a thorough comparative evaluation using numerous assessment measurements, such as accuracy, recall, precision, confusion matrix, top 1 accuracy, top 2 accuracy, and the F-score.
5. Pre-trained networks' weights are fine-tuned with the help of the HAM10000 dataset and a modified version of Resnet-50.

6.   The recommended technique's overall effectiveness has been enhanced due to this change. Overfitting is prevented by using an alternative training process supported by applying various training strategies (e.g., batch size, learning rate, validation patience, and data augmentation).

This study provides an optimization strategy incorporating a CNN model a transfer learning model for detecting multiple skin lesions. Additionally, we utilized a revised form of Resnet-50 to train the weights of each Model before using it. Comparing the models' output using images of skin lesions from the HAM10000 dataset is necessary. The dataset has a class imbalance, necessitating an oversampling approach. The paper will proceed in accordance with this arrangement. Section 2 describes the relevant research work; after that, Section 3 illustrates the dataset and the proposed approach. The following Section 4 provides and analyzes the outcomes of the suggested technique described in Section 3; this study concludes with Section 5.

2. Related Work

The development of a CAD procedure for skin cancer has been the basis of several investigations [21,22]. CAD systems have followed the standard medical image analysis pipeline using classical machine learning approaches for skin lesion image processing [21]. In this pipeline, image preparation, fragmentation, extraction of features, and classifications have all been tried numerous times with little success. In skin cancer research, image processing, machine learning, CNN, and DL have all been used [23] in the past. Traditional image identification algorithms necessitate feature estimate and extraction, whereas deep learning can automatically exploit the images' deep nonlinear relationships [24,25]. CNN was the first DL model employed for skin lesion image processing. Some of the most recent deep learning studies are summarized in the following lines.

For instance, Haenssle et al. [26] analyzed a Google Inception V4 deep learning model against 58 dermatologists' diagnoses. The data collection includes one hundred patients' images (dermoscopic and digitalized) and medical records. Additional research presented by Albahar [24] generated an improved DL model for detecting malignant Melanoma. Model results were compared to dermatologist diagnoses from 12 German hospitals, where 145 dermatologists used the Model to arrive at their conclusions. Li et al. [27] reviewed CNN deep learning models with 99.5 percent of the time; residual learning and separable convolution are the greatest methods for constructing the most accurate Model. This level of precision, however, was only possible since the problem was binary in nature.

For automated Diagnosis, Pacheco et al. [25] developed a smartphone app that used images of skin lesions and clinical data to identify them. The study looked at the skin lesions of 1641 persons with six types of cancer. An experimental three-layer convolutional neural network, GoogleNet, ResNet, VGGNet, and MobileNet, was compared by researchers. Initially, images of lesions taken with smartphones were used as teaching aids, but later, images of both sorts of lesions were included (clinical descriptions and images of skin lesions). The original Model's accuracy was 0.69 percent, but clinical data increased that to 0.764 percent. To improve upon Pacheco's findings, a new study was proposed. Based on dermal cell images, a model-driven framework for melanoma diagnosis was created by Kadampur and Riyaee [27]. With the help of the HAM10000 dataset, several deep-learning models attained an area under the curve (AUC) of 0.99. To categorize malignant and benign skin lesions, two CNN models were employed by Jinnai et al. [28]. Results of the Model were compared to dermatologists' diagnoses and found to have a superior classification accuracy than dermatologists, according to the results.

Furthermore, Prassanna et al. [29] proposed a deep learning-based system for high-level skin lesion segmentation and malignancy detection by building a neural network. It accurately recognizes the edge of a significant lesion and designs a mobile phone model using deep neural network transfer learning and fine-tuning to improve prediction accuracy. Another approach presented by Panja et al. [30] classifies skin cancer as melanoma or benign; feature extraction was used to retrieve damaged skin cell features using a CNN model after segmenting skin images. In [31], researchers classify ISIC 2019 Dataset photos into eight classes. ResNet-50 was used to train the Model by evaluating initial parameter values and altering them using transfer training. Images outside these eight classifications are classified as unknown.

Skin cancer detection relied heavily on the transfer learning idea. According to Kassem et al. [32], a study utilizing the GoogleNet pre-trained model for eight categories of skin cancer lesions produced an accuracy of 0.949. This time, a dermatoscope, a medical device used to examine skin lesions, was used to test the proposed YOLOv2-SquuezeNet's segmentation and drawback performance. Using the equipment considerably improved the capacity to make an early diagnosis. Table 1 shows that several deep-learning models have been implemented to categorize skin cancer in current history.

Table 1. Methods, data, and results for skin cancer detection available nowadays.

Notable Designs	Size	Dataset	Methods	# Classes
[3]	2298	PAD-UFES-20	EfficientNetB3 + Extreme Gradient Boosting (XGB)	6
[19]	1600	ISIC-2017	swarm intelligence (SI)	2
	1600	ISIC-2018		
	1000	PH-2		
[33]	300	HAM10000	CNN + XGBoost	5
[34]	1323	HAM10000	InSiNet	2
[35]	7470	HAM10000	ResNet50	7
[36]	1000	ISIC	RF + Support Vector Machine (SVM)	8
[37]	6705	HAM10000	CNN	2
[38]	10,015	HAM10000	AlexNet	7
[39]	10,015	HAM10000	CNN	7
[40]	4753	Atlas	ResNet-152	12
[41]	10,015	HAM10000	MASK-RCNN	7
[42]	10,015	HAM10000	DenseNet121	7

3. Research Methodology

The authors of this study developed a smart classification algorithm and an automated skin lesion segmentation based on dermoscopic images. We used Resnet-50 and a CNN to perform machine learning in this case.

3.1. Dataset Overview

Skin Cancer MNIST: HAM10000 [20] provided the benchmark datasets used in this investigation. The CC-BY-NC-SA-4.0 licensed dataset is a reliable source of information for skin cancer diagnosis. Kaggle's public Imaging Archive was used to gather the data. A total of 10,015 JPEG skin cancer training images from two locations, one in Vienna, Austria, and the other in Queensland, Australia, were just compiled into a single dataset for training purposes. The Australian site used PowerPoint files and Excel databases to hold images and metadata. The Austrian site started collecting images with pre-digital cameras and preserved them in several formats. Based on the research, a variety of approaches are endorsed [31–40]. Using data from this benchmark, the Resnet-50 and the suggested CNN are trained to identify skin cancer in this study. In this dataset, all of the essential diagnostic categories for pigmented lesions were included, such as: akiec, benign keratosis-like lesions (bkl), bcc, dermatofibroma (df), melanocytic nevi (nv), mel, and vascular lesions (vasc). The HAM10000 dataset is presented in the illustrative form Figure 2.

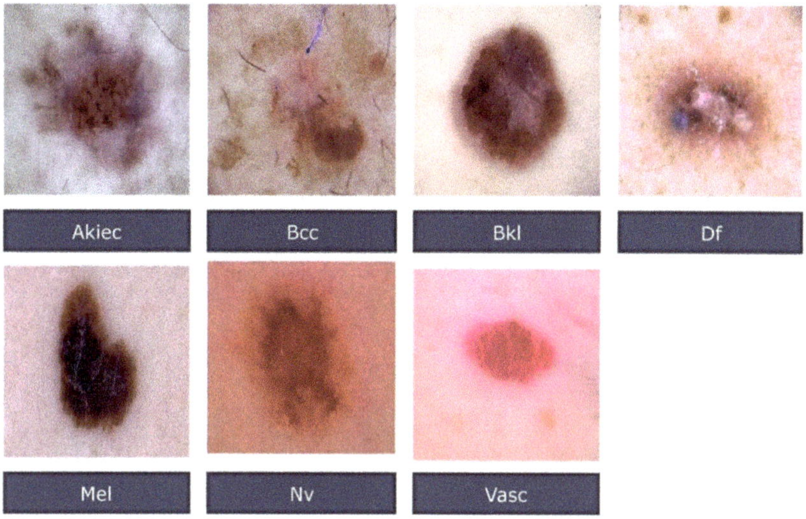

Akiec Bcc Bkl Df

Mel Nv Vasc

Figure 2. Examples of HAM10000 Dataset.

3.2. Proposed Methodology

Figure 3 depicts the overall process of the suggested method, based on the dataset mentioned in this article, which was used to develop an automatic skin lesion classification model. Dermoscopic skin lesion images are utilized to aid in the Classification of skin cancer, and the proposed Model's entire operational approach displays the functional architecture of that module. After preprocessing, Classification and Resnet-50/CNN-based training are the primary steps in the given Model's functioning. ESRGAN is used to perform the initial preprocessing step, which includes image quality improvement. Ground truth images are then used to determine an augmented image's region of interest (ROI) for each segmented lesion. Lastly, the dermoscopy image is sent to the Resnet-50/CNN models for instantaneous skin lesion and smart classification training and exposure. An intelligent classification model and an automated procedure for segmenting skin lesions are used to create the following sections of the research study, which are described in depth on each stage in the process.

3.2.1. ESRGAN Preprocessing

It was important to improve the quality of dermoscopic images and eliminate multiple kinds of noise from skin lesion images in order to carry out the proposed strategy. Ensuring that the image is as clear as possible is critical to creating a reliable skin lesion categorization model. In this step, first, we perform ESRGAN to improve the overall accuracy of the image; after that, Augmentation of data is used to overcome the problem of class unbalanced; then, all the images are resized to $224 \times 224 \times 3$, and, finally, normalization is performed.

SRGAN [43], Enhanced SRGAN, and other approaches can help improve skin lesions. The Enhanced Super Resolution GAN is an improved version of the Super Resolution GAN [44]. Regarding Model micro gradients, a Convolution trunk or a basic Residual Network is unnecessary. In addition, there is no batch normalization layer in the Model to smooth out the image. As a result, ESRGAN images can better resemble the sharp edges of image artifacts. ESRGAN employs a Relativistic Discriminator to decide whether an image is true or false [45]. The results are more accurate using this strategy. Relativistic Average Loss and Pixelwise Absolute Difference are used as loss functions in training data. The abilities of the generator can be honed through a two-stage training process. Local minima can be avoided by reducing the pixelwise L_1 distance among the source and targeting high images. Second, the smallest artifacts are to be improved and refined in the second step. It is interpolated between the adversarially trained models and the L_1 loss for a photo-realistic reconstruction of the original scene.

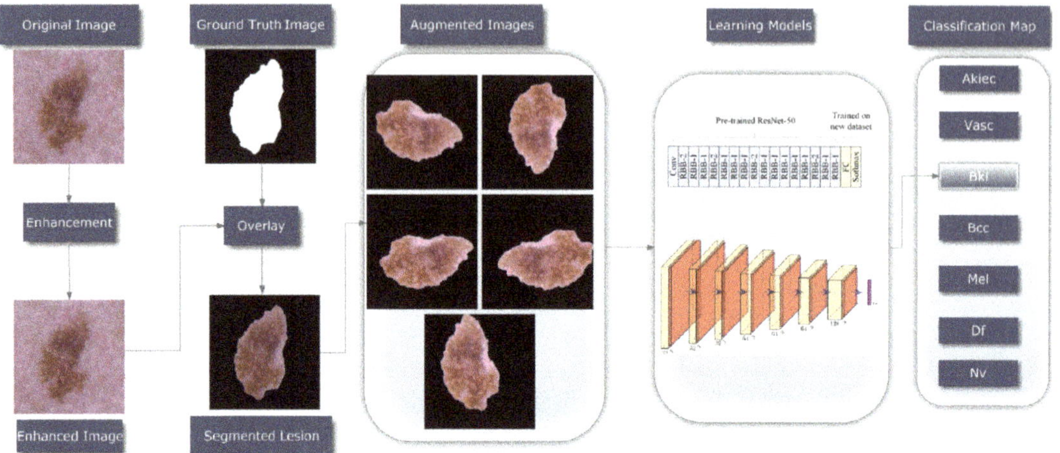

Figure 3. An overall process of how to recognize skin cancer.

In order to discriminate between super-resolved images and genuine photo images, a discriminator network was trained. Lesion images were improved by rearranging brightness values in the histogram of the original image using an adaptive contrast enhancement technique. As a result, the procedure in Figure 4 improves the appearance of the picture's borders and arcs while also raising the image's contrast.

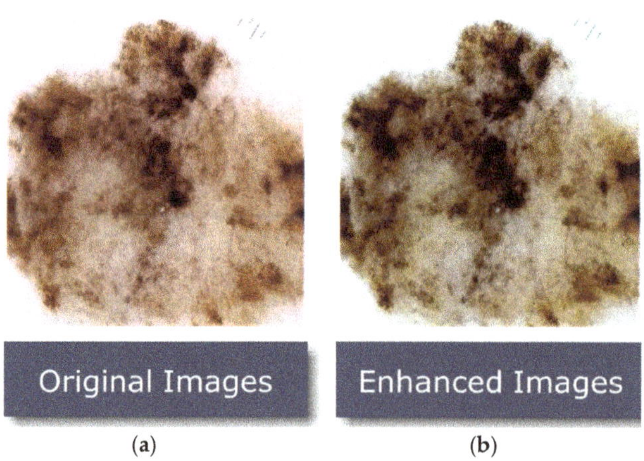

Figure 4. Proposed image-enhancement algorithm results; (**a**) image in its raw form; (**b**) an enhanced version of that image.

3.2.2. Segmentation

Following the protocol for preparing images, ROI from the dermoscopy image is segmented. To generate ROI in each image, a ground truth mask, which was provided by the HAM10000 dataset for general purpose usage, would be applied to the enhanced image, as demonstrated in Figure 5.

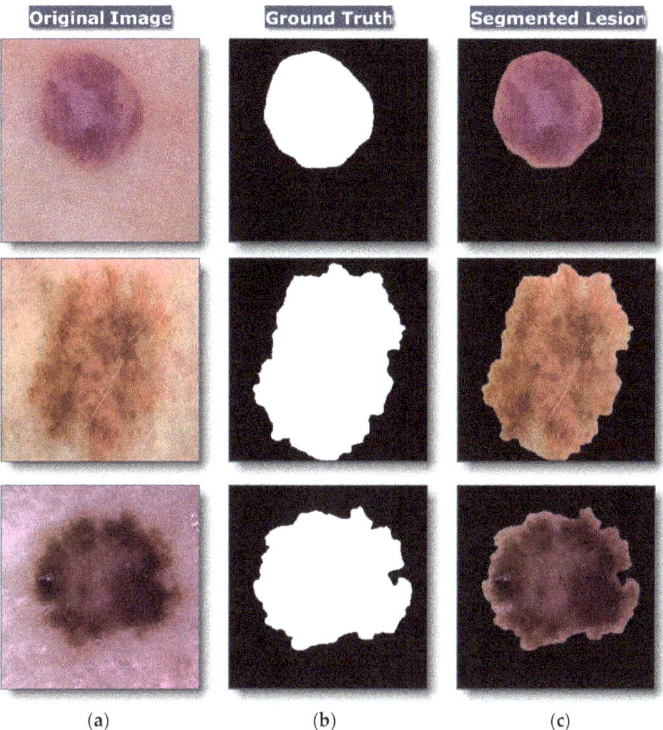

Figure 5. Samples of (**a**) original Image, (**b**) ground truth, and (**c**) the segmented ROI.

3.2.3. Data Augmentation

We performed data augmentation on the training set before exposing the deep neural network to the original dataset images in order to boost the dataset's image number and address the issue of an imbalanced dataset. Adding more training data to deep learning models improves their overall performance. We can use the nature of dermatological images to apply many alterations to each image. The deep neural network does not suffer if the image is magnified, flipped horizontally/vertically, or rotated in a specific number of degrees. Regularizing the data and reducing overfitting are two goals of data augmentation, as well as addressing the dataset imbalance issue. The horizontal shift augmentation is one of the transformations used in this study; it adjusts the image pixels horizontally while maintaining the image dimension using an integer between zero and one indicating the step size for this process. Rotation is another transformation; a rotation angle between 0 and 180 is selected, and then the image is rotated randomly. The images were resized with a zoom range of 0.1, a rescale of 1.0/255, and a recommended input size of 244 × 244 × 3. In order to generate new samples for the network, all previous modifications are applied to the training set's images. Figure 6 demonstrates how adding slightly changed copies of either current data or new synthetic data produced from the existing data is the primary goal of data augmentation.

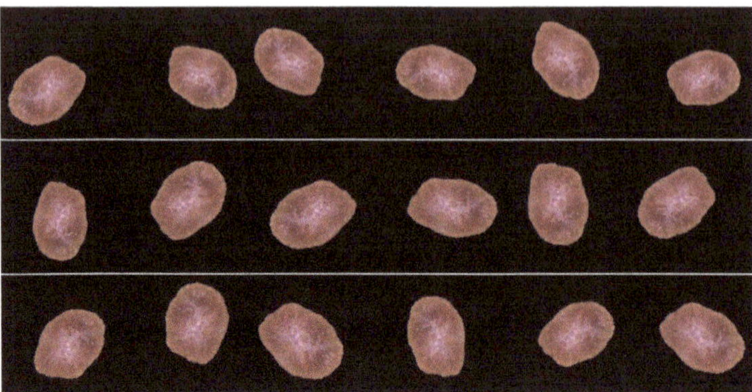

Figure 6. Samples of image augmentation for the same image.

Using data augmentation approaches, researchers can overcome the problem of inconsistent sample sizes and complex classifications. This dataset, the HAM dataset, clearly illustrates the term "imbalanced class", which refers to the unequal distribution of samples across distinct classes, as described in Table 2 and Figure 7. Following the augmentation approaches, the new dataset is shown in Figure 8. The classes are clearly balanced after using augmentation techniques on the dataset.

Table 2. A balanced dataset resulting from applying Augmentation (oversampling) techniques. As part of the data expansion, segmented photos were included.

Class	Number of Training Images
Akiec	5684
Bcc	5668
Mel	5886
Vasc	5570
Nv	5979
Df	4747
Bkl	5896
Total	39,430

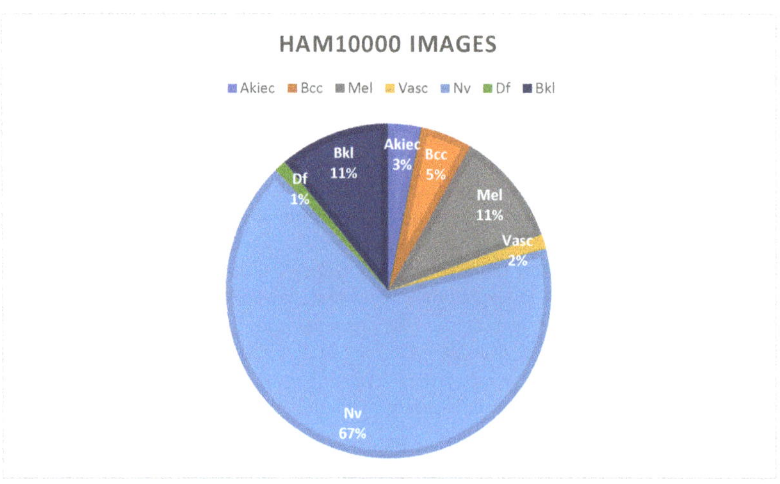

Figure 7. Unbalanced dataset before applying augmentation techniques.

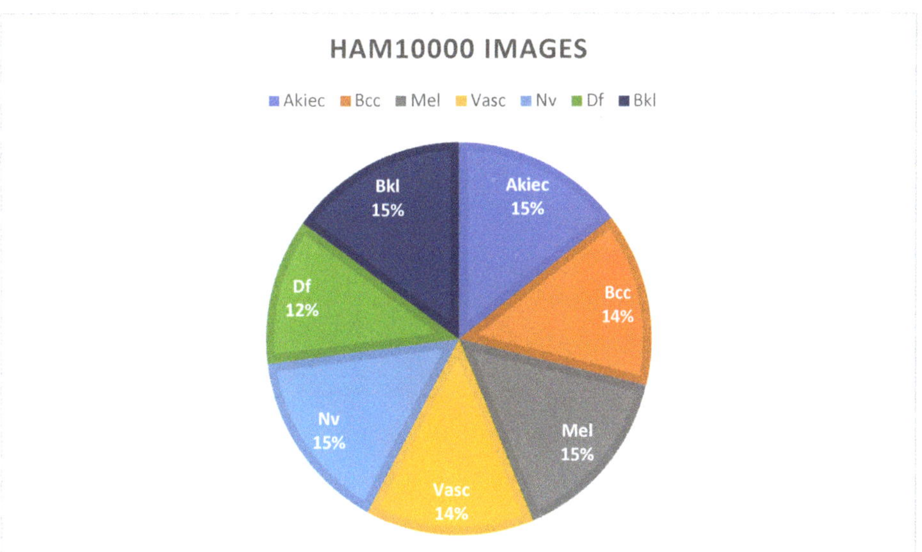

Figure 8. Balanced dataset after applying augmentation techniques.

3.2.4. Learning Models

This section describes the basic theory of the adopted approaches, and the proposed DL approach is presented in the next sections.

Model Training Using CNN

Dermoscopic images of a single skin lesion were utilized for training the Model using a CNN classifier. A suitable input set for CNN is made up of many skin cancers, such as melanomas and nonmelanomas, basal cell carcinomas and squamous cell carcinomas and Melanoma, Merkel cell carcinomas and cutaneous T-cell lymphomas, as well as Kaposi sarcoma.

As depicted in Figure 9, the proposed CNN architecture includes a proposed classification model that aids in strengthening the accuracy of the proposed mechanism's Classification. In terms of artificial neural networks, CNNs are the most advanced, thanks to their deep architectures-based architecture (ANNs). It was not until 1989 that LeCun et al. [46,47] presented the notion of CNN, an enhanced and more complex version of ANN with a deep architectural structure, as presented in Figure 9. The segmented ROIs are sent as source data to the convolutional layer of CNN when they are thrown into a convolution with a set of trainable filters to plot out the attributes.

Convolution, activation, pooling, and fully interconnected layers are all part of the basic structure of CNN as depicted in Figure 9. The proposed CNN model has four main layers and an output layer; each of these layers is composed of three convolution layers with a kernel size of three for the first two convolution layers and a kernel size of five for the final convolution layer. Stride equal to one for the first two convolution layers and stride equal to two for the final convolution layer are used; the relu activation function is used for all layers; and, finally, there are three maxpooling layers with a pool size of three and a stride of one. The convolution layer acts as a "filter", taking the observed pixel values from the input image and transforming them into a single value using the convolution process. When the convolution layer is applied, the original images will be reduced to a smaller matrix. In order to improve the filtered images, backpropagation training will be used. Down-sampling and shrinking the matrix size will help speed up training, as the pooling layer has this purpose. After that, the classification results are output by the completely linked layer (a typical multilayer perceptron).

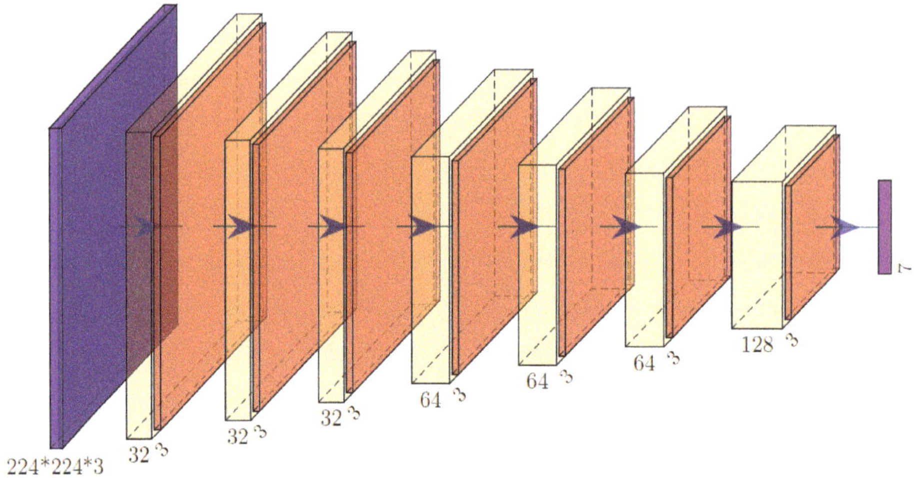

Figure 9. Proposed CNN architecture.

Model Training Using Modified Resnet-50

The Fundamental architecture of the proposed system is founded on the Resnet-50 Model. DL models must account for a staggering amount of structures and hyperparameters (e.g., number of frozen layers, batch size, epochs, and learning rate, etc.). The effect of numerous hyperparameter settings on system functioning is investigated. The Resnet-50 [48] model is updated in this part to serve as a basis for a possible solution. A novel residual learning attribute of the CNN design was created in 2015 by He K. et al. [48]. A standard layer compensates for the residual unit with a missing connection. By connecting to the layer's output, the skip connection makes it possible for an input signal to pass throughout the network.

A 152-layer model was created due to the residual units, which achieved the 2015 LSVRC2015 competition. Its new residual architecture makes gradient flow and training easier and more efficient thanks to its novel residual structure. A mistake rate of less than 3.6 percent is among the best in the industry. Other variants of ResNet have 34, 50, or 101 layers. Figure 10 shows the original Resnet-50 Model and its modified variants, which we analyze in this study. Figure 10a shows the initial Resnet-50 Model.

Figure 10b demonstrates how the proposed two versions are built: We add a fully connected (FC) layer and two more FC layers, replacing the existing FC and softmax layers in both versions. This Model's first two layers were trained using the ImageNet dataset [49]. That is why at the beginning the additional layers' weights will be chosen at random. The weights of all models are then updated using backpropagation, the key algorithm for training neural network architecture. Figure 10b shows how Resnet-50's initial FC layer, which was already deleted and substituted by the new FC layer of size 512, was swapped with another FC layer of size three and a new softmax layer that was replaced with a novel softmax layer (Figure 10b). The system needs more FC layers for tiny datasets than that for larger ones [50,51].

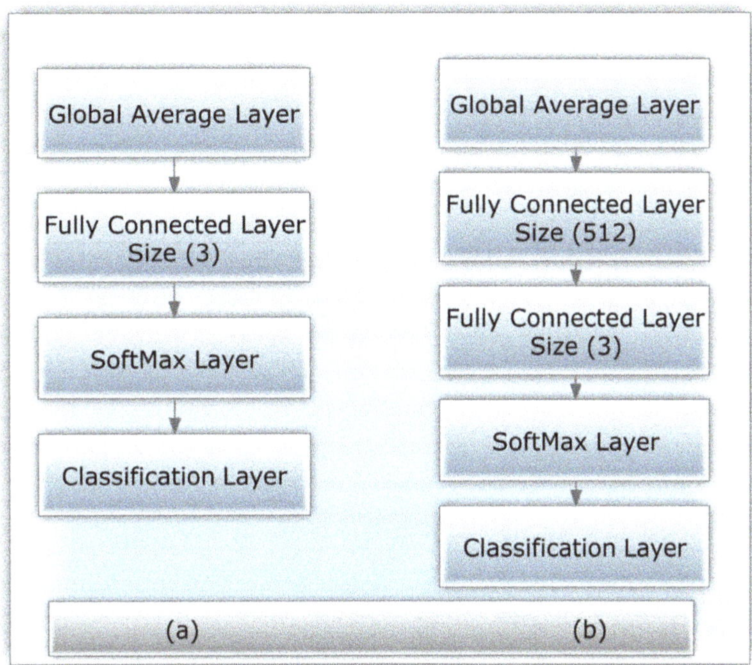

Figure 10. Versions of the Resnet-50 model that were modified; (**a**) the initial pre-trained model; (**b**) the addition of one FC.

In the completely linked layer, all neurons are coupled to all other neurons in the layer above and below it. Grading is determined by an activation function that accepts the output from the final FC layer. One of the most popular classifiers in DNN is Softmax, which uses its equations to calculate the probability dissemination of the n output sets. Only the high computational cost of adding a single FC layer prevents this approach from being widely adopted.

One thousand twenty-four bytes make up the first FC layer; three bytes make up the third FC layer. We employ batch normalization to combat network overfitting; this takes place when a model does a great job of retaining information from its training data but lacks the ability to transfer that knowledge to novel testing data. To put it another way, this problem is more likely to arise when the training dataset is small. To account for the inherent unpredictability of the algorithm's numerous phases, deep neural networks (DNNs) always produce somewhat variable results [52]. Ensemble learning can be used to maximize the functioning of DNN algorithms. We present the "many-runs ensemble" as a means to achieve stacking generalization through numerous training iterations of the same framework.

4. Experimental Results

4.1. Training and Configuration of Resnet-50 and the Proposed CNN

DL systems have been tested on the HAM10000 dataset to see how well they work and to see how they compare to current best practices. There are two groups of data: 90% for training (9016 images) and 10% for testing (984 images). A total of 10% of the training set is utilized for validation (992). All images were scaled to $227 \times 227 \times 3$ and increased to 39,430 images in the training method. Linux PC with RTX3060 and 8 GB of RAM were used to test the TensorFlow Keras application on this machine. A random image set of 80 percent served as the basis of the suggested DL systems' training. After training,

10 percent of training data was used as a validation set in which the most accurate weight combinations were saved for future use. The HAM10000 dataset is used to pre-train the suggested framework, which employs the Adam optimizer and a learning rate technique that slows down learning when it becomes stagnant for a prolonged span of time (i.e., validation patience). The subsequent hyperparameters were fed into the Adam optimizer during the training process: Batch sizes range from 2 to 64 with a move of two times the former value; epochs are 50; patience is 10; and momentum is 0.9 for this simulation. An infection form dissemination approach known as "batching" rounds out our arsenal of anti-infective measures.

4.2. Set of Criteria for Evaluation

This study section provides an in-depth description of the evaluation metrics and their results. A popular metric for gauging classification efficiency is classifier accuracy (Ac). The number of instances (images) correctly classified divided by the dataset's total number of examples (images) is the equation's definition (1). When analyzing the efficiency of image categorization algorithms, precision (Pre) and recall (Rec) are the two most commonly utilized criteria. The greater the number of accurately labeled images, the greater the degree of precision in the Equation (2). The ratio of photographs in the database was successfully categorized to those associated numerically in Equation (3). Having a higher F-score indicates that the system is better at forecasting the future than if it has a lower one. A system's effectiveness cannot be measured solely on the basis of accuracy or recall. Explanation (4) shows how to calculate the F-score mathematically (Fsc). The last metric is Top N accuracy, where the model N's highest probability answers must match the expected softmax distribution to be considered "top N accuracy". A classification is considered correct if at least one of the N predictions matches the label being sought.

$$\mathrm{Ac} = \frac{\mathrm{T^p + T^n}}{\mathrm{T^p + T^n + F^p + F^n}} \tag{1}$$

$$\mathrm{Pre} = \frac{\mathrm{T^p}}{\mathrm{T^p + F^p}} \tag{2}$$

$$\mathrm{Rec} = \frac{\mathrm{T^p}}{\mathrm{T^p + F^n}} \tag{3}$$

$$\mathrm{Fsc} = 2 * \left(\frac{\mathrm{Pre * Rec}}{\mathrm{Pre + Rec}} \right) \tag{4}$$

True positives are denoted by the symbol ($\mathrm{T^p}$) and are positive cases that were successfully predicted, while true negatives ($\mathrm{T^n}$) are negative situations that were accurately predicted. False positives ($\mathrm{F^p}$) are positive situations that were mistakenly predicted, and false negatives ($\mathrm{F^n}$) are negative examples that were wrongly forecasted.

4.3. Performance of Various DCNN Models

Data from the HAM10000 skin lesion categorization challenge dataset are being used to train and evaluate a variety of DCNNs (including CNN and Resnet-50). The results of multiple assessments of the HAM100000 dataset for the suggested systems are shown using a 90–10 split between training and testing. In order to minimize the time it takes to complete the project, this division was decided. Models were trained for 50 epochs using 10% of the training set as a validation set, a batch size of 2 to 64, and learning rates ranging from 1×10^4, 1×10^5, and 1×10^6 for CNN and Resnet-50, respectively. Resnet-50 was further fine-tuned by freezing varying numbers of layers to reach the useful accuracy possible. A model ensemble was created by running a number of runs on the same Model with the same parameters. Because the weights are created randomly for each run, the accuracy varies from run to run. Only the highest run outcome is stored and illustrated in Tables 3 and 4, one for CNN and one for Resnet-50 training on HAM10000 datasets, respectively. It demonstrates that the best result obtained using CNN and Resnet-50 is

86% and 85.3%, respectively. Figures 11 and 12 demonstrate the confusion matrix using CNN and Resnet-50, respectively. By applying the proposed approach to the test set, the confusion matrix was obtained. According to the confusion matrix, the suggested technique can identify nv lesions with 97% accuracy (770 correctly classified image out of 790 total images), which is extremely desirable for real-world applications using the CNN model and 94% (749 correctly classified image out of 790 total images) using the modified version of Resnet-50.

Table 3. Best accuracy using CNN learning model.

Acc	Top-2 Accuracy	Top-3 Accuracy	Pre	Rec	Fsc
0.8598	0.9400	0.9726	0.84	0.86	0.8598

Table 4. Best accuracy after fine-tuning using modified Resnet-50 transfer learning model.

Acc	Top-2 Accuracy	Top-3 Accuracy	Pre	Rec	Fsc
0.8526	0.9329	0.9695	0.86	0.85	0.8526

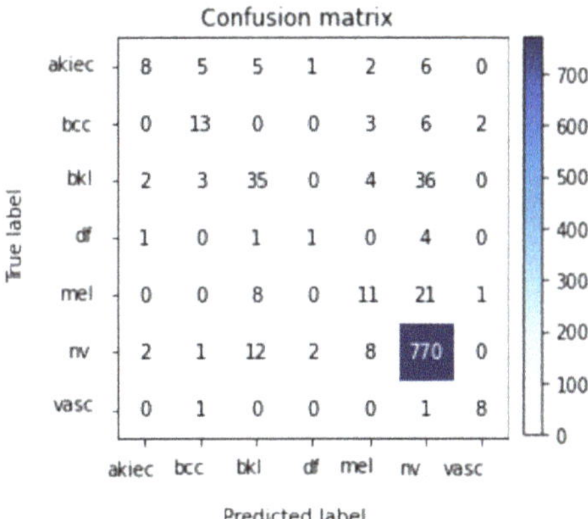

Figure 11. Best confusion matrix of CNN.

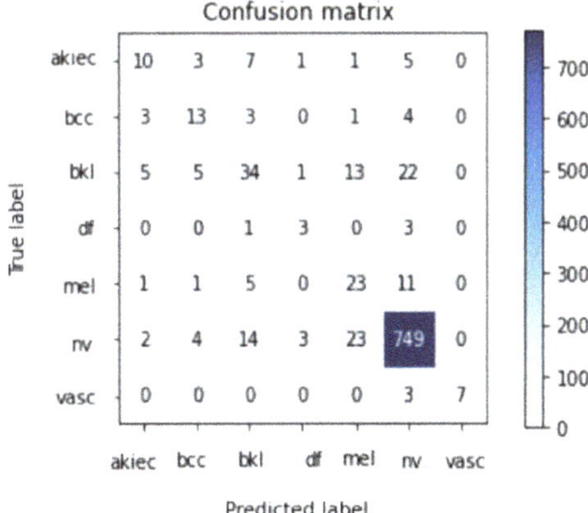

Figure 12. Best confusion matrix of Resnet-50.

Figure 13 shows two successful examples of classifying two images, one belonging to the Nv class and the other to the Akiec class. A total number of images used for each class in the Ham10000 dataset is shown in Tables 5 and 6, which reveal the number of images used for testing in each class. According to the results, it is obvious that the Nv class has the biggest number of images with 795; its pre, rec, and Fsc are all very high, equal to 91 percent, 97 percent, and 94 percent, respectively, using the CNN model. The values of these parameters are 94 percent, 94 percent, and 94 percent, respectively, using the modified Resnet-50 model.

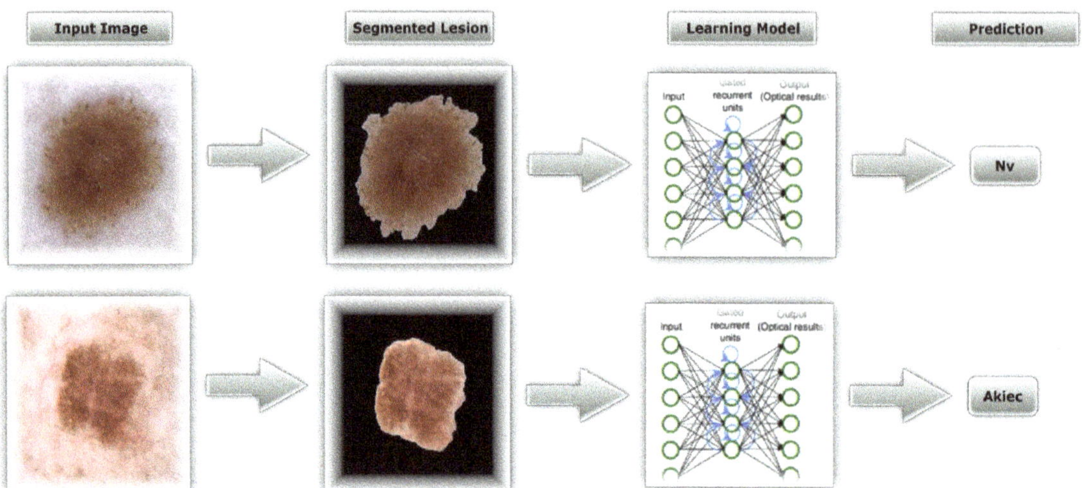

Figure 13. Example of testing classification phase.

Table 5. Detailed results for each class using CNN learning model.

	Pre	Rec	Fsc	Total Images
Akiec	0.62	0.30	0.4	27
Bcc	0.57	0.54	0.55	24
Bkl	0.57	0.44	0.50	80
Df	0.25	0.14	0.18	7
Mel	0.39	0.27	0.32	41
Nv	0.91	0.97	0.94	795
Vasc	0.73	0.80	0.76	10
Average	0.84	0.86	0.86	984

Table 6. Detailed results for each class using modified Resnet-50 learning model.

	Pre	Rec	Fsc	Total Images
Akiec	0.48	0.37	0.42	27
Bcc	0.48	0.54	0.51	24
Bkl	0.55	0.42	0.48	80
Df	0.38	0.43	0.40	7
Mel	0.37	0.59	0.45	41
Nv	0.94	0.94	0.94	795
Vasc	1.00	0.70	0.82	10
Average	0.86	0.85	0.85	984

Using lesion images to help dermatologists diagnose infections more accurately and reduce their workload has now been proven feasible in real-world settings.

4.4. Evaluation with Other Methods

Efficacy to that of other approaches is conducted. Table 7 indicates that our technique outperforms other approaches in terms of efficiency and effectiveness. Overall, the proposed inception model achieves an 86 percent accuracy rate, transcending the current methods.

Table 7. Comparison with other methods

Reference	Dataset	Model	Accuracy
[14]	HAM10000	RegNetY-3.2GF	85.8%
[49]	HAM10000	AlexNet	84%
[50]	HAM10000	MobileNet	83.9%
[51]	ISIC2018	CNN	83.1%
[51]	ISIC2018	Resnet-50	83.6%
[52]	HAM10000	MobileNet, VGG-16	80.61%
[53]	ISIC2018	Resnet-50	85%
[54]	HAM10000	Support Vector Machine (SVM), Logistic Regression (LR), Random Forest (RF), AdaBoost (Adaptive Boosting), Balanced Bagging (BB) and Balanced Random Forest (BRF)	74.75%
[55]	HAM10000	CNN	77%
[56]	HAM10000	ResNet, Xception, and DenseNet	78%, 82%, 82%
[57]	HAM10000	MobileNet and LSTM	85%
Proposed	HAM10000	CNN	86%
Proposed	HAM10000	Modified Resnet-50	85.3%

4.5. Discussion

As we discovered, other methods could not meet our degree of accuracy. One of three contributing elements is the general resolution enhancement of ESRGAN, which we believe is responsible for this. In addition, we deploy a variety of architectures, each with a varied ability to generalize and adapt to diverse types of data. Transfer learning architectures could not classify medical images more accurately due to a lack of distinctive features. Resnet-50's classification accuracy was worse than the proposed CNN when applied to medical images, even though it was better at identifying natural images. More generalizable qualities of CNN's shorter networks suggest that they can be used for a wider range of images. Deeper networks such as Resnet-50, on the other hand, can learn abstract properties that can be used in any sector. CNN features are more generalizable and adaptable for medical imaging because they lack semantic relevance to natural images (compared to Resnet-50). Fine-tuning networks, in turn, made the two models more accurate. CNN's accuracy improved the greatest compared to Resnet-50. Deep networks, as opposed to shallow ones, were found to be more likely to pick up significant information when trained on a smaller dataset. Shown in Figures 11 and 12 are the results of the indicated processes, which were adequate. Table 7 displays that ResNet and CNN, in references [55,56], yielded 77% and 78% accuracy, respectively. Researchers evaluated the accuracy of their model against the results of these two research projects that used the same dataset and trained their models using the same methods (Convolutional Neural Networks and Resnet-50) so that comparisons could be made easily. To witness its robustness further, the proposed CNN model outperforms two other referenced works [14,57] while being trained on a significantly smaller dataset (9016 images vs. 100,000 in the ImageNet Dataset).

5. Conclusions

Researchers devised a method for promptly and accurately diagnosing seven different types of cancer by analyzing skin lesions. The suggested method uses image-enhancing techniques to brighten the lesion image and remove noise. Preprocessed lesion medical imaging was used to train CNN and modified Resnet-50 to avoid overfitting and to boost the overall competence of the suggested DL approaches. The proposed approach was challenged using a dataset of lesion images known as the HAM10000 dataset. When employing CNN and a modified Resnet-50, the conception model had an accuracy rate of 85.3 percent and 85.98 percent $\approx$ 86 percent, respectively, comparable to the accuracy rate of professional dermatologists, as proposed. In addition, the research's originality and contribution lie in its use of ESRGAN as a pre-processing step with the various models (designed CNN and modified Resnet50) and in its contribution to the field. Compared to the pre-trained Model, our new Model performs similarly. Current models are outperformed by the proposed system, as demonstrated by comparison studies. Experiments on a big and complicated dataset, including future cancer cases, are required to demonstrate the efficacy of the suggested method. In the future, DenseNet, VGG, or AlexNet may be utilized to evaluate the cancer dataset. Lesion-less skin and lesioned skin are not always caused by skin cancer; it may also be a confounding factor in clinical diagnosis. In future, we will add this into the dataset to test the effectiveness of the model further.

Author Contributions: Conceptualization, W.G., G.A., M.H. and N.U.S..; methodology, W.G., G.A., M.H. and N.U.S.; software, W.G., G.A., M.H. and N.U.S.; validation, W.G., G.A., M.H. and N.U.S.; formal analysis, W.G., G.A., M.H. and N.U.S.; investigation, W.G., G.A., M.H. and N.U.S.; resources, W.G., G.A., M.H. and N.U.S.; data curation, W.G., G.A., M.H. and N.U.S.; writing—original draft preparation, W.G., G.A., M.H. and N.U.S.; writing—review and editing, W.G., G.A., M.H. and N.U.S.; visualization, W.G., G.A., M.H. and N.U.S.; supervision, W.G., G.A., M.H. and N.U.S.; project administration, W.G., G.A., M.H. and N.U.S.; funding acquisition, W.G., G.A. All authors have read and agreed to the published version of the manuscript.

Funding: This work was funded by the Deanship of Scientific Research at Jouf University under grant No (DSR2022-NF-04).

Institutional Review Board Statement: Not applicable.

Informed Consent Statement: Not applicable.

Data Availability Statement: Publicly available datasets were analyzed in this study. These data can be found here: (https://www.kaggle.com/datasets/kmader/skin-cancer-mnist-ham10000?select=HAM10000_metadata.csv (accessed on 13 April 2022)).

Acknowledgments: The authors extend their appreciation to the Deanship of Scientific Research at Jouf University for funding this work through Research Grant No (DSR2022-NF-04).

Conflicts of Interest: The authors declare no conflict of interest.

References

1. Saeed, J.; Zeebaree, S. Skin Lesion Classification Based on Deep Convolutional Neural Networks Architectures. *J. Appl. Sci. Technol. Trends* **2021**, *2*, 41–51. [CrossRef]
2. Albahar, M.A. Skin Lesion Classification Using Convolutional Neural Network with Novel Regularizer. *IEEE Access* **2019**, *7*, 38306–38313. [CrossRef]
3. Khan, I.U.; Aslam, N.; Anwar, T.; Aljameel, S.S.; Ullah, M.; Khan, R.; Rehman, A.; Akhtar, N. Remote Diagnosis and Tri-aging Model for Skin Cancer Using EfficientNet and Extreme Gradient Boosting. *Complexity* **2021**, *2021*, 5591614. [CrossRef]
4. Nikitkina, A.I.; Bikmulina, P.Y.; Gafarova, E.R.; Kosheleva, N.V.; Efremov, Y.M.; Bezrukov, E.A.; Butnaru, D.V.; Dolganova, I.N.; Chernomyrdin, N.V.; Cherkasova, O.P.; et al. Terahertz radiation and the skin: A review. *J. Biomed. Opt.* **2021**, *26*, 043005. [CrossRef]
5. Xu, H.; Lu, C.; Berendt, R.; Jha, N.; Mandal, M. Automated analysis and classification of melanocytic tumor on skin whole slide images. *Comput. Med. Imaging Graph.* **2018**, *66*, 124–134. [CrossRef]
6. Namozov, A.; Im Cho, Y. Convolutional neural network algorithm with parameterized activation function for mela-noma classification. In Proceedings of the 2018 International Conference on Information and Communication Technology Convergence (ICTC), Jeju Island, Republic of Korea, 17–19 October 2018.

7. Ozkan, I.A.; KOKLU, M. Skin lesion classification using machine learning algorithms. *Int. J. Intelli-Gent Syst. Appl. Eng.* **2017**, *5*, 285–289. [CrossRef]

8. Thamizhamuthu, R.; Manjula, D. Skin Melanoma Classification System Using Deep Learning. *Comput. Mater. Contin.* **2021**, *68*, 1147–1160. [CrossRef]

9. Stolz, W. ABCD rule of dermatoscopy: A new practical method for early recognition of malignant melanoma. *Eur. J. Der-Matol.* **1994**, *4*, 521–527.

10. Argenziano, G.; Fabbrocini, G.; Carli, P.; De Giorgi, V.; Sammarco, E.; Delfino, M. Epiluminescence microscopy for the diagnosis of doubtful melanocytic skin lesions: Comparison of the ABCD rule of dermatoscopy and a new 7-point checklist based on pattern analysis. *Arch. Dermatol.* **1998**, *134*, 1563–1570. [CrossRef]

11. Pehamberger, H.; Steiner, A.; Wolff, K. In vivo epiluminescence microscopy of pigmented skin lesions. I. Pattern analysis of pigmented skin lesions. *J. Am. Acad. Dermatol.* **1987**, *17*, 571–583. [CrossRef]

12. Reshma, G.; Al-Atroshi, C.; Nassa, V.K.; Geetha, B.; Sunitha, G.; Galety, M.G.; Neelakandan, S. Deep Learning-Based Skin Lesion Diagnosis Model Using Dermoscopic Images. *Intell. Autom. Soft Comput.* **2022**, *31*, 621–634. [CrossRef]

13. Litjens, G.; Kooi, T.; Bejnordi, B.E.; Setio, A.A.A.; Ciompi, F.; Ghafoorian, M.; van der Laak, J.A.W.M.; van Ginneken, B.; Sánchez, C.I. A survey on deep learning in medical image analysis. *Med. Image Anal.* **2017**, *42*, 60–88. [CrossRef] [PubMed]

14. Yao, P.; Shen, S.; Xu, M.; Liu, P.; Zhang, F.; Xing, J.; Shao, P.; Kaffenberger, B.; Xu, R.X. Single model deep learning on im-balanced small datasets for skin lesion classification. *arXiv* **2021**, arXiv:2102.01284.

15. Adegun, A.; Viriri, S. Deep learning techniques for skin lesion analysis and melanoma cancer detection: A survey of state-of-the-art. *Artif. Intell. Rev.* **2020**, *54*, 811–841. [CrossRef]

16. Yang, J.; Sun, X.; Liang, J.; Rosin, P.L. Clinical skin lesion diagnosis using representations inspired by dermatologist cri-teria. In Proceedings of the IEEE Conference on Computer Vision and Pattern Recognition 2018, Salt Lake City, UT, USA, 18–23 June 2018.

17. Satheesha, T.Y.; Satyanarayana, D.; Prasad, M.N.G.; Dhruve, K.D. Melanoma Is Skin Deep: A 3D Reconstruction Technique for Computerized Dermoscopic Skin Lesion Classification. *IEEE J. Transl. Eng. Health Med.* **2017**, *5*, 1–17. [CrossRef] [PubMed]

18. Tschandl, P.; Rosendahl, C.; Kittler, H. The HAM10000 dataset, a large collection of multi-source dermatoscopic images of common pigmented skin lesions. *Sci. Data* **2018**, *5*, 180161. [CrossRef] [PubMed]

19. Smith, L.; MacNeil, S. State of the art in non-invasive imaging of cutaneous melanoma. *Ski. Res. Technol.* **2011**, *17*, 257–269. [CrossRef]

20. Masood, A.; Ali Al-Jumaily, A. Computer aided diagnostic support system for skin cancer: A review of techniques and algorithms. *Int. J. Biomed. Imaging* **2013**, *2013*, 323268. [CrossRef]

21. Efimenko, M.; Ignatev, A.; Koshechkin, K. Review of medical image recognition technologies to detect melanomas us-ing neural networks. *BMC Bioinform.* **2020**, *21*, 270. [CrossRef]

22. Brinker, T.J.; Hekler, A.; Enk, A.H.; Klode, J.; Hauschild, A.; Berking, C.; Schilling, B.; Haferkamp, S.; Schadendorf, D.; Fröhling, S.; et al. A convolutional neural network trained with dermoscopic images performed on par with 145 derma-tologists in a clinical melanoma image classification task. *Eur. J. Cancer* **2019**, *111*, 148–154. [CrossRef]

23. Pacheco, A.G.; Krohling, R.A. The impact of patient clinical information on automated skin cancer detection. *Comput. Biol. Med.* **2020**, *116*, 103545. [CrossRef] [PubMed]

24. Haenssle, H.A.; Fink, C.; Schneiderbauer, R.; Toberer, F.; Buhl, T.; Blum, A.; Kalloo, A.; Hassen, A.B.H.; Thomas, L.; Enk, A.; et al. Man against machine: Diagnostic performance of a deep learning convolutional neural network for dermoscopic melanoma recognition in comparison to 58 dermatologists. *Ann. Oncol. Off. J. Eur. Soc. Med. Oncol.* **2018**, *29*, 1836–1842. [CrossRef] [PubMed]

25. Li, L.F.; Wang, X.; Hu, W.J.; Xiong, N.N.; Du, Y.X.; Li, B.S. Deep learning in skin disease image recognition: A review. *IEEE Access* **2020**, *8*, 208264–208280. [CrossRef]

26. Kadampur, M.A.; Al Riyaee, S. Skin cancer detection: Applying a deep learning based model driven architecture in the cloud for classifying dermal cell images. *Inform. Med. Unlocked* **2020**, *18*, 100282. [CrossRef]

27. Jinnai, S.; Yamazaki, N.; Hirano, Y.; Sugawara, Y.; Ohe, Y.; Hamamoto, R. The Development of a Skin Cancer Classification System for Pigmented Skin Lesions Using Deep Learning. *Biomolecules* **2020**, *10*, 1123. [CrossRef]

28. Kassem, M.A.; Hosny, K.M.; Fouad, M.M. Skin lesions classification into eight classes for ISIC 2019 using deep convolu-tional neural network and transfer learning. *IEEE Access* **2020**, *8*, 114822–114832. [CrossRef]

29. Hekler, A.; Utikal, J.S.; Enk, A.H.; Hauschild, A.; Weichenthal, M.; Maron, R.C.; Berking, C.; Haferkamp, S.; Klode, J.; Schadendorf, D.; et al. Superior skin cancer classification by the combination of human and artificial intelligence. *Eur. J. Cancer* **2019**, *120*, 114–121. [CrossRef]

30. Reis, H.C.; Turk, V.; Khoshelham, K.; Kaya, S. InSiNet: A deep convolutional approach to skin cancer detection and seg-mentation. *Med. Biol. Eng. Comput.* **2022**, *60*, 643–662. [CrossRef]

31. Le, D.N.; Le, H.X.; Ngo, L.T.; Ngo, H.T. Transfer learning with class-weighted and focal loss function for automatic skin cancer classification. *arXiv* **2020**, arXiv:2009.05977.

32. Murugan, A.; Nair, S.A.H.; Preethi, A.A.P.; Kumar, K.P.S. Diagnosis of skin cancer using machine learning techniques. *Microprocess. Microsystems* **2020**, *81*, 103727. [CrossRef]

33. Ali, M.S.; Miah, M.S.; Haque, J.; Rahman, M.M.; Islam, M.K. An enhanced technique of skin cancer classification using deep convolutional neural network with transfer learning models. *Mach. Learn. Appl.* **2021**, *5*, 100036. [CrossRef]

34. Rajput, G.; Agrawal, S.; Raut, G.; Vishvakarma, S.K. An accurate and noninvasive skin cancer screening based on imaging technique. *Int. J. Imaging Syst. Technol.* **2022**, *32*, 354–368. [CrossRef]

35. Kanani, P.; Padole, M. Deep learning to detect skin cancer using google colab. *Int. J. Eng. Adv. Technol. Regul. Issue* **2019**, *8*, 2176–2183. [CrossRef]

36. Mendes, D.B.; da Silva, N.C. Skin lesions classification using convolutional neural networks in clinical images. *arXiv* **2018**, arXiv:1812.02316.

37. Khan, M.A.; Akram, T.; Zhang, Y.-D.; Sharif, M. Attributes based skin lesion detection and recognition: A mask RCNN and transfer learning-based deep learning framework. *Pattern Recognit. Lett.* **2021**, *143*, 58–66. [CrossRef]

38. Zare, R.; Pourkazemi, A. DenseNet approach to segmentation and classification of dermatoscopic skin lesions images. *arXiv* **2021**, arXiv:2110.04632.

39. Thapar, P.; Rakhra, M.; Cazzato, G.; Hossain, M.S. A novel hybrid deep learning approach for skin lesion segmentation and classification. *J. Healthc. Eng.* **2022**, *2022*, 1709842. [CrossRef]

40. Ledig, C.; Theis, L.; Huszár, F.; Caballero, J.; Cunningham, A.; Acosta, A.; Aitken, A.; Tejani, A.; Totz, J.; Wang, Z.; et al. Photo-realistic single image super-resolution using a generative adversarial network. In Proceedings of the IEEE conference on computer vision and pattern recognition. In Proceedings of the 2017 IEEE Conference on Computer Vision and Pattern Recognition (CVPR), Honolulu, HI, USA, 21–26 July 2017.

41. Wang, X.; Yu, K.; Wu, S.; Gu, J.; Liu, Y.; Dong, C.; Qiao, Y.; Change Loy, C. Esrgan: Enhanced super-resolution generative adversarial networks. In Proceedings of the European Conference on Computer Vision (ECCV) Workshops 2018, Munich, Germany, 8–14 September 2018.

42. Jolicoeur-Martineau, A. The relativistic discriminator: A key element missing from standard GAN. *arXiv* **2018**, arXiv:1807.00734.

43. LeCun, Y.; Bengio, Y. Convolutional networks for images, speech, and time series. *Handb. Brain Theory Neural Netw.* **1995**, *3361*, 1995.

44. LeCun, Y.; Boser, B.; Denker, J.S.; Henderson, D.; Howard, R.E.; Hubbard, W.; Jackel, L.D. Backpropagation Applied to Handwritten Zip Code Recognition. *Neural Comput.* **1989**, *1*, 541–551. [CrossRef]

45. He, K.; Zhang, X.; Ren, S.; Sun, J. Deep residual learning for image recognition. In Proceedings of the IEEE Conference on Computer Vision and Pattern Recognition 2016, Las Vegas, NV, USA, 27–30 June 2016.

46. Russakovsky, O.; Deng, J.; Su, H.; Krause, J.; Satheesh, S.; Ma, S.; Huang, Z.; Karpathy, A.; Khosla, A.; Bernstein, M.; et al. Imagenet large scale visual recognition challenge. *Int. J. Comput. Vis.* **2015**, *115*, 211–252. [CrossRef]

47. Basha, S.S.; Dubey, S.R.; Pulabaigari, V.; Mukherjee, S. Impact of fully connected layers on performance of convolutional neural networks for image classification. *Neurocomputing* **2019**, *378*, 112–119. [CrossRef]

48. Renard, F.; Guedria, S.; De Palma, N.; Vuillerme, N. Variability and reproducibility in deep learning for medical image segmentation. *Sci. Rep.* **2020**, *10*, 13724. [CrossRef] [PubMed]

49. Ameri, A. A deep learning approach to skin cancer detection in dermoscopy images. *J. Biomed. Phys. Eng.* **2020**, *10*, 801. [CrossRef] [PubMed]

50. Sae-Lim, W.; Wettayaprasit, W.; Aiyarak, P. Convolutional neural networks using MobileNet for skin lesion classification. In Proceedings of the 2019 16th International Joint Conference on Computer Science and Software Engineering (JCSSE), Chonburi, Thailand, 10–12 July 2019.

51. Gouda, W.; Almurafeh, M.; Humayun, M.; Jhanjhi, N.Z. Detection of COVID-19 Based on Chest X-rays Using Deep Learning. *Healthcare* **2022**, *10*, 343. [CrossRef]

52. Salian, A.C.; Vaze, S.; Singh, P.; Shaikh, G.N.; Chapaneri, S.; Jayaswal, D. Skin lesion classification using deep learning architectures. In Proceedings of the 2020 3rd International Conference on Communication System, Computing and IT Applications (CSCITA), Mumbai, India, 3–4 April 2020.

53. Li, X.; Wu, J.; Chen, E.Z.; Jiang, H. From deep learning towards finding skin lesion biomarkers. In Proceedings of the 2019 41st Annual International Conference of the IEEE Engineering in Medicine and Biology Society (EMBC), Berlin, Germany, 23–27 July 2019.

54. Pham, T.C.; Tran, G.S.; Nghiem, T.P.; Doucet, A.; Luong, C.M.; Hoang, V.D. A comparative study for classification of skin cancer. In Proceedings of the 2019 International Conference on System Science and Engineering (ICSSE), Dong Hoi, Vietnam, 20–21 July 2019.

55. Polat, K.; Koc, K.O. Detection of skin diseases from dermoscopy image using the combination of convolutional neural network and one-versus-all. *J. Artif. Intell. Syst.* **2020**, *2*, 80–97. [CrossRef]

56. Rahman, Z.; Ami, A.M. A transfer learning based approach for skin lesion classification from imbalanced data. In Proceedings of the 2020 11th International Conference on Electrical and Computer Engineering (ICECE), Dhaka, Bangladesh, 17–19 December 2020.

57. Srinivasu, P.N.; SivaSai, J.G.; Ijaz, M.F.; Bhoi, A.K.; Kim, W.; Kang, J.J. Classification of skin disease using deep learning neural networks with MobileNet V2 and LSTM. *Sensors* **2021**, *21*, 2852. [CrossRef]

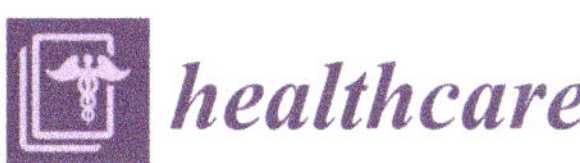 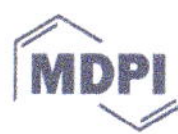

Article

Using Deep Neural Network Approach for Multiple-Class Assessment of Digital Mammography

Shih-Yen Hsu [1], Chi-Yuan Wang [2], Yi-Kai Kao [3], Kuo-Ying Liu [4], Ming-Chia Lin [5], Li-Ren Yeh [6,7], Yi-Ming Wang [1,8], Chih-I Chen [9,10,11,12,*] and Feng-Chen Kao [11,13,14,*]

1 Department of Information Engineering, I-Shou University, Kaohsiung City 84001, Taiwan
2 Department of Medical Imaging and Radiological Science, I-Shou University, Kaohsiung City 82445, Taiwan
3 Division of Colorectal Surgery, Department of Surgery, E-DA Hospital, Kaohsiung City 82445, Taiwan
4 Department of Radiology, E-DA Cancer Hospital, I-Shou University, Kaohsiung City 82445, Taiwan
5 Department of Nuclear Medicine, E-DA Hospital, I-Shou University, Kaohsiung City 82445, Taiwan
6 Department of Anesthesiology, E-DA Cancer Hospital, I-Shou University, Kaohsiung City 82445, Taiwan
7 Department of Medical Imaging and Radiology, Shu-Zen College of Medicine and Management, Kaohsiung City 82144, Taiwan
8 Department of Critical Care Medicine, E-DA Hospital, I-Shou University, Kaohsiung City 82445, Taiwan
9 Division of Colon and Rectal Surgery, Department of Surgery, E-DA Hospital, Kaohsiung City 82445, Taiwan
10 Division of General Medicine Surgery, Department of Surgery, E-DA Hospital, Kaohsiung City 82445, Taiwan
11 School of Medicine, College of Medicine, I-Shou University, Kaohsiung City 82445, Taiwan
12 The School of Chinese Medicine for Post Baccalaureate, I-Shou University, Kaohsiung City 82445, Taiwan
13 Department of Orthopedics, E-DA Hospital, Kaohsiung City 82445, Taiwan
14 Department of Orthopedics, Dachang Hospital, Kaohsiung City 82445, Taiwan
* Correspondence: ed106687@edah.org.tw (C.-I.C.); kaofengchen@gmail.com (F.-C.K.)

Citation: Hsu, S.-Y.; Wang, C.-Y.; Kao, Y.-K.; Liu, K.-Y.; Lin, M.-C.; Yeh, L.-R.; Wang, Y.-M.; Chen, C.-I.; Kao, F.-C. Using Deep Neural Network Approach for Multiple-Class Assessment of Digital Mammography. *Healthcare* **2022**, *10*, 2382. https://doi.org/10.3390/healthcare10122382

Academic Editor: Mahmudur Rahman

Received: 17 October 2022
Accepted: 25 November 2022
Published: 27 November 2022

Publisher's Note: MDPI stays neutral with regard to jurisdictional claims in published maps and institutional affiliations.

Abstract: According to the Health Promotion Administration in the Ministry of Health and Welfare statistics in Taiwan, over ten thousand women have breast cancer every year. Mammography is widely used to detect breast cancer. However, it is limited by the operator's technique, the cooperation of the subjects, and the subjective interpretation by the physician. It results in inconsistent identification. Therefore, this study explores the use of a deep neural network algorithm for the classification of mammography images. In the experimental design, a retrospective study was used to collect imaging data from actual clinical cases. The mammography images were collected and classified according to the breast image reporting and data-analyzing system (BI-RADS). In terms of model building, a fully convolutional dense connection network (FC-DCN) is used for the network backbone. All the images were obtained through image preprocessing, a data augmentation method, and transfer learning technology to build a mammography image classification model. The research results show the model's accuracy, sensitivity, and specificity were 86.37%, 100%, and 72.73%, respectively. Based on the FC-DCN model framework, it can effectively reduce the number of training parameters and successfully obtain a reasonable image classification model for mammography.

Keywords: mammography; deep neural network; classification

1. Introduction

The incidence and mortality of female breast cancer are 69.1 and 12.0 per 100,000, respectively, based on the Taiwan Health Promotion Administration in the Ministry of Health and Welfare. Among the stages of breast cancer, I and II are the most common, and the peak incidence tends to be in the younger population. Meanwhile, female cancer is headed by Breast Cancer, and its peak incidence is in forty-five-year-old to sixty-year-old female patients [1]. Furthermore, female breast cancer ranks fourth in the top ten cancer causes of death, and the mortality rate has been increasing year by year, with the mortality rate per 100,000 population increasing from 13.5% to 20.1% from 2008 to 2020. Clinically, in addition to self-examination, there are many different tools of imaging diagnosis for breast diseases, such as mammography, breast ultrasound, and breast magnetic resonance imaging [2–4]. In mammography, different lesions, such as breast calcifications, tumors, and cysts, can be detected using low-dose X-rays to penetrate the human body for imaging. The false-negative rate of mammography is about 10%. Small tumors may be obscured by dense tissue, resulting in the possibility that the tumor image overlaps with a large amount of normal tissue, making it difficult to distinguish. Similarly, there are also a few cases of patients with false positives. Breast ultrasound without radiation is the preferred inspection tool, especially for female cases younger than 40 years old, patients suspected of having breast lumps [5], cases with a BIRADS-0 score, or female cases of dense breasts, pregnancy, and lactation. The subject is placed in a lying position and scanned clockwise or counterclockwise with a probe at a high frequency of 7–10 MHz, which can distinguish cysts or parenchymatous tumors [6]. In the case of cysts with irregular margins or complex and recurrent ones, there is a high probability of malignancy, and further examination is required. In breast magnetic resonance imaging, a high-level examination method without radiation [7], a contrast agent containing Gadolinium (Gd) is injected into the patient's intravenous veins to facilitate the observation of the distribution of breast blood vessels on the image.

Based on a literature review, there is feasible and challenging technology for computer-vision-assisted detection and analysis of breast cancer. In traditional technology, the study published by Arden Sagiterry Setiawan et al. in 2015 proposed to use LTEM (Law's Texture Energy Measure) as the method of texture feature extraction [8]. The study adopted an Artificial Neural Network (ANN) using two-layer feedforward backpropagation for breast imaging classification. The results of the study show that LAWS provides better accuracy compared to other similar methods (such as GLCM). LAWS provides 83.30% accuracy for benign or malignant images classification. The GLCM has only 72.20% accuracy for normal/abnormal classification and 53.06% for benign/malignant classification. In the 2017 study by Yuchen Qiu et al. [9], the study report shows total 560 regions of interest (ROI) mammography images that were extracted, the input image is 512 × 512 pixels, and the 64 × 64 pixels of ROI are taken out as the targets of image feature extraction. It is followed by the 8 layers of the designed deep learning network layer, including 3 max pooling layers for automatic feature extraction and a multilayer perceptron (MLP) as a classifier to process ROI. The results showed that the AUC of the model obtained was 0.790 ± 0.019. A computer-aided diagnosis (CAD) system is an affordable, readily available, fast, and reliable source of early diagnosis [10,11].

Mammography is one of the most commonly used clinical methods for screening breast-related diseases. In studies, there are many applications in the domain of artificial intelligence. Meanwhile, different architectures of convolutional networks have also been developed to interpret different types of images [12,13] such as those obtained by computed tomography, magnetic resonance imaging, and ultrasound. In recent years, the methods of image recognition by artificial intelligence have been actively developed with higher sensitivity and specificity than CAD [14–17]. This not only enables radiologists to reduce errors in diagnosis results but also reduces the time for interpretation. In 2019, Alejandro Rodriguez-Ruiz et al. used deep learning convolution neural networks to classify and detect calcification and soft tissue lesions [18]. In 2020, Thomas Schaffter et al. developed a deep learning model called Vanilla U-Net, using U-Net as a base model, for tiny segment lesions in mammography images [19]. In 2021, José Luis Raya-Povedano et al. used artificial intelligence in digital mammography (DM) and digital breast tomosynthesis (DBT), using the system to detect suspicious lesions and mark them on each image [20].

This study uses the clinically collected mammograms and the BIRADS grading report as image datasets to establish the classification model with artificial intelligence technology. The main aim is to adopt the fully convolutional dense connection network (FC-DCN) to create the classification model. Then, the model performance can be evaluated in the small-sample-size mammography images. It can provide appropriate classification results to assist clinicians and reduce the time required for clinical interpretations.

2. Methodology

2.1. Mammography Image Collection and Description

This study was designed as a retrospective group experiment and collected mammography cases and diagnostic reports from 2016–2017, which had been reviewed by the Medical Ethics Committee of E-DA Hospital (EMRP-107-031). The imaging instrument used was Hologic Lorad Selenia. Each case in the study was irradiated with four images from multiple angles. These were the right craniocaudal view (RCC), the left craniocaudal view (LCC), the right mediolateral oblique view (RMLO), and the left mediolateral oblique view (LMLO) (Figure 1). Most breast tissue can be sighted in a single image with MLO View, such as pectoralis major and axillary lymph nodes. The CC view can avoid medial tissue missed with the MLO view.

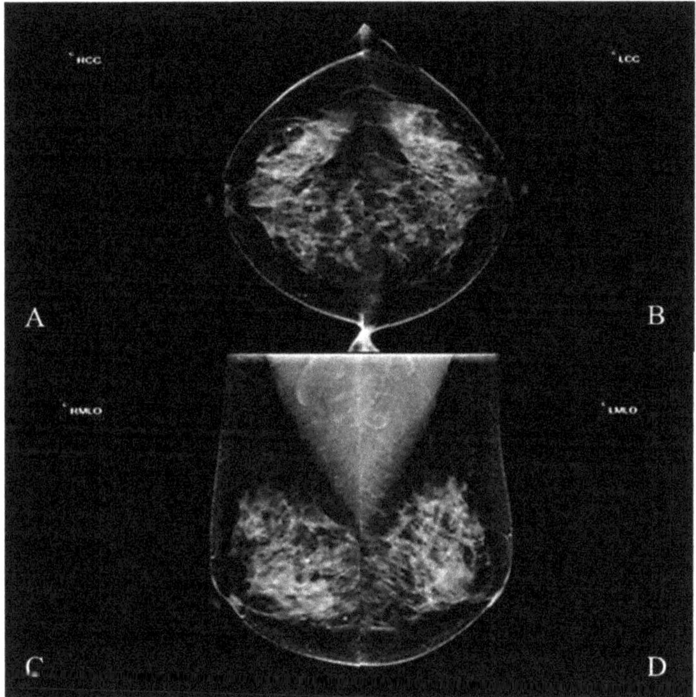

Figure 1. The mammographic image. (**A**) Right craniocaudal view (RCC), (**B**) left craniocaudal view (LCC), (**C**) right mediolateral oblique view (RMLO), (**D**) left mediolateral oblique view (LMLO).

In clinical practice, the American College of Radiology (ACR) established the Breast Image Reporting and Data Analyzing System (BI-RADS), in order to ensure the consistency of inspection reports and facilitate the collection and comparison of inspection results. The grading of results is based on the image characteristics of the tumor, including shape, appearance, density, edge, calcification pattern, distribution, and the symmetry of the breast tissue on both sides determined by mammography. The cases of BIRADS-0 were excluded from the conditions for acceptance of this study. Cases of incomplete examinations and additional images required for interpretation were also excluded. This study takes cases of BIRADS-4 and 5 as the subjects. Most cases of BIRADS-6, diagnosed with breast cancer, had surgery on or under treatment. They were also excluded. The tissue of the subjects being operated on might be destroyed and affect feature extraction and texture analysis.

In the study, different pieces of images of mammography on the left and right are extracted, which excluded local surgical resection and obvious skin folds. The study included the images from 150 cases based on the pathology report diagnosed by the radiologist, including 50 negative cases (BIRADS-1) and 100 positive cases (BIRADS-4 and BIRADS-5), and the data were expanded to 5400 images through data augmentation technology [16,21]. Each image was augmented by rotating, horizontally flipping, and vertically flipping. DICOM was the file format of the mammography image, and the pixel size was resized to 1024 × 1024. All the images are split into 7:3 and 5:5 to be the training set and the testing set, respectively. This split percentage was considered based on a review of the relevant literature [22–25]. In the positive cases, the lesions included calcifications, well-defined or localized masses, radially shaped masses, other and uncertain defined masses, structural distortions, and asymmetry tissue.

2.2. Experimental Design

A fully convolutional densely connected network (FC-DCN) model was developed for mammography image classification. The experimental design included image preprocessing, pre-trained model, transfer learning, model weighted calculation, etc. The research process is shown in Figure 2, and the practical steps are as follows.

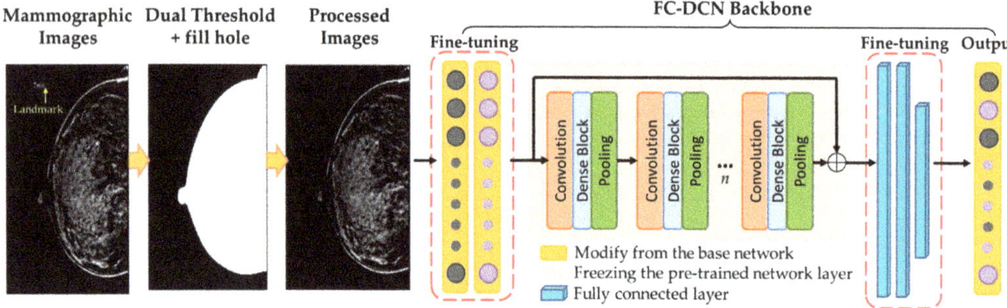

Figure 2. The classification architecture for mammography image.

Step 1. Collecting mammography images.
Step 2. Removing the imaging marker (such as right/left side notation) and embedding the image-processing technique.
Step 3. Dividing collected images of breasts into training group and test group randomly.
Step 4. Training the classified model by FC-DCN with transfer learning technology and fine-tuning the model weight.
Step 5. Testing different parameters by FC-DCN model to find the best parameters for mammography image interpretation.
Step 6. Using the accuracy, sensitivity, and specificity of the testing set as the indicators of validation performance.

After importing the mammography images, the background markers of patient data and location labels were removed. The unnecessary factors that might interfere with the model analysis in the region of breast image must be removed, including the radiologist's code, the markers on the left and right, the name of hospital, and dose values used. To remove the background marker, the double-threshold method was used [26,27]. The image intensity values less than five and higher than 4090 were removed. Most of the subjects with values above 4090 were artificial markers. After thresholding, there were small holes in the screen. Therefore, the hollow space in the image was filled with the image fill technology [28]. Then, the filled-in image was the region of interest to specify the area in the image and achieve removal of background marker. Next, the model training was completed with the preprocess images input into the architecture of the FC-DCN.

2.3. Deep Transfer Learning Model

In 2017, Huang et al. published a research report at the IEEE Conference on Computer Vision and Pattern Recognition (CVPR) [29]; the method they published mainly solves the issues of the vanishing gradient problem, feature propagation, feature recyclability, and reducing the number of parameters. Hence, it can be used on personal computer or NB platforms. The authors named the architecture of their network as a dense convolutional network on account of its densely connected nature. All information input is allowed to be used among layers, and the information in any layer could be connected to subsequent layers.

This study's pre-trained model was used as the network backbone and was also built with the transfer learning technique. There are three emphases in transfer learning: first, modifying the input layer; second, retraining the weights; third, modifying the output layer. It included image input layer, convolution layer, pooling layer, dense block and transition layer, and classification layer. Each layer's design structure is introduced below. The training parameter is listed in Table 1.

Table 1. The investigated training model.

Item	Content
Ratio for training	70%, 50%
Batch Size	20, 30, 40, 50, 60, 70, 100
Epoch Size	50, 60, 70, 100, 150, 200, 250
Learning rate	0.0001
Optimizer	sgdm

In the input layer of the image, the image pixel size is adjusted from 1024×1024 to 224×224 pixels, and the image is input to the next layer, which is the first convolutional layer, for which convolution kernel size is 7×7, the stride is 2, and the output image size is 112×112. The eigenvalues of each region in the image are collected by the convolution layer, and the weights of each point in the convolution kernel are multiplied based on the specified convolution kernel size and stride to obtain the feature map. The pooling layer, for which the kernel size is 3×3, the stride is 2, and the size of output image is 56×56, is connected after the convolution layer (in this study, we used max pooling). Pooling is another important concept in convolutional networks and is actually a form of downsampling, which reduces the dimensionality of each feature map and retains eigen features by reducing the size of the input image—most often by half—and avoids redundant calculations and speeds up the efficiency of system operation by decreasing the parameters required for subsequent layers. It does not affect the results, with minor differences in the adjacent areas of pixels in the image to improve the consistency of the output and reduce the situation of overfitting.

In FC-DCN, it is most important to design many dense blocks in the architecture to improve the compactness of the model further and reduce the number of feature maps in the transition layer. The dense block contains the number of m characteristic mapping. It lets the lower transition layer generate the number of $[\theta m]$ output feature maps, where $0 < \theta \leq 1$, which is called the compressibility factor. As $\theta = 1$, the number of feature maps remains unchanged, and it crosses the transition layer. In this study, the network structure with four dense blocks is used. A batch normalization layer (BN Layer), a rectified linear unit layer (ReLU Layer), and a convolutional layer with a kernel size of 3×3 are contained in dense blocks. For convolutional layers with a kernel size of 3×3, each side of the input is zero stuffing in order to keep the feature map size fixed. The final output layer includes the global average pooling layer (GAP Layer), fully connected layer, and normalization layer. As mentioned, adopting the fully connected layer to integrate the results of the convolution and pooling operations makes it possible to extract features. It can reduce image parameters separately and input the feature information into the fully connected layer for classification. Each connection has its own independent and different weight value. The softmax function transforms the vector z into another K-dimensional vector σ(z) to make each element in the range of (0, 1), and the sum of all elements is 1 (Equation (1)). The softmax function is usually placed in the last layer of the neural network.

$$\sigma\left(z_j\right) = \frac{e^{z_j}}{\sum_{k=1}^{K} e^{z_k}} \quad for\ j = 1, \ldots, k \tag{1}$$

The output value of the parameter value in a neural node is represented by "z_j" after performing the weight calculation of class j, and σ(z)j is the probability that the sample vector Z belongs to the *j*th class; that is to say, the input of the function is obtained from different linear functions of K as a result, when the input is Z, the probability that the predicted class is j is σ, and the sum of the probabilities of all predicted classes is 1. The softmax function is usually placed in the last layer of the neural network. The outputs of all nodes in the last layer are passed through the exponential function, the results are added as the denominator, and the individual outputs are used as the numerator. The cross-entropy loss of the multi-class classification problems with mutually exclusive classes is calculated with the classification layer, which is also the last output layer in the network layer. In addition, the output of the function value is based on the softmax layer as the classification basis to classify it to the correct category. Meanwhile, the cross-entropy function is used to assign each input to one of the K mutually exclusive classes for the output result of 1-K encoding scheme. This function uses its backpropagation to correct the weights and biases in the hidden layer. This correction and optimization improve the accuracy of neural network classification. In Equation (2), "N" is the number of samples, "K" is the number of species, t_{ij} is the indication that the ith sample belongs to the jth species, and y_{ij} is the output of sample i of species j, which in this case is the value of the softmax function. That is, it is the probability that the ith input to the network is associated with category j.

$$loss = -\sum_{i=1}^{N} \sum_{j=1}^{K} t_{ij} ln(y_{ij}) \tag{2}$$

2.4. Evaluation Criteria

The image samples are randomly obtained for each iteration to build a model, with 7:3 and 5:5 as training and testing sets. Furthermore, the sensitivity and specificity of the test set are used as validation performance indicators.

(1) Sensitivity: it is defined as TP/(TP + FN). It represents the proportion of positive samples in the test set when the model predicts that the samples are positive in the true judgment. It is also known as true-positive rate (TPR); the opposite is false-positive rate (FPR), which is defined as FP/(FP + TN).
(2) Specificity: it is defined as TN/(TN + FP), which represents the proportion of the true-negative samples in the test set when the model predicts that the samples are negative; it is also known as true-negative rate (TNR); its opposite is false-negative rate (FNR), which is defined as FN/(TP + FN).
(3) Accuracy: it is defined as (TP + TN)/(TP + FN + FP + TN), which represents the proportion of true positives and true negatives in all samples when the model predicts that the samples in the test set are true positives and true negatives.

The sensitivity and specificity are used to measure the effectiveness of the classifier. In above, TP means true-positive fraction, TN means true-negative fraction, FN means false-negative fraction, and FP means false-positive fraction. For the mentioned criteria, higher values indicate better classification performance.

3. Results

In this study, FC-DCN was used to classify the positive and negative lesions based on BIRADS grades of breast images. Meanwhile, 5:5 and 7:3 of the data were used as the training and testing sets, respectively. In each iteration, image samples were randomly obtained to build a model, and then the test set was used to verify the model. Sensitivity, specificity, and accuracy were used as the indicators of the validation performance.

The interaction between batch size and the number of iterations is discussed separately, when the training and testing dataset is set to 7:3. According to the experimental data, the batch sizes of 20, 30, 40, 50, 60, 70, and 100 and iteration times of 100, 50, 100, 50, 50, 50, and 100 have better results, and their accuracies are 0.818, 0.864, 0.727, 0.727, 0.682, 0.773, and 0.727, respectively (Table 2). The results show that increasing the number of iterations does not actually improve the performance of the model, for the model reached the condition (state) of convergence. In addition, in the case where the two-fold cross validation method is used and the training and testing dataset is set to 5:5, the connection between the batch size and the number of iterations was ambiguous. According to the data in the experiment, the accuracies are 0.658, 0.632, 0.684, 0.684, 0.684, 0.684, and 0.789 for batch sizes of 20, 30, 40, 50, 60, 70, and 100 with the iteration times of 60, 60, 60, 50, 60, 50, and 50, respectively (Table 3). The result does not show a higher batch size that can obtain a better result.

Table 2. The experiment results in investigated batch size by split percentage 7:3.

Batch Size	Accuracy	Sensitivity	Specificity	Kappa	AUC
20	0.818	0.909	0.727	0.634	0.885
30	0.864	1.000	0.727	0.657	0.907
40	0.727	0.546	0.909	0.631	0.886
50	0.727	0.909	0.546	0.654	0.896
60	0.682	0.727	0.636	0.625	0.892
70	0.773	0.818	0.727	0.619	0.869
100	0.727	0.818	0.636	0.627	0.884

Table 3. The experiment results in investigated batch size by split percentage 5:5.

Batch Size	Accuracy	Sensitivity	Specificity	Kappa	AUC
20	0.658	0.526	0.790	0.631	0.855
30	0.632	0.790	0.474	0.613	0.872
40	0.684	0.737	0.632	0.606	0.857
50	0.684	0.895	0.474	0.576	0.862
60	0.684	0.737	0.632	0.630	0.862
70	0.684	0.579	0.790	0.621	0.853
100	0.789	0.789	0.789	0.615	0.876

The performance of this multi-class classification issue can be illustrated utilizing the receiver operating characteristics (ROC) curve. The performance of a classification model at all classification thresholds can be shown on a graph called a ROC curve. This curve outlines two different parameters such as true-positive rate and false-positive rate. The term true-positive rate is used to represent sensitivity. The term false-positive rate is used to represent 1-specificity. The ROC curve is plotted with 1-specificity on the y-axis against the sensitivity on the x-axis. In Figure 3, ROC curves are plotted for every model. The best AUC achieved by the FC-DCN model at a ratio equal to 70% is 0.907, and the best AUC at a ratio equal to 50% is 0.876. This shows our model has excellent discrimination.

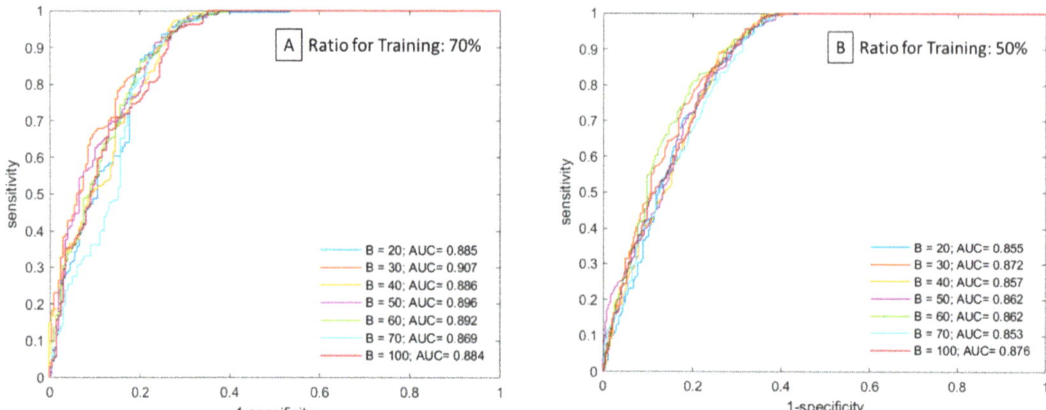

Figure 3. Receiver operating characteristic curves of the classified model on each batch size. Picture (**A**) presents by split ratio of 7:3. Picture (**B**) presents by split ratio of 5:5.

According to the statistical indicators, different batch sizes and iterations were used for training and testing in 7:3 and 5:5 of the data. The experiments were conducted to compare the interactions among 7 batch sizes and 7 iteration parameter combinations. In 7:3 of the data, the best parameter-construction model is to use batch size 30 and iterations 50, for which sensitivity is 100%, specificity is 72.73%, and accuracy is 86.37%. In 5:5 of the data, the best parameter construction model is to use a batch size 100 and iterations 50, for which sensitivity is 78.95%, the specificity is 78.95%, and the accuracy is 78.95%. Figures 4 and 5 show each accuracy of batch size from 20~100. The experimental results show that it does not improve sensitivity, specificity, or accuracy to increase the number of iterations or batch size. However, it will be related to the split ratio.

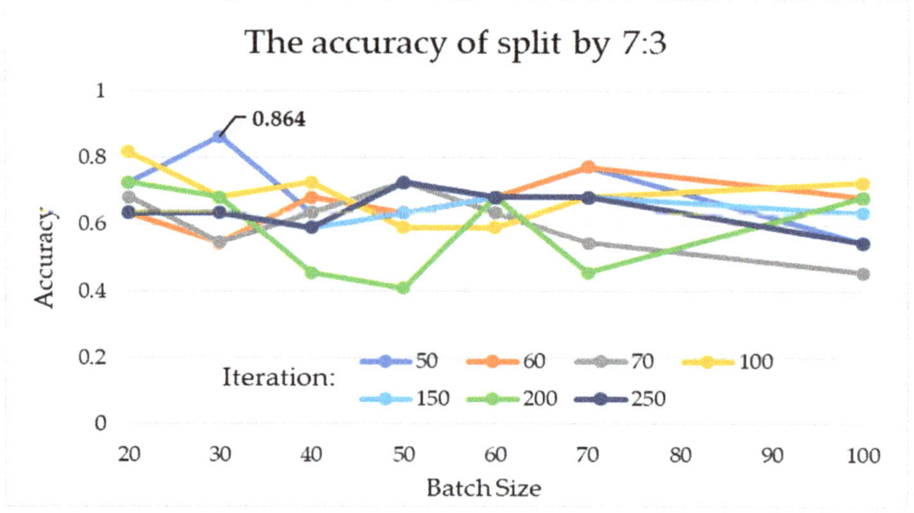

Figure 4. Experimental results for different batch sizes and iterations at a split ratio of 7:3.

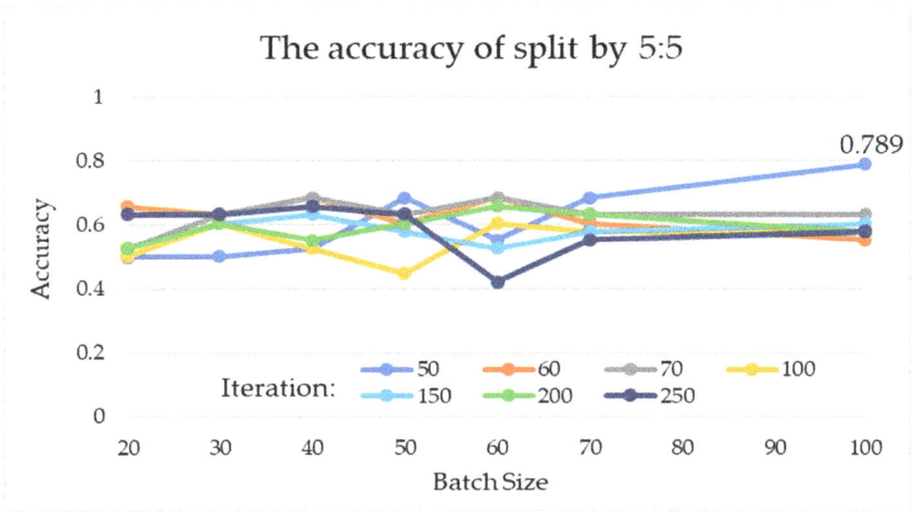

Figure 5. Experimental results for different batch sizes and iterations at a split ratio of 5:5.

4. Discussion

Based on the above experiments, 7:3 and 5:5 of each group were divided into the training set and the testing set. In each iteration, image samples were randomly obtained to build a model, and the confusion matrix was used to calculate the sensitivity and specificity of the test set as the indicator of the verification performance. When the training set is 7:3 to use mini-batch size 30 and iterations 50, the sensitivity is 100%, the specificity is 72.73%, and the accuracy is 86.37%.

This study found that in the model training of mammography data, even increasing the number of iterations does not actually increase the accuracy, so there is no existing overfitting problem. In the experimental results, the batch size is relatively important. Increasing the batch size can more effectively provide more information for the model, so that better results can be obtained.

This study confirms that FC-DCN can successfully achieve good performance with a small number of parameters and a small amount of computation; moreover, it is an effective method to use FC-DCN to identify specific breast images. FC-DCN introduces direct connections between any two layers with the same characteristic mapping size. It can be found that FC-DCN does not show optimization difficulties when it is extended to hundreds of layers. In the relevant literature (Table 4), the model established in this study can be used for small-sample-size data to obtain over 85% classification accuracy. In addition, regarding the ratio of data split, this research method can still obtain nearly 80% accuracy under the condition that the data split ratio is 5:5.

Table 4 compares the same model architecture with Medeiros et al. The authors used the ROI selection method for dataset preprocessing. ROI extraction is an accepted technique. This study still considers using the entire image for model training. The whole image can provide more feature information. Hence, the model can have more data to learn during training. Therefore, it can obtain better performance. However, the disadvantage is the need to spend more training time. Furthermore, the sample size is also one of the reasons to use the whole image. Based on simple connection rules, FC-DCN integrates the properties of feature maps and learns deeply with diverse depths. In addition, it allows features to be reused throughout the network; hence, learning can be more compact. FC-DCN is a good feature extractor due to its compact internal representation and reduced feature redundancy. For this reason, CNN models developed by artificial intelligence can be widely used clinically in mammography images, even for different image tools.

Table 4. Comparison with other works for mammography image classification.

Reference	Categories	Cases/Extend	Split Scale	Model	Accuracy
Medeiros et al. [30]	2	10239/no	8:2	DenseNet201-MLP	0.634
Lenin et al. [31]	6	18000/no	8:2	nasnet-m-TL	0.812
Yang et al. [32]	2	384/1173	8:2	MommiNet-v2	0.910(AUC)
Boumaraf et al. [33]	4	500/2620	6:4	–	0.845
Our	3	150/5400	7:3	FC-DCN	0.864
			5:5		0.789

In this paper, the deep learning algorithm designed belongs to "weak AI" in the field of artificial intelligence. In weak AI, human intervention is relied on to define the parameters of learning algorithms and provide relevant training data to ensure accuracy. In recent years, scientists have worked hard to move towards "strong AI". In the future, this research can introduce semi-automatic analysis methods. First, the model will be used for the preliminary classification, and then experts will conduct secondary screening. In addition to reducing the degree of human intervention, it will gradually lead to stronger AI development.

5. Conclusions

This study proposes a deep learning FC-DNN method for stage classification from mammography images. Since deep learning methods do not require manual feature processing, the model performs exceptionally well compared to traditional image-processing techniques. The excellent performance of mammography detection is supported by accurate classification results. As a result, this technology can help during image interpretation screening, reducing the error rate and decreasing the computational time. Meanwhile, this study can be used to provide a theoretical framework for an assisted diagnosis system.

The deep neural network can be categorized into supervised learning, unsupervised learning, and semi-supervised learning. The supervised learning task is mostly accomplished by classifying predefined labeled training data (also known as "ground truth"). On the other hand, unsupervised learning is quite automated, as the network can automatically learn the correct answers from a huge amount of data, without requiring predefined labels [34]. Semi-supervised learning is the combination of two approaches by relatively smaller amounts of unlabeled data. In this study, supervised machine learning approach is used.

According to this research, using a pre-trained model could reduce the time spent on the new CNN model development. However, to use the pre-trained model, it needs to conform to the model architecture, and the model weight must be fine-tuned. The fine-tuning needs to be carried out before training. In fine-tuning, the image size of source data and the number of output categories need to be corrected.

In this paper, the dense block is selected as the model base architecture. The reason is that dense block can effectively alleviate the problem of model gradient vanishing [35–37], making backpropagation easier and the model convergence effect better. FC-DCN retains important features more comprehensively from the initial layer to the final output through feature reuse. Finally, fewer model training parameters exist because the old feature maps do not need to be relearned.

Based on the above, the method developed in this study can be applied to data types with a small number of samples. The established model can provide clinically useful reference information, speed up clinical operations, and reduce human misjudgment. In addition, the research also tested the stability of the model architecture through different data split ratios and found that even in 50% of the cases, an accuracy of nearly 80% can be obtained. In the future, we will continue to develop lightweight models to increase the possibility of clinical application.

Author Contributions: Data curation, Y.-K.K.; Methodology, S.-Y.H.; Resources, K.-Y.L. and M.-C.L.; Supervision, C.-I.C. and F.-C.K.; Validation, C.-Y.W.; Writing—original draft, S.-Y.H.; Writing—review and editing, L.-R.Y. and Y.-M.W. All authors have read and agreed to the published version of the manuscript.

Funding: This research received no external funding.

Institutional Review Board Statement: The enrolled data was also approved by the hospital research ethics committee and the Institutional Review Board (IRB), under protocol number: EMRP-107-031, E-DA Hospital, Taiwan.

Informed Consent Statement: Informed consent was obtained from all subjects involved in the study.

Data Availability Statement: Not applicable.

Acknowledgments: The authors would like to thank E-DA Hospital for providing the data source for this research. And also want to thank the E-DA Hospital for partially financially supporting this research under Contract No. EDAHP110031.

Conflicts of Interest: The authors declare no conflict of interest.

References

1. Ho, M.L.; Hsiao, Y.H.; Su, S.Y.; Chou, M.C.; Liaw, Y.P. Mortality of breast cancer in Taiwan, 1971–2010: Temporal changes and an age-period-cohort analysis. *J. Obstet. Gynaecol.* **2015**, *35*, 60–63. [CrossRef] [PubMed]
2. Khodjaeva, D.I. Magnetic-resonance imaging in the diagnosis of breast cancer and its metastasis to the spinal column. *Sci. Prog.* **2021**, *2*, 540–547.
3. Murtaza, G.; Shuib, L.; Abdul Wahab, A.W.; Mujtaba, G.; Nweke, H.F.; Al-garadi, M.A.; Zulfiqar, F.; Raza, G.; Azmi, N.A. Deep learning-based breast cancer classification through medical imaging modalities: State of the art and research challenges. *Artif. Intell. Rev.* **2020**, *53*, 1655–1720. [CrossRef]
4. Beutel, J.; Kundel, H.L.; Kim, Y.; Van Metter, R.L.; Horii, S.C. *Handbook of medical imaging*; SPIE Press: Bellingham, WA, USA, 2000; Volume 3.
5. Sehgal, C.M.; Weinstein, S.P.; Arger, P.H.; Conant, E.F. A review of breast ultrasound. *J. Mammary Gland. Biol. Neoplasia* **2006**, *11*, 113–123. [CrossRef] [PubMed]
6. Brem, R.F.; Lenihan, M.J.; Lieberman, J.; Torrente, J. Screening breast ultrasound: Past, present, and future. *Am. J. Roentgenol.* **2015**, *204*, 234–240. [CrossRef]
7. Gallagher, F.A.; Woitek, R.; McLean, M.A.; Gill, A.B.; Manzano Garcia, R.; Provenzano, E.; Riemer, F.; Kaggie, J.; Chhabra, A.; Ursprung, S.; et al. Imaging breast cancer using hyperpolarized carbon-13 MRI. *Proc. Natl. Acad. Sci. USA* **2020**, *117*, 2092–2098. [CrossRef]
8. Setiawan, A.S.; Wesley, J.; Purnama, Y. Mammogram classification using law's texture energy measure and neural networks. *Procedia Comput. Sci.* **2015**, *59*, 92–97. [CrossRef]
9. Qiu, Y.; Yan, S.; Gundreddy, R.R.; Wang, Y.; Cheng, S.; Liu, H.; Zheng, B. A new approach to develop computer-aided diagnosis scheme of breast mass classification using deep learning technology. *J. X-ray Sci. Technol.* **2017**, *25*, 751–763. [CrossRef]
10. Doi, K. Computer-aided diagnosis in medical imaging: Historical review, current status and future potential. *Comput. Med. Imaging Graph.* **2007**, *31*, 198–211. [CrossRef] [PubMed]
11. Sadaf, A.; Crystal, P.; Scaranelo, A.; Helbich, T. Performance of computer-aided detection applied to full-field digital mammography in detection of breast cancers. *Eur. J. Radiol.* **2011**, *77*, 457–461. [CrossRef]
12. Kale, M.C.; Fleig, J.D.; İmal, N. Assessment of feasibility to use computer aided texture analysis based tool for parametric images of suspicious lesions in DCE-MR mammography. *Comput. Math. Methods Med.* **2013**, *2013*. [CrossRef]
13. Norman, B.; Pedoia, V.; Noworolski, A.; Link, T.M.; Majumdar, S. Applying densely connected convolutional neural networks for staging osteoarthritis severity from plain radiographs. *J. Digit. Imaging* **2019**, *32*, 471–477. [CrossRef] [PubMed]
14. Huang, S.; Yang, J.; Fong, S.; Zhao, Q. Artificial intelligence in the diagnosis of COVID-19: Challenges and perspectives. *Int. J. Biol. Sci.* **2021**, *17*, 1581. [CrossRef] [PubMed]
15. Balasubramaniam, V. Artificial intelligence algorithm with SVM classification using dermascopic images for melanoma diagnosis. *J. Artif. Intell. Capsul. Netw.* **2021**, *3*, 34–42. [CrossRef]
16. Chlap, P.; Min, H.; Vandenberg, N.; Dowling, J.; Holloway, L.; Haworth, A. A review of medical image data augmentation techniques for deep learning applications. *J. Med. Imaging Radiat. Oncol.* **2021**, *65*, 545–563. [CrossRef]
17. Kontos, D.; Conant, E.F. Can AI help make screening mammography "lean"? *Radiology* **2019**, *293*, 47. [CrossRef] [PubMed]
18. Rodriguez-Ruiz, A.; Lång, K.; Gubern-Merida, A.; Broeders, M.; Gennaro, G.; Clauser, P.; Helbich, T.H.; Chevalier, M.; Tan, T.; Mertelmeier, T.; et al. Stand-alone artificial intelligence for breast cancer detection in mammography: Comparison with 101 radiologists. *JNCI J. Natl. Cancer Inst.* **2019**, *111*, 916–922. [CrossRef] [PubMed]

19. Schaffter, T.; Buist, D.S.; Lee, C.I.; Nikulin, Y.; Ribli, D.; Guan, Y.; Lotter, W.; Jie, Z.; Du, H.; Wang, S.; et al. Evaluation of combined artificial intelligence and radiologist assessment to interpret screening mammograms. *JAMA Netw. Open* **2020**, *3*, e200265. [CrossRef] [PubMed]

20. Raya-Povedano, J.L.; Romero-Martín, S.; Elías-Cabot, E.; Gubern-Mérida, A.; Rodríguez-Ruiz, A.; Álvarez-Benito, M. AI-based strategies to reduce workload in breast cancer screening with mammography and tomosynthesis: A retrospective evaluation. *Radiology* **2021**, *300*, 57–65. [CrossRef]

21. Zhao, T.; Liu, Y.; Neves, L.; Woodford, O.; Jiang, M.; Shah, N. Data augmentation for graph neural networks. In Proceedings of the AAAI Conference on Artificial Intelligence, Virtually, 2–9 February 2021; pp. 11015–11023.

22. Boudouh, S.S.; Bouakkaz, M. Breast Cancer: Using Deep Transfer Learning Techniques AlexNet Convolutional Neural Network For Breast Tumor Detection in Mammography Images. In Proceedings of the 2022 7th International Conference on Image and Signal Processing and their Applications (ISPA), Mostaganem, Algeria, 8–9 May 2022; pp. 1–7.

23. Rehman, K.U.; Li, J.; Pei, Y.; Yasin, A.; Ali, S.; Saeed, Y. Architectural Distortion-Based Digital Mammograms Classification Using Depth Wise Convolutional Neural Network. *Biology* **2021**, *11*, 15. [CrossRef]

24. Wang, Y.; Qi, Y.; Xu, C.; Lou, M.; Ma, Y. Learning multi-frequency features in convolutional network for mammography classification. *Med. Biol. Eng. Comput.* **2022**, *60*, 2051–2062. [CrossRef] [PubMed]

25. Rehman, K.U.; Li, J.; Pei, Y.; Yasin, A.; Ali, S.; Mahmood, T. Computer vision-based microcalcification detection in digital mammograms using fully connected depthwise separable convolutional neural network. *Sensors* **2021**, *21*, 4854. [CrossRef] [PubMed]

26. Hou, W.; Zhang, D.; Wei, Y.; Guo, J.; Zhang, X. Review on computer aided weld defect detection from radiography images. *Appl. Sci.* **2020**, *10*, 1878. [CrossRef]

27. Zhang, J.; Guo, Z.; Jiao, T.; Wang, M. Defect detection of aluminum alloy wheels in radiography images using adaptive threshold and morphological reconstruction. *Appl. Sci.* **2018**, *8*, 2365. [CrossRef]

28. Soille, P. *Morphological Image Analysis: Principles and Applications*; Springer: Berlin/Heidelberg, Germany, 1999; Volume 2.

29. Hu, J.; Shen, L.; Sun, G. Squeeze-and-excitation networks. In Proceedings of the IEEE Conference on Computer Vision and Pattern Recognition (CVPR), Salt Lake City, UT, USA, 18–23 June 2018; pp. 7132–7141.

30. Medeiros, A.; Ohata, E.F.; Silva, F.H.; Rego, P.A.; Reboucas Filho, P.P. An approach to BI-RADS uncertainty levels classification via deep learning with transfer learning technique. In Proceedings of the 2020 IEEE 33rd International Symposium on Computer-Based Medical Systems (CBMS), Rochester, MN, USA, 28–30 July 2020; pp. 603–608.

31. Falconí, L.; Pérez, M.; Aguilar, W.; Conci, A. Transfer learning and fine tuning in mammogram bi-rads classification. In Proceedings of the 2020 IEEE 33rd International Symposium on Computer-Based Medical Systems (CBMS), Rochester, MN, USA, 28–30 July 2020; pp. 475–480.

32. Yang, Z.; Cao, Z.; Zhang, Y.; Tang, Z.; Lin, X.; Ouyang, R.; Wu, M.; Han, M.; Xiao, J.; Huang, L.; et al. MommiNet-v2: Mammographic multi-view mass identification networks. *Med. Image Anal.* **2021**, *73*, 102204. [CrossRef]

33. Boumaraf, S.; Liu, X.; Ferkous, C.; Ma, X. A new computer-aided diagnosis system with modified genetic feature selection for bi-RADS classification of breast masses in mammograms. *BioMed Res. Int.* **2020**, *2020*. [CrossRef]

34. Suen, H.-Y.; Hung, K.-E.; Lin, C.-L. TensorFlow-based automatic personality recognition used in asynchronous video interviews. *IEEE Access* **2019**, *7*, 61018–61023. [CrossRef]

35. Priya, K.; Peter, J.D. A federated approach for detecting the chest diseases using DenseNet for multi-label classification. *Complex Intell. Syst.* **2022**, *8*, 3121x3129. [CrossRef]

36. Rathore, Y.K.; Janghel, R.R. Prediction of Stage of Alzheimer's Disease DenseNet Deep Learning Model. In *Next Generation Healthcare Systems Using Soft Computing Techniques*; CRC Press: Boca Raton, FL, USA, 2022; pp. 105–121.

37. Girdhar, P.; Johri, P.; Virmani, D. Deep Learning in Image Classification: Its Evolution, Methods, Challenges and Architectures. In *Advances in Distributed Computing and Machine Learning*; Springer: Berlin/Heidelberg, Germany, 2022; pp. 381–392.

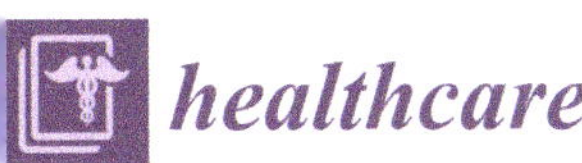
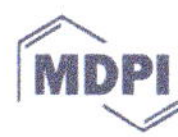

Article

Uncertainty Ordinal Multi-Instance Learning for Breast Cancer Diagnosis

Xinzheng Xu [1,*]**, Qiaoyu Guo** [1]**, Zhongnian Li** [1] **and Dechun Li** [2]

[1] School of Computer Science and Technology, China University of Mining and Technology, Xuzhou 221116, China

[2] Xuzhou Central Hospital, Xuzhou 221116, China

* Correspondence: xxzheng@cumt.edu.cn

Abstract: Ordinal multi-instance learning (OMIL) deals with the weak supervision scenario wherein instances in each training bag are not only multi-class but also have rank order relationships between classes, such as breast cancer, which has become one of the most frequent diseases in women. Most of the existing work has generally been to classify the region of interest (mass or microcalcification) on the mammogram as either benign or malignant, while ignoring the normal mammogram classification. Early screening for breast disease is particularly important for further diagnosis. Since early benign lesion areas on a mammogram are very similar to normal tissue, three classifications of mammograms for the improved screening of early benign lesions are necessary. In OMIL, an expert will only label the set of instances (bag), instead of labeling every instance. When labeling efforts are focused on the class of bags, ordinal classes of the instance inside the bag are not labeled. However, recent work on ordinal multi-instance has used the traditional support vector machine to solve the multi-classification problem without utilizing the ordinal information regarding the instances in the bag. In this paper, we propose a method that explicitly models the ordinal class information for bags and instances in bags. Specifically, we specify a key instance from the bag as a positive instance of bags, and design ordinal minimum uncertainty loss to iteratively optimize the selected key instances from the bags. The extensive experimental results clearly prove the effectiveness of the proposed ordinal instance-learning approach, which achieves 52.021% accuracy, 61.471% sensitivity, 47.206% specificity, 57.895% precision, and an 59.629% F1 score on a DDSM dataset.

Keywords: ordinal classification; multi-instance learning; weak supervision; breast cancer; key instance; uncertainty select

Citation: Xu, X.; Guo, Q.; Li, Z.; Li, D. Uncertainty Ordinal Multi-Instance Learning for Breast Cancer Diagnosis. *Healthcare* **2022**, *10*, 2300. https://doi.org/10.3390/healthcare10112300

Academic Editor: Mahmudur Rahman

Received: 17 October 2022
Accepted: 15 November 2022
Published: 17 November 2022

Publisher's Note: MDPI stays neutral with regard to jurisdictional claims in published maps and institutional affiliations.

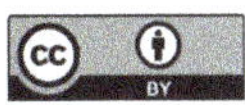

1. Introduction

Breast cancer is one of the most fatal diseases among women. The study of the benign and malignant classifications of breast cancer has been quite extensive. Elmoufidi [1] proposed a framework that uses a modified K-means algorithm to segment the ROI and extract textural features from the ROI for classification. Fahssi et al. [2] presented a novel CAD system for mammography diagnosis. The ROIs are detected by dividing the mammogram into regions and MIL algorithms are applied to identify malignant regions to label the whole mammogram. Most of the existing work has solved the binary classification problem of breast cancer, but there are more normal breast images than abnormal ones. Although the classification of benign and malignant regions of interest in abnormal breast images can achieve good performance, when the classification category becomes normal, benign, or malignant, the classification performance tends to decline. Lamard et al. [3] carried out experiments on binary classification and three-class classification. The experimental results show that the accuracy of the three-class classification is 30% lower than that of the two-class classification, which undoubtedly shows that the three-class classification of breast cancer is more challenging than the two-class classification. Moreover, we found that the classification of normal and benign regions is much more difficult than benign and malignant. The effective screening of early benign lesions is of great importance for further diagnosis and treatment. Since there is a certain order of lesions in the normal, benign, and malignant categories, we transform the general multi-instance learning problem into an orderly multi-instance-learning technique.

Multi-instance learning (MIL) [4–6] is a popular learning framework in weakly supervised learning [7–10]. Different from supervised learning, the data sample for MIL is a bag that consists of a set of instances. In the MIL setting, bags are labeled, while instances in bags are unlabeled. The researchers have studied various paradigms for MIL, including, but not limited to, multiple instance classification(MIC) [11], multiple instance regression, multi-instance clustering, imbalanced multi-instance learning, and multi-instance multi-labeling.

Here, we consider another typical scenario of MIL-ordinal multiple instance learning [12] (OMIL): the classes of bags are not only ordered, but the instances in the bag are also in a certain rank order. Moreover, the highest level of instance label cannot exceed the label of the bag. For example, in the medical diagnosis of breast cancer, the class of lesion in a mammogram is not only normal, benign, and malignant, but also a rank order among these categories, namely, normal < benign < cancer, as shown in Figure 1. To solve the OMIL problem, previous works have mainly focused on settling one of issues, which could be roughly divided into two problems: one is multiple instance classification, and the other is the ordinal classification problem.

Multi-instance classification is the most widely used MIL paradigm. Zhou et al. [4] proposed a MIEN-metric method that learns discriminative metrics for classifying samples from the observed classes and recognizing the samples from the novel class, which solves the emerging novel class problem concerning muti-instance learning in open and changing complex scenarios. Subsequently, in the study of multi-instance classification, Zhou et al. [5] found that samples in multi-instance learning are described by multiple instances and associated with multiple class labels. Based on a simple degeneration strategy with MIMLBOOST and MIMLSVM algorithms, the proposed multi-instance multi-label framework can deal with problems involving complex objects with multiple semantic meanings. Class imbalance is also a persistent problem in multi-instance classification tasks. Javad et al. [13] proposed a new instance reduction method that preserves the between-class distribution in the balanced data and handles minority class instance reduction in two-class imbalanced data.

The method of multi-instance learning for classification problems generally assumes that the class value is unordered. However, in many practical applications, a natural ordered relationship exists between the categories of instances. Frank et al. [14] proposed a simple method involving the incorporation of a decision tree. Accordingly, the standard classifier algorithm made full use of the ordered information between the class attributes. Different from most of the previous works that employ a loss function based on the absolute difference between the predicted and ground truth class labels, Joan et al. [15] argues that the label values in ordinal classification may be arbitrary, and proposed a network architecture that produces not a single class prediction but an ordered vector.

The recent work by Evan [12] used OMIL in the estimation of ulcerative colitis severity. However, their method transformed the multi-classification problem of OMIL into multiple binary classifiers, which fails to directly model multi-class instance bags and loses the ordered information between classes. To tackle this problem, we propose a discriminative solution to directly model ordinal multi-instance bags, which obviously learns ordered information between classes. Specifically, we exact key instances from the bag as positive instances of bags, and design ordinal minimum uncertainty loss to iteratively optimize the selected key instances from the bags. This study's main contributions are summarized as follows:

1. We select a key instance as a positive instance of the bags and send the key instance, which has a bag label, to the network for training. The instances selected from the bag at each iteration are uncertain but incur minimal loss.
2. We employ ordinal minimum uncertainty loss to take advantage of the ordered information in classes.
3. We carry out experiments on a DDSM dataset to evaluate the OMIL method. The experimental results demonstrate that our OMIL approach achieves better performance than the existing OMIL method.

The rest of the paper is organized as follows. In Section 2, we introduce some related works about key instances, multi-instance learning, and ordinal classification. The proposed OMIL method and model architecture are proposed in Section 3. In Section 4, the processing of the DDSM dataset and experimental setup are introduced in detail. The experimental results are also presented. In Section 5, in order to verify the effectiveness of our proposed method, we conduct some ablation studies. Finally, Section 6 presents the conclusions of this paper.

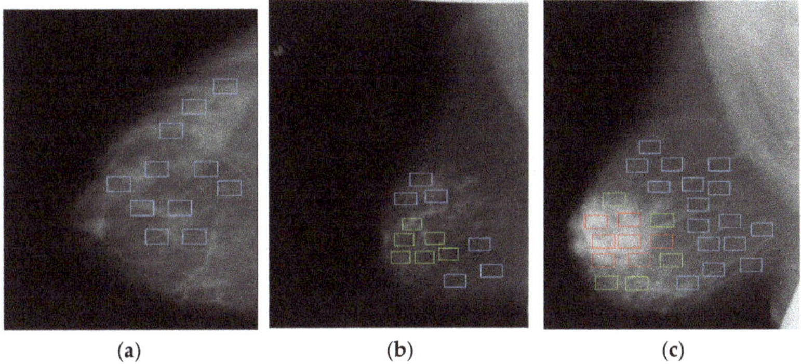

(a)   (b)   (c)

Figure 1. We show images of three types of breast disease lesions: (**a**) normal, (**b**) benign, and (**c**) cancerous. Specifically, the image (bag) consists of several patches (instances). The instances marked by blue rectangles denote normal lesion, green rectangles denote benign lesion, and red rectangles denote cancer. More importantly, the lesion level of the instance in each bag cannot exceed the lesion intensity of the bag.

2. Related Works

This section defines the basis for and reviews the related works on key instances, multi-instance learning, and ordinal classification.

2.1. Key Instance

Key instances [16–18] play a key role in multi-instance learning, and their labels can trigger the label of the bag. To solve the key instance detection (KID) problem, Liu et al. [16] proposed a voting framework (VF) solution to KID, which utilizes the relationship among instances to form a citer KNN graph, and uses them to define the confidences of the votes of the training instances. However, when encountering a more complex situation, key instance detection may fail. Traditional max pooling cannot make full use of the information from input examples. Yan et al. [19] proposed a novel dynamic-pooling function for MIL that can iteratively update the instance contribution to its bag and highlights the key instance. Inspired by this work, the key instance of our model selected from each bag is constantly optimized. In order to incorporate interpretability into the MIL approach, Ilse et al. [20] proposed an "Attention-based Multiple Instance Learning" method, which pays more attention to positive instances during training. Hence, the attention weights allow us to find a key instance. Notably, this approach makes it clear how each instance contributes to the bag. Nonetheless, shin et al. [17] argued that the performance of the model with respect to key instance detection is limited; that is, an attention-based model [20] focuses on the weight of the positive instance yet the difference between positive and negative instances in the positive bag is not obvious, which may influence performance. To improve the performance of the attention-based model in a KID task, they apply a neural network inversion with a sparseness constraint that updates the instances in a positive bag. In this way, the key instance is better highlighted by using optimized instances.

2.2. Multiple Instance Learning

Multi-instance learning [5,6,20–22] was proposed by early researchers when studying drug activity prediction. The standard assumption for multi-instance learning is that if a bag is labeled positive, there is at least one positive instance in it. Otherwise, the bag will be labeled negative. The traditional multi-instance hypothesis assumes that the class label of a bag is determined by the key instances in the bag. Multi-instance classification is the most common task in multi-instance learning. Furthermore, it has promoted the emergence of many classification algorithms, such as DD, Citation-KNN, BP-MIP, MI-SVM, mi-SVM, etc. All these MIL algorithms [21] assume that the bag is a binary classification problem, namely, positive and negative bag.

However, in general scenarios, multiple classification tasks are more common than binary classification tasks. Over the last few years, the multi-instance multi-classification task has also attracted the attention of many researchers. Different from ordinary multi-instance learning, which assumes each observation belongs to a class, a framework of multi-instance multi-label learning (MIMIL) can better describe complex objects with several classes. Zhou et al. [5] proposed the MIMLBOOST and MIMLSVM algorithms to solve problems involving complex objects associated with multiple class labels. Following this work, Pham et al. [23] extended the MIMIL problem to the setting wherein a novel class instance is present. They proposed a maximum likelihood method to optimize the model and trained an instance-level classifier for all classes as well as the novel class. Nonetheless, the ground-truth label of the sample is difficult to obtain in the real world. To alleviate this problem, Ishida et al. [24] proposed a novel setting called complementary label learning [24,25] to implement multi-class classification tasks, which only requires the provision of complementary data labels.

In this paper, we focus on the ordinal multi-instance-learning problem. The most similar work to ours is the ordinal multi-instance-learning approach proposed by Evan et al. [12]. One difference is that we directly model the bag as multi-class and select the instance with minimum loss from the bags as a positive instance of the bags to update the model parameters. In this way, each key instance we select from the bag is uncertain and optimal. Nevertheless, they transformed the multi-classification problem of bags into several binary classifiers to deal with, rather than explicitly modeling the bag.

2.3. Ordinal Classification

Ordinal classification problems [15,26–28] can be viewed as an intermediate problem between classification and regression, where the target variable is both categorical and ordinal. In general classification problems, the categorical variables are taken from a finite set, and there is no metric relationship between the categories, although they are represented numerically. Examples of categorical variables are gender, race, nationality, types of animals, etc. When there is a naturally ordered relationship between categorical variables, the ordinary classification problem transforms into an ordinal classification problem. Some common scenarios include bank credit-rating assessments, determining income level, the lesion grade of cancer, users' evaluation of service, etc.

Gutierrez et al. [28] assessed the performance of five different methods under different representations of ordinal input variables. The results show that both the Num and Num-CDR methods perform well and the Num method directly maps each class to a consecutive natural number. Considering that the misclassification loss of ordinal classification should be different, Beckham et al. [27] proposed a simple modification of the squared error loss, which utilizes the characteristic of the sensitivity of class ordering and guarantees that the possibility of distribution over the classes is discrete. Different from most previous works that compute the absolute difference between the predicted and ground-truth class labels to optimize the loss function, Joan et al. [15] argued that label values in ordinal classification may be arbitrary and replace a single class prediction with an ordered vector.

3. Proposed Approach

In this section, we will briefly formalize the OMIL problem and describe several crucial concepts of OMIL. In addition, we introduce a discriminative model for OMIL data wherein the instances in each bag are ordered.

3.1. Problem Formalization of OMIL

In the problem definition of OMIL, the training set is represented as: $D = \{(X_1, y_1), \ldots, (X_i, y_i), (X_N, y_N)\}$, where X_i denotes a bag, which contains n_i instances, and each instance is described by a d-dimensional vector, i.e., $X_i = \{x_i^1, x_i^2, \ldots, x_i^{n_i}\}, x_i \in R^d$. The labels of the bags are not only multi-class but also have a certain rank order [12] among classes. Simultaneously, the labeling of the instances in the bag cannot exceed the label of the bag. The formal definition is as follows: bag-level class label $y_i \in y = \{0, 1, \ldots, C\}, (0 < 1 < \cdots < C)$, and instance-level class label $y_{ij} \in y = \{0, 1, \cdots, C_1\}, (0 < 1 < \cdots < C_1 \leq y_i)$. It is supposed that: (1) If a bag X_i is labeled as the cth class $\Leftrightarrow$ The instance-level label of X_i belongs to the set $y' = \{0, 1, \ldots, C\}, (0 < 1 < \ldots < C)$. The strongest label-level of instances must be the same as the bag label, where the strongest instance-level label is cth class. (2) A label for a bag X_i is not assigned to the cth class. $\Leftrightarrow$ None of the instances in bag X_i belong to the cth class. We give a full description of the three important concepts of OMIL in Table 1.

Table 1. Three relevant, important concepts of OMIL.

Concepts	Descriptions
Bags	The data unit of OMIL dataset that has labels. Each bag contains several ordinal instances without label information.
Instance	The label class of instances in a bag is ordered, and the largest category belongs to the bag category.
Key instance	The instance with minimum loss, which is selected from bag X_i. Bag-level label is provided for the instance to participate in the model-training process.

3.2. Model

The proposed model addresses the OMIL problem in two basic steps: (1) after the model outputs the loss of all the instances in the bag, the instance with the least amount of loss is selected as the key instance of the bag. (2) The selected key instances serve as a positive instance of the bag, assign the label of the bag, and participate in the training and optimization of the model.

Our model is presented in Figure 2. The training sample set is composed of a multi-class bag, which has a class label but the instances in it do not possess label information. The convolutional neural network [29] consists of two convolutional layers with a 5×5 and 3×3 filter, one pooling layer, and two fully connected layers [30]. The specific structural design of the CNN is shown in Table 2. In the model-training phase, not all instances in a bag participate in training, but the selected key instance [6,17] from the bags can be fed into the network to optimize parameters. In addition, the selected key instances from the bags are not constant, and they will further approach the true positive instances under each optimization of the network.

Table 2. Setting of the parameters of convolutional neural network (CNN) in the model structure diagram.

Network Layer	Input	Output	Filter	Stride	Padding	Parameter
Input	$224 \times 224 \times 1$	$224 \times 224 \times 1$	-	-	-	0
Conv1	$224 \times 224 \times 1$	$220 \times 220 \times 10$	$5 \times 5 \times 10$	1	0	260
Relu	$220 \times 220 \times 10$	$220 \times 220 \times 10$	-	-	-	0
MaxPool	$220 \times 220 \times 10$	$110 \times 110 \times 10$	2×2	2	0	0
Conv2	$110 \times 110 \times 10$	$108 \times 108 \times 20$	$3 \times 3 \times 20$	1	0	1820
Relu	$108 \times 108 \times 20$	$108 \times 108 \times 20$	-	-	-	0
FC1	$108 \times 108 \times 20$	500	-	-	-	116,640,500
FC2	500	1	-	-	-	501

We illustrate the use of our notation, for example, of OMIL in Table 3, where $Y_b \in \mathrm{argmax}\{0, 1, \cdots, C\}$. This model indicates that the bag label Y_b is obtained from the strongest-level label in the instance labels $Y_b^{n_b}$. Hence, Y_b can reveal information about the ordinal class of instances in the bag.

Table 3. Instance labels and bag labels of the proposed model.

Bag 1	Bag 2	Bag 3
$n_1 = 1$	$n_2 = 2$	$n_3 = 3$
$y_{11} = \mathrm{normal}$	$y_{21} = \mathrm{normal}$	$y_{31} = \mathrm{normal}$
$y_{12} = \mathrm{normal}$	$y_{22} = \mathrm{normal}$	$y_{32} = \mathrm{benign}$
$\vdots$	$\vdots$	$\vdots$
$y_{1n} = \mathrm{normal}$	$y_{2n} = \mathrm{benign}$	$y_{3n} = \mathrm{cancer}$
$Y_1^1 = \{\mathrm{normal}\}$	$Y_2^2 = \{\mathrm{normal, benign}\}$	$Y_3^3 = \{\mathrm{normal, benign, cancer}\}$
$Y_1 = \{\mathrm{normal}\}$	$Y_2 = \{\mathrm{benign}\}$	$Y_3 = \{\mathrm{cancer}\}$

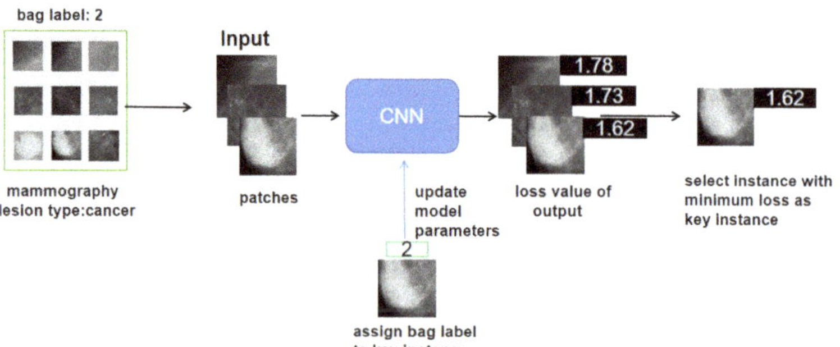

Figure 2. Overall model structure of OOMIL. Mammograms are split into patches, and then fed to the model to select the minimum-loss patch. The key instance-assigned bag labels participate in model training.

4. Experiments

In this section, we evaluate the performance of the proposed novel OOMIL approach against the original OMIL approach, and the results of the comparison when applied to a DDSM dataset are shown in Table 4. Further on, to increase the interpretability of the model, we visualize the process of the model's selection of key instances from a bag, which is displayed in Figure 3.

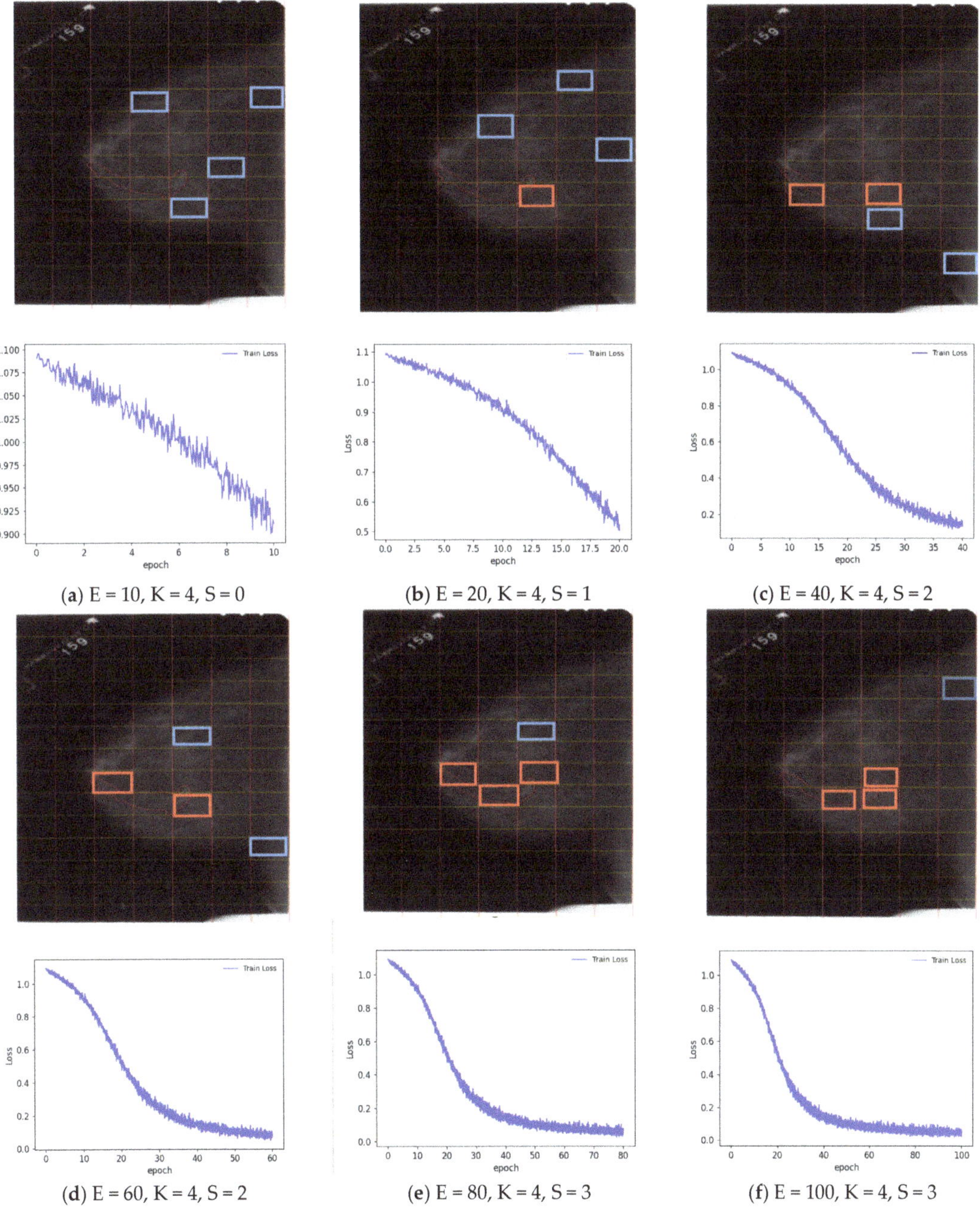

(**a**) E = 10, K = 4, S = 0

(**b**) E = 20, K = 4, S = 1

(**c**) E = 40, K = 4, S = 2

(**d**) E = 60, K = 4, S = 2

(**e**) E = 80, K = 4, S = 3

(**f**) E = 100, K = 4, S = 3

Figure 3. When the key instance K value is 4, the number of positive instances S in the key instances selected by the model and the model training loss change as the epoch E increases E, K, and S represent epoch times, key instance, and positive instance in key instance, respectively. The key instances marked with a blue rectangle denote false instances, whereas the red rectangles represent true instances.

Table 4. Test accuracy comparison results for OMIL and OOMIL (our) method.

Dataset	OMIL	OOMIL (Our Method)
DDSM	49.882	52.021

4.1. Datasets

DDSM [31] is a widely used mammography dataset in computer-aided medical diagnosis. DDSM includes four types of data, namely, normal, benign, benign-without-callback, and cancer, which comprise 10,420 images from 2605 breast cancer cases. For benign and cancer cases, only the images with the lesion area marked by a physician are selected. Hence, our dataset employs 1700 images from normal, benign, and cancer cases. We selected 1360 images from each type of case to form the training set and 340 images to form the test set.

Some processing operations must be performed on the training set. We first divide each image into grids [32–34] with an aspect ratio of 14:7 to obtain 98 patches so that each bag (image) consists of 98 instances (patches). Since some instances come from the noisy region of the image, we use a threshold-processing operation [35,36] to further filter the instances in the bag. To ensure a balanced number of instances per bag, we again expand the dataset with horizontal and vertical flipping as well as rotating image enhancement techniques [37,38], and resize each instance to 224×224. Finally, our training set consists of 4080 bags (1360 per lesion type), each containing 70 instances with a 224×224 size. To verify the effectiveness of the instance-level classifier trained by our proposed method, we crop the region of interest from each image in the test set as a test example, which has a specific class label.

4.2. Experimental Setup

In our experiments, our network is composed of two convolution layers with a 5×5 and 3×3 filters, a pooling layer with a 2×2 kernel, and two fully connected layers [30] with 500 neurons and 1 neuron, respectively. The weights and biases are initialized to be 0. In addition, the k value of the selected key instance is assigned to 4. We employ the approach developed by Adam [39] to optimize our network. Detailed hyper-parameters such as the learning rate, weight decay, eps, and betas are set to 0.0001, 0.0005, and 1×10^{-6}, (0.9, 0.99). We choose pytorch as the deep-learning framework [40] and write the code in python. The experiments are run on a PC with AMD EPYC-7302 CPU and 64 GB RAM.

4.3. Empirical Results of OMIL

Here, we present the comparison results for our novel OOMIL method and existing OMIL method. The experimental results in Table 4 show that our method performs better than the OMIL when applied to the DDSM dataset. In order to intuitively show the effectiveness of our proposed method, we visualize the process of the model selecting the key instances from a bag. The process is shown in Figure 3. The letter E represents the training epoch of the model, K represents the number of key instances to pick from the bag, and S denotes the number of key instances that represent positive instances. Instances with a blue rectangle represent the key instances that are not selected correctly. On the contrary, the red rectangles represent key instances that are selected correctly. As is vividly shown in Figure 3, when the training epoch increases, the number of real key instances that are selected out also increases. Thus, the effectiveness of our proposed method has been proven.

5. Ablation Study and Discussion

In this section, we conduct some ablation studies regarding the effect of the k value of the key instance on each class prediction and different loss functions across the DDSM dataset. In addition, the evaluation metrics of the model are presented in Table 5.

Table 5. Different performance measurements of our model.

Proposed Method	Sensitivity (%)	Specificity (%)	Precision (%)	F1 (%)
OOMIL	61.471	47.206	57.895	59.629

Each class accuracy on different k values of the key instances. As mentioned in Section 3, a key instance [16,18] is an instance with minimum loss, which is closest to the positive instance in the bag. The accuracy of the key instance's selection further affects the effectiveness of the model's ability to learn. To reduce the probability of the erroneous selection of key instances, we select the first k instances with minimum loss as the key instances of the bag. Hence, we carry out comparison experiments to study the influence of different k values. In Table 6, we show each class result of the different k values on the DDSM dataset. In addition, we can see that as the number of key instances selected increases, each category has a more even prediction probability instead of being inclined towards selecting a certain class. That is, the model performs well overall.

Table 6. Class accuracy comparison of number set K for key instances in the model. K takes values from 1 to 5, which denote different values of selected key instances.

Class	K				
	1	2	3	4	5
0	20.294	43.529	57.059	52.059	71.765
1	26.176	32.941	22.059	42.353	35.882
2	85.294	54.706	60.000	49.118	22.353

Different loss functions' accuracies on different k values of key instance. Through previous MIL tasks [4,23], cross entropy loss [41] has proven to be one of the most commonly used loss functions in MIL methods. Instead, our OMIL uses the ordinal minimum uncertainty loss during training. To discuss the influence of different loss functions, we conduct ample comparative experiments on cross entropy loss and minimum uncertainty ordinal loss. In order to apply the Cross Entropy loss to our OMIL, we change the network architecture by replacing the last fully connected layer, which has one neuron, with a fully connected layer, which has three neurons and employs a SoftMax function. Then, combining the bag label with the instance probability, we can calculate the Cross Entropy loss. Finally, we can obtain the loss of each instance from the bag and obtain the instance with minimum loss. Table 7 indicates that, with respect to the DDSM dataset, the results based on the minimum uncertainty ordinal loss are better than cross entropy loss. This proves the effectiveness of the minimum uncertainty ordinal loss to our OMIL.

Table 7. Average test accuracy comparison of different loss functions on number set K for key instances. K ranges from 1 to 5.

Loss	K				
	1	2	3	4	5
cross entropy (OOMIL)	47.255	47.059	49.706	51.176	47.667
min-uncertainty ordinal (OOMIL)	48.529	47.451	49.679	52.021	47.983
cross entropy (OMIL)	46.972	47.183	48.127	48.743	46.430
min-uncertainty ordinal (OMIL)	47.943	47.372	49.232	49.882	46.846

The experimental results in Table 7 show that the accuracy of the model does not always rise with the number of key instances (K). A possible reason is that the sample imbalance affects the improvement of the model's performance. In our training bags, the number of normal instances is much greater than that of benign and cancer instances, which is due to the limitations of the mammogram itself. The lesion regions in the mammogram may account for only 4% of the whole image. The model performs well and the prediction accuracy for each class is relatively average when the value of K is 4. The model tends to predict class 0 in the case of K being 5. The reason is that it is difficult to pick the correct instances in the early stage of model training, and the model's fault tolerance rate is low if the number of key instances is too small. However, when the number of key instances is too large, false key instances are far larger in number than true key instances, which also leads to the degradation of the model's performance.

Currently, most of the existing work on breast cancer classification addresses the binary classification problem, that is, judging whether the ROI (mass or calcification) is benign or malignant. Elmoufidi [1] proposed a framework comprising two steps of ROI segmentation and feature extraction from ROI for classification. The experimental results regarding the method's sensitivity, specificity, and accuracy are 94.46%, 94.40%, and 94.43%. Fahssi et al. [2] presented a novel CAD system for mammography diagnosis. They first partition the mammogram into regions and detect the ROI, and then use MIL algorithms to identify malignant regions in order to assign the label to the whole mammogram. This achieves 90.84% sensitivity, 90.17% specificity, and 90.33% accuracy. However, in practical situations, normal cases are generally more frequent than abnormal cases in the diagnosis of breast disease. There is no doubt that screening for abnormal mammograms from large numbers of normal mammograms is energy-consuming work for physicians. Accordingly, the classifier we trained was three-class, classifying mammograms as normal, benign, or malignant. The three-class task is more challenging than ordinary binary classification, as the instance features of normal and benign categories are very similar, especially with respect to benign lesions in early breast cancer. Lamard et al. [3] carried out experiments on binary classification, which achieved an accuracy of 91.1%, while the accuracy of the three-class classification was only 62.1%, a drop of almost 30%, which strongly suggests that three-class classification tasks are more difficult than binary classification tasks. Although our experiment achieved only 52.021% accuracy, to the best of our knowledge, we are the first to propose a novel OMIL method to directly model multi-category bags rather than transforming them into multiple binary classifiers for multi-categories. During the experiment, we found that the accuracy of malignant classification is generally higher than normal and benign, while the accuracy of normal and benign categories is similar. How to more effectively classify normal and benign mammograms and improve the accuracy of model prediction is the key point to consider in our next experiment.

6. Conclusions

In this paper, we addressed the ordinal multi-instance-learning problem in breast cancer diagnosis using mammograms. Compared with the binary classification of mammograms, the three-classification task provides superior support for the screening of early breast cancer, as the features of normal tissues and benign lesion areas are very similar. During the experiment, we found that the predictive accuracy with respect to the malignant categories is generally higher than that of the normal and benign categories. Simultaneously, the accuracy gap between the normal and benign categories is small. This also shows that benign lesions can easily be predicted as normal categories, which is very influential in preventing further deterioration in early breast cancer. Hence, we propose a method that directly models the ordinal class information for bags and the instances in the bags. Moreover, to ensure that the key instance selected in the bag is closer to the real positive instances, we employed minimum uncertainty ordinal loss to iteratively optimize the selected key instances from the bags. To increase the interpretability of the model, the simple grid segmentation method acted as the generator of bags, which allowed for the convenient recording of the specific location of instances in the bag to visualize the process of the model's instance selection. Other more elaborate bag generation methods such as

SBN, ImaBag, BlobBag, etc., may improve the performance of the model. The problem of sample imbalance is also not addressed by our current work. The number of normal samples is much higher than benign and cancer samples, leading to the higher prediction accuracy of the model for normal instances. A model with strong generalizability is trained by introducing cost-sensitive methods that impose different penalties for different numbers of samples, which is the focus of our future work. Overall, our method breaks down the barrier that medical images are difficult to label and supply help for breast cancer diagnosis in the future.

Author Contributions: Conception and design of the study, X.X. and Q.G.; collection of the data, Q.G. and D.L.; analysis of the data and contribution to the writing of the manuscript, X.X., Q.G., Z.L. and D.L. All authors have read and agreed to the published version of the manuscript.

Funding: This work was supported by the National Natural Science Foundation of China (No. 61976217), the Fundamental Research Funds of Central Universities (No. 2019XKQYMS87), and the Science and Technology Planning Project of Xuzhou (No. KC21193).

Institutional Review Board Statement: Not applicable.

Informed Consent Statement: Not applicable.

Data Availability Statement: Not applicable.

Conflicts of Interest: The authors declare no conflict of interest.

References

1. Elmoufidi, A. Deep Multiple Instance Learning for Automatic Breast Cancer Assessment Using Digital Mammography. *IEEE Trans. Instrum. Meas.* **2022**, *71*, 4503813. [CrossRef]
2. Elmoufidi, A.; El Fahssi, K.; Jai-andaloussi, S.; Sekkaki, A.; Gwenole, Q.; Lamard, M. Anomaly Classification in Digital Mammography Based on Multiple-Instance Learning. *IET Image Process.* **2018**, *12*, 320–328. [CrossRef]
3. Sánchez de la Rosa, R.; Lamard, M.; Cazuguel, G.; Coatrieux, G.; Cozic, M.; Quellec, G. Multiple-Instance Learning for Breast Cancer Detection in Mammograms. In Proceedings of the 2015 37th Annual International Conference of the IEEE Engineering in Medicine and Biology Society (EMBC), Milan, Italy, 25–29 August 2015; pp. 7055–7058.
4. Wei, X.-S.; Ye, H.-J.; Mu, X.; Wu, J.; Shen, C.; Zhou, Z.-H. Multiple Instance Learning with Emerging Novel Class. *IEEE Trans. Knowl. Data Eng.* **2019**, *33*, 2109–2120. [CrossRef]
5. Zhou, Z.-H.; Zhang, M.-L.; Huang, S.-J.; Li, Y.-F. Multi-Instance Multi-Label Learning. *Artif. Intell.* **2012**, *176*, 2291–2320. [CrossRef]
6. Zhou, Z.-H. *Multi-Instance Learning: A Survey*; Technical Report; Department of Computer Science & Technology, Nanjing University: Nanjing, China, 2004.
7. Bilen, H.; Vedaldi, A. Weakly Supervised Deep Detection Networks. In Proceedings of the IEEE Conference on Computer Vision and Pattern Recognition (CVPR), Las Vegas, NV, USA, 27–30 June 2016; pp. 2846–2854. [CrossRef]
8. Campanella, G.; Hanna, M.G.; Geneslaw, L.; Miraflor, A.; Werneck Krauss Silva, V.; Busam, K.J.; Brogi, E.; Reuter, V.E.; Klimstra, D.S.; Fuchs, T.J. Clinical-Grade Computational Pathology Using Weakly Supervised Deep Learning on Whole Slide Images. *Nat. Med.* **2019**, *25*, 1301–1309. [CrossRef] [PubMed]
9. Kim, J.; Kim, H.J.; Kim, C.; Lee, J.H.; Kim, K.W.; Park, Y.M.; Kim, H.W.; Ki, S.Y.; Kim, Y.M.; Kim, W.H. Weakly-Supervised Deep Learning for Ultrasound Diagnosis of Breast Cancer. *Sci. Rep.* **2021**, *11*, 24382. [CrossRef] [PubMed]
10. Zhou, Z.-H. A Brief Introduction to Weakly Supervised Learning. *Natl. Sci. Rev.* **2018**, *5*, 44–53. [CrossRef]
11. Alpaydın, E.; Cheplygina, V.; Loog, M.; Tax, D.M.J. Single- vs. Multiple-Instance Classification. *Pattern Recognit.* **2015**, *48*, 2831–2838. [CrossRef]
12. Schwab, E.; Cula, G.O.; Standish, K.; Yip, S.S.F.; Stojmirovic, A.; Ghanem, L.; Chehoud, C. Automatic Estimation of Ulcerative Colitis Severity from Endoscopy Videos Using Ordinal Multi-Instance Learning. *Comput. Methods Biomech. Biomed. Eng. Imaging Vis.* **2022**, *10*, 425–433. [CrossRef]
13. Hamidzadeh, J.; Kashefi, N.; Moradi, M. Combined Weighted Multi-Objective Optimizer for Instance Reduction in Two-Class Imbalanced Data Problem. *Eng. Appl. Artif. Intell.* **2020**, *90*, 103500. [CrossRef]
14. Frank, E.; Hall, M. A Simple Approach to Ordinal Classification. In *Machine Learning: ECML 2001*; De Raedt, L., Flach, P., Eds.; Lecture Notes in Computer Science; Springer: Berlin/Heidelberg, Germany, 2001; Volume 2167, pp. 145–156.
15. Serrat, J.; Ruiz, I. Rank-Based Ordinal Classification. In Proceedings of the 2020 25th International Conference on Pattern Recognition (ICPR), Milan, Italy, 10–15 January 2021; pp. 8069–8076.
16. Liu, G.; Wu, J.; Zhou, Z.-H. Key Instance Detection in Multi-Instance Learning. In Proceedings of the Asian Conference on Machine Learning, PMLR, Singapore, 17 November 2012; pp. 253–268.
17. Shin, B.; Cho, J.; Yu, H.; Choi, S. Sparse Network Inversion for Key Instance Detection in Multiple Instance Learning. In Proceedings of the 2020 25th International Conference on Pattern Recognition (ICPR), Milan, Italy, 10–15 January 2021; pp. 4083–4090.

18. Zhang, Y.-L.; Zhou, Z.-H. Multi-Instance Learning with Key Instance Shift. In Proceedings of the Twenty-Sixth International Joint Conference on Artificial Intelligence; International Joint Conferences on Artificial Intelligence Organization, Melbourne, Australia, 19–25 August 2017; pp. 3441–3447.
19. Yan, Y.; Wang, X.; Guo, X.; Fang, J.; Liu, W.; Huang, J. Deep Multi-Instance Learning with Dynamic Pooling. In Proceedings of the 10th Asian Conference on Machine Learning, PMLR, Beijing, China, 14–16 November 2018; pp. 662–677.
20. Ilse, M.; Tomczak, J.; Welling, M. Attention-Based Deep Multiple Instance Learning. In Proceedings of the 35th International Conference on Machine Learning, PMLR, Stockholm, Sweden, 10–15 July 2018; pp. 2127–2136.
21. Astorino, A.; Fuduli, A.; Gaudioso, M.; Vocaturo, E. Multiple Instance Learning Algorithm for Medical Image Classification. *SEBD* **2019**, *2400*, 1–8.
22. Zhou, Z.-H.; Zhang, M.-L. Neural Networks for Multi-Instance Learning. In Proceedings of the International Conference on Intelligent Information Technology, Beijing, China, 22–25 September 2002; pp. 455–459.
23. Pham, A.T.; Raich, R.; Fern, X.Z.; Arriaga, J.P. Multi-Instance Multi-Label Learning in the Presence of Novel Class Instances. In Proceedings of the International Conference on Machine Learning(ICML), Lille, France, 7–9 July 2015; pp. 2427–2435.
24. Ishida, T.; Niu, G.; Hu, W.; Sugiyama, M. Learning from Complementary Labels. In Proceedings of the Advances in Neural Information Processing Systems, Long Beach, CA, USA, 4–9 December 2017; Curran Associates, Inc.: New York, NY, USA, 2017; Volume 30.
25. Gao, Y.; Zhang, M.-L. Discriminative Complementary-Label Learning with Weighted Loss. In Proceedings of the International Conference on Machine Learning(ICML). PMLR, Virtual, 18–24 July 2021; pp. 3587–3597.
26. Albuquerque, T.; Cruz, R.; Cardoso, J.S. Ordinal Losses for Classification of Cervical Cancer Risk. *PeerJ Comput. Sci.* **2021**, *7*, e457. [CrossRef] [PubMed]
27. Beckham, C.; Pal, C. A Simple Squared-Error Reformulation for Ordinal Classification 2017. *arXiv* **2016**, arXiv:1612.00775.
28. Gutiérrez, P.A.; Pérez-Ortiz, M.; Sánchez-Monedero, J.; Hervás-Martínez, C. Representing Ordinal Input Variables in the Context of Ordinal Classification. In Proceedings of the 2016 International Joint Conference on Neural Networks (IJCNN), Vancouver, BC, Canada, 24–29 July 2016; pp. 2174–2181.
29. Lecun, Y.; Bottou, L.; Bengio, Y.; Haffner, P. Gradient-Based Learning Applied to Document Recognition. *Proc. IEEE* **1998**, *86*, 2278–2324. [CrossRef]
30. Jegou, S.; Drozdzal, M.; Vazquez, D.; Romero, A.; Bengio, Y. The One Hundred Layers Tiramisu: Fully Convolutional DenseNets for Semantic Segmentation. In Proceedings of the IEEE Conference on Computer Vision and Pattern Recognition Workshops, Honolulu, HI, USA, 21–26 July 2017; pp. 11–19.
31. Lekamlage, C.D.; Afzal, F.; Westerberg, E.; Chaddad, A. Mini-DDSM: Mammography-Based Automatic Age Estimation. In Proceedings of the 2020 3rd International Conference on Digital Medicine and Image Processing, ACM, Kyoto Japan, 6–9 November 2020; pp. 1–6.
32. Bhagat, P.K.; Choudhary, P.; Singh, K.M. Two Efficient Image Bag Generators for Multi-Instance Multi-Label Learning. In Proceedings of the Computer Vision and Image Processing, Jaipur, India, 27–29 September 2019; Nain, N., Vipparthi, S.K., Raman, B., Eds.; Springer: Singapore, 2020; pp. 407–418.
33. Wei, X.-S.; Zhou, Z.-H. An Empirical Study on Image Bag Generators for Multi-Instance Learning. *Mach. Learn.* **2016**, *105*, 155–198. [CrossRef]
34. Zhou, Z.-H.; Zhang, M.-L.; Chen, K.-J. A Novel Bag Generator for Image Database Retrieval with Multi-Instance Learning Techniques. In Proceedings of the 15th IEEE International Conference on Tools with Artificial Intelligence, Sacramento, CA, USA, 3–5 November 2003; pp. 565–569.
35. Jyothi, S.; Bhargavi, K. A Survey on Threshold Based Segmentation Technique in Image Processing. 26 K Bhargavi Jyothi. *Int. J. Innov. Res. Dev.* **2014**, *3*, 234–239.
36. Middleton, D. Channel Modeling and Threshold Signal Processing in Underwater Acoustics: An Analytical Overview. *IEEE J. Ocean. Eng.* **1987**, *12*, 4–28. [CrossRef]
37. Hong, L.; Wan, Y.; Jain, A. Fingerprint Image Enhancement: Algorithm and Performance Evaluation. *IEEE Trans. Pattern Anal. Mach. Intell.* **1998**, *20*, 777–789. [CrossRef]
38. Maini, R.; Aggarwal, H. A Comprehensive Review of Image Enhancement Techniques 2010. *arXiv* **2010**, arXiv:1003.4053.
39. Kingma, D.P.; Ba, J. Adam: A Method for Stochastic Optimization 2017. *arXiv* **2014**, arXiv:1412.6980.
40. Jaafar, B.; Mahersia, H.; Lachiri, Z. A Survey on Deep Learning Techniques Used for Breast Cancer Detection. In Proceedings of the 2020 5th International Conference on Advanced Technologies for Signal and Image Processing (ATSIP), Sfax, Tunisia, 2–5 September 2020; pp. 1–6.
41. Zhang, Z.; Sabuncu, M. Generalized Cross Entropy Loss for Training Deep Neural Networks with Noisy Labels. In Proceedings of the Advances in Neural Information Processing Systems, Montreal, QC, Canada, 3–8 December 2018; Curran Associates, Inc.: New York, NY, USA, 2018; Volume 31.

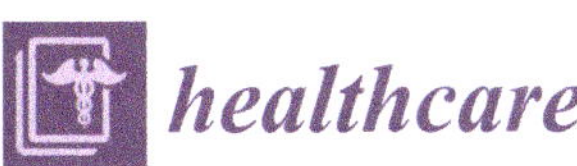

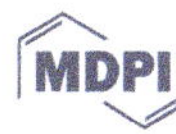

Article

Dysarthria Speech Detection Using Convolutional Neural Networks with Gated Recurrent Unit

Dong-Her Shih [1], Ching-Hsien Liao [1], Ting-Wei Wu [1,*], Xiao-Yin Xu [1] and Ming-Hung Shih [2]

[1] Department of Information Management, National Yunlin University of Science and Technology, Douliu 64002, Taiwan
[2] Department of Electrical and Computer Engineering, Iowa State University, 2520 Osborn Drive, Ames, IA 50011, USA
* Correspondence: wutingw@yuntech.edu.tw

Abstract: In recent years, due to the rise in the population and aging, the prevalence of neurological diseases is also increasing year by year. Among these patients with Parkinson's disease, stroke, cerebral palsy, and other neurological symptoms, dysarthria often appears. If these dysarthria patients are not quickly detected and treated, it is easy to cause difficulties in disease course management. When the symptoms worsen, they can also affect the patient's psychology and physiology. Most of the past studies on dysarthria detection used machine learning or deep learning models as classification models. This study proposes an integrated CNN-GRU model with convolutional neural networks and gated recurrent units to detect dysarthria. The experimental results show that the CNN-GRU model proposed in this study has the highest accuracy of 98.38%, which is superior to other research models.

Keywords: dysarthria; deep learning; convolutional neural network; gated recurrent units

Citation: Shih, D.-H.; Liao, C.-H.; Wu, T.-W.; Xu, X.-Y.; Shih, M.-H. Dysarthria Speech Detection Using Convolutional Neural Networks with Gated Recurrent Unit. *Healthcare* **2022**, *10*, 1956. https://doi.org/10.3390/healthcare10101956

Academic Editors: Mahmudur Rahman and Daniele Giansanti

Received: 12 September 2022
Accepted: 5 October 2022
Published: 7 October 2022

Publisher's Note: MDPI stays neutral with regard to jurisdictional claims in published maps and institutional affiliations.

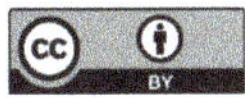

1. Introduction

Speech is an essential medium of communication between people. Once the medium of communication is abnormal, it increases the difficulty of communication. Furthermore, many people with neurological diseases often have this condition, which is called dysarthria. Dysarthria is mainly a symptom caused by neuromuscular control disorders that affect breathing, vocalization, resonance, articulation, and prosody [1]. Sounds can be too loud or too low due to damage to the central and peripheral nervous system, such as stroke, Parkinson's disease, brain trauma, brain tumors, cerebral palsy, amyotrophic lateral sclerosis, multiple sclerosis, muscular dystrophy, and other neurological diseases. The voice will also appear hoarse and lack tone changes. Hence, dysarthria patients are more likely to have abnormal speech characteristics [2].

Dysarthria may lead to social difficulties, a sense of isolation, and even world-weariness, depression, and other psychological problems [3]. Therefore, if there is no timely intervention and early rehabilitation training, it is easy to cause difficulties in disease course management, and the disease will continue to worsen. Doctors can subjectively diagnose dysarthria, but it is generally considered an expensive, laborious, and time-consuming test [4]. Therefore, having an objective and immediate automatic backing test is extremely important.

Deep learning has recently been popular and widely used in medical treatment. In order to objectively and accurately diagnose patients with dysarthria, more and more researchers are using deep learning to develop automatic detection of dysarthria. Many researchers use words for speech detection and different feature extraction methods to extract features from speech signals. For example, Vashkevich et al. [5] use pitch period entropy (PPE) based on acoustic features. Muhammad et al. [6] use glottal to noise excitation (GNE) and formant frequency or use spectrum and cepstrum for feature extraction. Other examples are mel-frequency cepstral coefficients (MFCC) [7], perception linear predictive coefficients (PLP), etc. [8]. After that, deep learning methods are used to detect dysarthria, such as convolutional neural network (CNN), CNN-LSTM (long short-term memory), and other models [9,10].

In the previous studies on the detection of dysarthria using the UA-Speech database, Narendra [10] selected the CNN-LSTM hybrid model as the classification model, but the accuracy of this model was only 77.57%. In order to improve the accuracy of the dysarthria detection model, this study used speech signals recorded by dysarthria patients and healthy people to undergo a short-time Fourier transform (STFT) and then convert the signals into spectrograms. After that, the signals were transformed into a spectral map, and mel-frequency cepstral coefficients (MFCC) were used to select the features. Finally, the accuracy in detecting dysarthria of the proposed CNN-GRU (gated recurrent unit) deep learning model was compared with three other models (CNN, LSTM, and CNN-LSTM).

2. Materials and Methods

2.1. Data Collection

Schlauch et al. [11] pointed out in their study that patients with dysarthria use words to make judgments with high recognition and low error rates. Therefore, this study chose words as the input audio samples for the subsequent studies. Our dataset was collected from the UA research database [12] (http://www.isle.illinois.edu/sst/data/UASpeech/, accessed on 18 February 2022). This database mainly contains the voice recordings of 15 dysarthria patients (4 women and 11 men) and 13 healthy subjects (4 women and 9 men), all of which were recorded by microphone and processed by noise removal. The subjects ranged in age from 18 to 58. A total of 455 words were recorded for each subject in the database, consisting of the numbers 1 to 10, the 26 letters, 19 computer command words, the 100 most common words from the Brown Corpus, and 300 words selected from the Project Gutenberg novel.

2.2. Method

The method proposed in this study consists of three stages, as shown in Figure 1. In the first stage, the original speech signal is transformed from the time domain to the frequency domain by a short-time Fourier transform. Second, the frequency domain data are extracted by mel-frequency cepstral coefficients. In the third stage, the features extracted from the mel spectrogram are used to detect and classify dysarthria patients and healthy people using the CNN-GRU model used in this study. In order to verify the excellence of the CNN-GRU deep learning model, this study also used the CNN model, LSTM model, and CNN-LSTM model to detect dysarthria and compare their results.

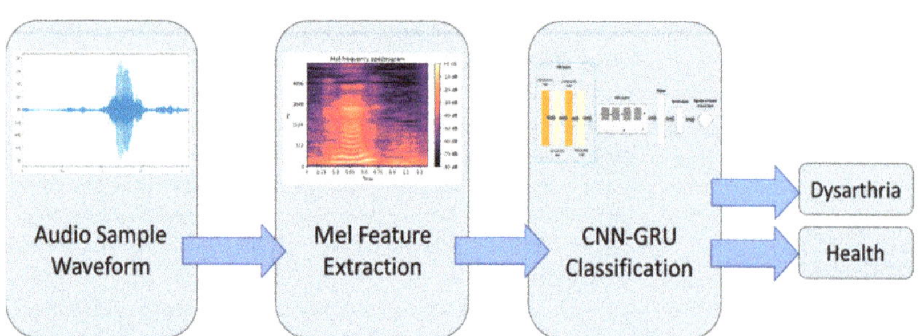

Figure 1. Flowchart of dysarthria detection.

2.3. Data Preprocessing

The audio could identify the amplitude waveform differences from the audio images of patients with dysarthria and healthy people through waveform images because people with dysarthria pronounce words more slowly and with a less steady pitch than healthy people. In general, the waveforms of the dysarthria patient (ID: dysarthria01) in Figure 2a are more irregular than the healthy subject (ID: healthy01) in Figure 2b. Audio waveforms can only show the relationship between amplitude and time. This study used Python Librosa to perform a short-time Fourier transform (STFT) of the audio. The short-time Fourier spectrograms of a dysarthria patient and a healthy subject are shown in Figure 3. From the spectrograms in Figure 3, it can be observed that the spectrum of subject dysarthria01 (Figure 3a) has more irregular frequencies and sudden higher decibels than the spectrum of subject healthy01 (Figure 3b).

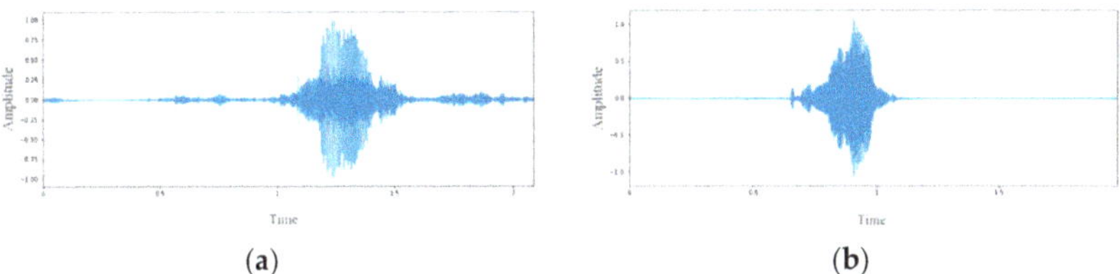

(a)   (b)

Figure 2. Amplitude waveforms of (**a**) dysarthria01 and (**b**) healthy01 subjects.

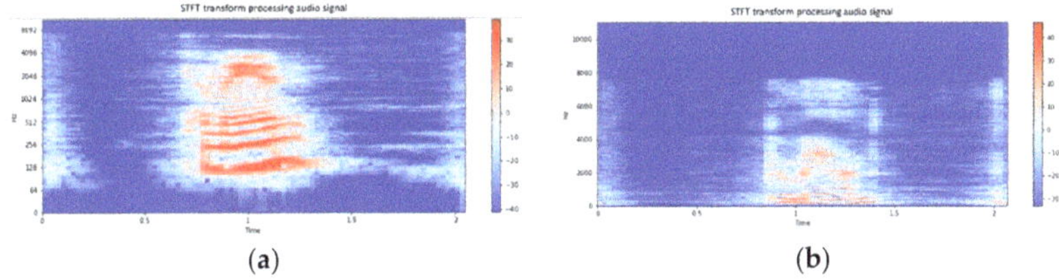

(a)   (b)

Figure 3. Short-time Fourier spectra of (**a**) dysarthria01 and (**b**) healthy01 subjects.

Short-time Fourier transform (STFT) was used to transform speech signals from the time domain to the frequency domain. The frame length of the speech in this study was between 10 and 30 ms, the sampling frequency was set to 8 KHz, and the window length was set to 128 to improve the resolution. The transformation of the STFT voice signal x(T) to the frequency domain is shown in Equation (1).

$$X(t, f) = \int_{-\infty}^{\infty} \omega(t - T)x(T)e^{-j2\pi fT}\, dT \tag{1}$$

2.4. Feature Selection

Mel-frequency cepstral coefficients (MFCC) are widely used in speech recognition. Mel is the scale of tone frequencies picked up by the human ear. The relationship between the mel spectrum (M) and frequency (Hz) is shown in Equations (2) and (3).

$$M(f) = 2595 \times \log_{10}(1 + f/700) \tag{2}$$

$$f = 700\left(10^{\frac{m}{2595}} - 1\right) \tag{3}$$

The power of spectrum, P(k), can be obtained from Equation (4).

$$P(k) = \frac{1}{N}\,|X(k)|^2 \tag{4}$$

The power of the spectrum, P(k), is passed through a series of mel-scale triangular filter windows to obtain the mel spectrum. The frequency, $H_m(k)$, of the triangular filter is calculated as shown in Equation (5).

$$H_m(k) = \begin{cases} 0, & \\ \dfrac{k-f(m-1)}{f(m)-f(m-1)} & \\ \dfrac{f(m+1)-k}{f(m+1)-f(m)}, & \\ 0, & \end{cases}$$
(5)

f(m) is the central frequency of the mel triangle filter. The logarithmic energy spectrum of each frame is S(m), which is obtained using a logarithmic process, as shown in Equation (6).

$$S(m) = \ln\left[\sum_{K=0}^{N-1} P(k)H_m(k)\right], 0 \leq m \leq M$$
(6)

$P(k)$ is the power spectrum, $H_m(k)$ is the filter window, and M is the number of filter windows.

This study used Librosa in Python software to extract the feature of the inverse coefficient of the mel frequency. Figure 4a is the voice signal. After extracting the speech signal samples and features, the mel spectrum is shown in Figure 4b.

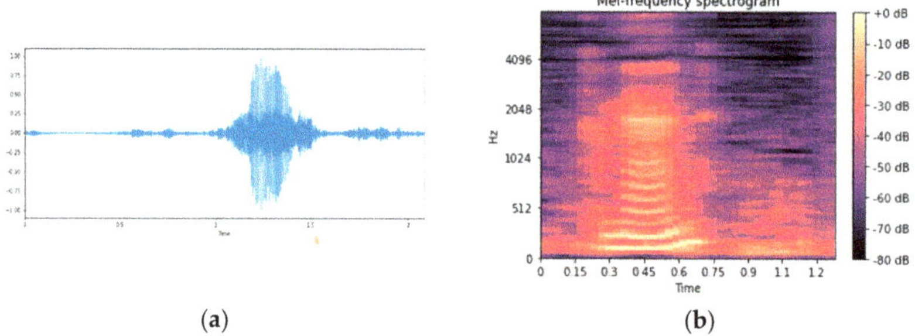

(**a**)   (**b**)

Figure 4. Feature extraction: (**a**) voice signal and (**b**) mel spectrum.

2.5. Deep Learning Algorithms

2.5.1. CNN Model

The CNN model can be used to detect the critical features of the audio in the audio message [13]. The CNN model's output and input architecture is shown in Figure 5, and the core CNN model is explained as follows.

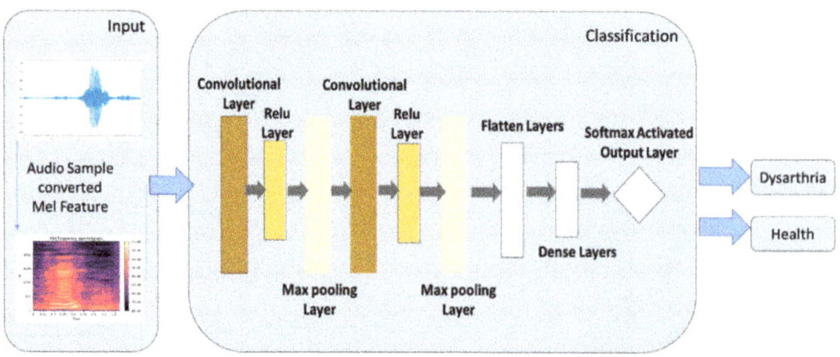

Figure 5. Architecture of CNN model.

The CNN model uses the convolution layer to retain the original feature arrangement of the image and obtain some essential features from the image. Then, the max pooling layer is used to select the more intense feature values from the essential features and shave the weak ones. This study adopted a rectified linear unit (Relu) to shave off the eigenvalues less than 0 at the site to speed up model training between the convolution layer and the max pooling layer. Then, the feature values are converted into one-dimensional data through the flatten layer to facilitate the subsequent use of the fully connected layer. Finally, the activation function of softmax is connected to the classification output. Table 1 shows the parameter settings of the CNN model in this study.

Table 1. Parameters of CNN model.

Network	Layer	No. of Activations	No. of Parameters
	Cov1	(27,27,32)	160
	Maxpooling1	(13,13,32)	0
CNN	Cov2	(12,12,64)	8256
	Maxpooling2	(6,6,64)	0
	Flatten	(2304)	0
	Dense	(3)	387

2.5.2. LSTM Model

Speech is a typical temporal signal because the LSTM (long short-term memory) model has a solid temporal ability [14]. The output and input architecture of the LSTM model is shown in Figure 6. In this study, a four-layer LSTM was used as the input layer, and a four-layer dropout was added to prevent the over-fitting problem of the model in the training process. A dense layer was used for dimensional transformation, and softmax was used for the classification output. Table 2 shows the parameter settings of the LSTM model in this study.

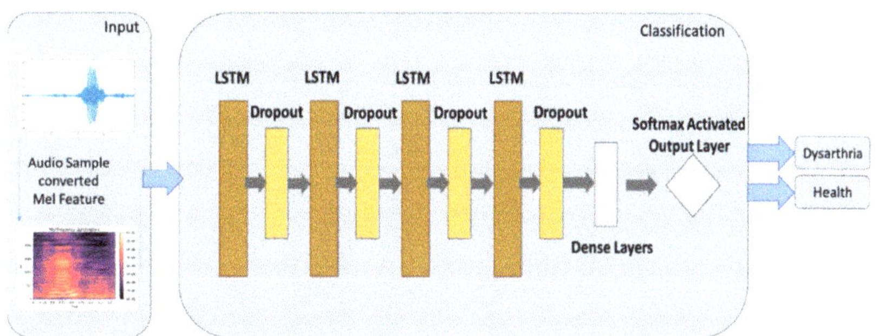

Figure 6. Architecture of LSTM model.

Table 2. Parameters of LSTM model.

Network	Layer	No. of Activations	No. of Parameters
	LSTM	(26,10)	480
	Dropout	(26,10)	0
	LSTM	(26,10)	840
	Dropout	(26,10)	0
LSTM	LSTM	(26,10)	840
	Dropout	(26,10)	0
	LSTM	(26,10)	840
	Dropout	(26,10)	0
	Dense	(26,2)	22

2.5.3. CNN-LSTM Model

CNN combined with LSTM for speech detection is an efficient and accurate hybrid model [15]. The CNN-LSTM model uses a CNN convolution layer to retain the original feature arrangement of an image and obtain some essential features from the image. Then, the max pooling layer is used to select the more intense feature values from the essential features and shave the weak ones. Between the convolution layer and the max pooling layer, the rectified linear unit (Relu) is provided to shave off feature values less than 0 to speed up model training. Then, the LSTM is connected to capture the temporal dynamics of the sequence, and the flatten layer is connected to convert the feature values into one-dimensional data. Finally, the activation function of softmax is connected for classification output. The output and input architecture of the CNN-LSTM model is shown in Figure 7. Table 3 shows the parameter settings of the CNN-LSTM model in this study.

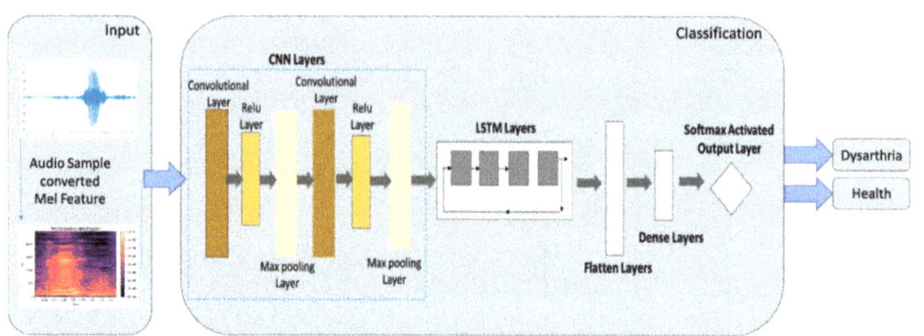

Figure 7. Architecture of CNN-LSTM model.

Table 3. Parameters of CNN-LSTM model.

Network	Layer	No. of Activations	No. of Parameters
	Cov1	(23,32)	320
	Maxpooling1	(11,32)	0
	Cov2	(11,64)	14,400
CNN-LSTM	Maxpooling2	(5,64)	0
	LSTM	(2,128)	20,608
	Flatten	(64)	0
	Dense	(44)	2860

2.5.4. CNN-GRU Model

CNN combined with GRU was used as a classifier in the study of speech enhancement [16] and android botnet detection [17]. In GRU architecture, fewer parameters need to be set, and it is simpler than LSTM architecture [18]. Therefore, it becomes natural to use GRU to optimize the CNN model. However, the combination of CNN and GRU is not always the same. This study combines the studies by Hasannezhad et al. [16] and Yerima et al. [17] into a different CNN-GRU model and writes programs through Python's Keras package for experiments. The output and input architecture of the CNN-GRU model proposed in this study is shown in Figure 8.

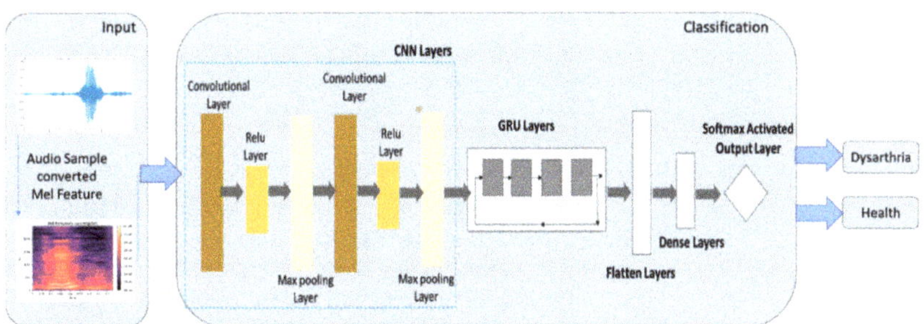

Figure 8. Architecture of CNN-GRU model.

The CNN-GRU model proposed in this study uses a CNN convolutional layer to retain the original feature arrangement of an image and obtains some essential features from the image. In addition, the max pooling layer is used to select more intense feature values from important features and shave the weak feature values, which can prevent the problem of over-fitting the model. Between the convolutional layer and the max pooling layer, this study also used a rectified linear unit to shave off the eigenvalues less than 0 to accelerate model training. Then, the eigenvalues are passed through the update gate and reset gate of the gated recurrent unit (GRU) to increase the calculation speed of the model so that the model can be more accurate. Then, the flattened layer is connected to convert the feature value into one-dimensional data, which is convenient for the subsequent use of the fully connected layer. Finally, softmax's activation function is connected as the output to determine whether the speech audio is dysarthria. Table 4 shows the parameter settings of the CNN-GRU model in this study.

Table 4. Parameters of CNN-GRU model.

Network	Layer	No. of Activations	No. of Parameters
	Cov1	(23,32)	320
	Maxpooling1	(11,32)	0
	Cov2	(11,64)	14,400
CNN-GRU	Maxpooling2	(5,64)	0
	GRU	(2,32)	15,552
	Flatten	(64)	0
	Dense	(44)	2860

2.6. Experimental Design

In this study, the word audio of dysarthria patients and healthy subjects was converted into the frequency domain by short-time Fourier transformation, and the mel spectrum image was extracted by the mel-frequency cepstral coefficient as the input of the four models, including CNN, LSTM, CNN-LSTM, and CNN-GRU, proposed in this study. The pros and cons of each model of dysarthria detection were compared by the training and validation sets and the test results. The dataset was divided into the training set, validation set, and test set, which were used for the training and testing of the four deep learning models. The distribution of data was based on the ratio of 0.7:0.15:0.15. In this study, after comprehensive area testing, these parameters had different batch sizes and learning rates to obtain the ideal solution. In the case of batch sizes of 32, 64, and 128, learning rates of 0.01, 0.001 and 0.0001, and Epoch = 10, the experimental results are described in detail in Section 3.

2.7. Model Evaluation

In this study, the effectiveness of the deep learning models was evaluated by the following evaluation indicators, which are generally divided into four types: (1) true positive (TP); (2) true negative (TN); (3) false positive (FP); and false negative (FN). The following evaluation metrics of the models can be calculated and learned based on those four results: accuracy, precision, recall, f1-score, and ROC curve [19,20].

3. Experimental Results

3.1. Experimental Results of CNN Model

The CNN model in this study adopted Keras in Python software for model training [21], and the classification results of the CNN model are shown in Table 5. If the CNN model parameter value of the batch size was set as 128 and the learning rate was set as 0.01, the highest accuracy of 94.36% of the CNN model could be obtained. In this study, Scikit-Learn [20] in Python software was used to draw the ROC curve of the CNN model in Figure 9, from which it can be seen that the AUC of the CNN model was 0.871 and the classification result of the model was good.

Table 5. Classification results of CNN model.

Model	Batch Size	Learning Rate	Accuracy%	Precision%	Recall	F1-Score
		0.1	70.00	70.01	0.7002	0.7010
	32	0.01	88.89	69.44	0.8334	0.7575
		0.001	75.00	75.50	0.7500	0.7506
		0.1	88.88	86.66	0.8333	0.8148
CNN	64	0.01	89.89	87.50	0.8333	0.8285
		0.001	86.67	79.99	0.666	0.6249
		0.1	93.33	87.50	0.8333	0.8285
	128	0.01	94.36	90.39	0.8913	0.8896
		0.001	94.35	86.66	0.8333	0.8148

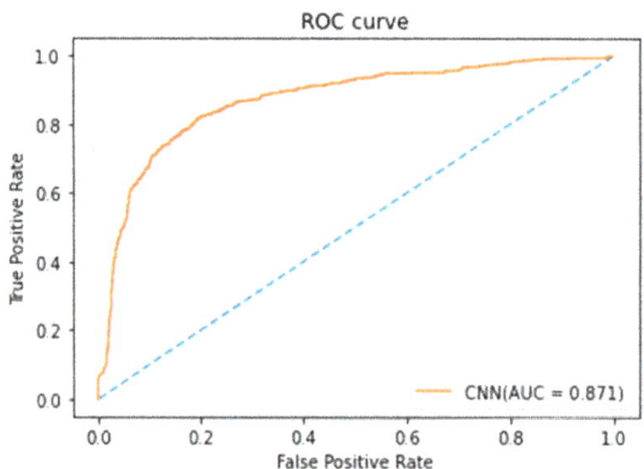

Figure 9. ROC curve of CNN model.

In this study, the epoch parameter value of the CNN model was set as 10, and the execution time, loss function, and accuracy of the CNN model can be observed from the training process in Table 6. The accuracy of the test set was 94.36%. It only took about 3 ms/epoch to train the CNN model. The accuracy of the final training set was 97.88%, and the loss function was 0.0638.

Table 6. Execution time, loss function, and accuracy of CNN model.

Epoch	Execution Time (ms)	Accuracy (Training) (%)	Loss Function	Accuracy (Validation) (%)	Accuracy (Testing) (%)
1	3	82.23	0.4972	45.40	79.20
2	3	91.26	0.2129	83.41	90.27
3	3	93.42	0.1674	90.35	91.27
4	3	94.18	0.1444	92.64	92.30
5	3	94.86	0.1314	93.90	93.24
6	3	95.77	0.1134	94.87	93.50
7	3	96.60	0.0931	95.48	93.52
8	3	96.52	0.0894	96.37	94.27
9	3	97.21	0.0757	97.13	94.20
10	3	**97.88**	**0.0638**	**97.53**	**94.36**

3.2. Experimental Results of LSTM Model

The LSTM model in this study adopted Keras in Python software for model training [21]. The classification results of the LSTM model are shown in Table 7. In the LSTM model, if the parameter value of the batch size was set as 64 and the learning rate was set as 0.001, the LSTM model could achieve the highest accuracy of 56.61%. In this study, Scikit-Learn [22] in Python software was used to draw the ROC curve of the LSTM model in Figure 10, from which it can be seen that the AUC of the LSTM model was 0.670 and the classification result of the model was, in general, poor. According to the area under an ROC curve (https://darwin.unmc.edu/dxtests/roc3.htm, accessed on 27 September 2022), AUC is divided into five grades: 0.9–1 = excellent (A), 0.80–0.90 = good (B), 0.70–0.80 = fair (C), 0.60–0.70 = poor (D), and 0.50–0.60 = fail (F). Since the AUC result of LSTM was 0.67, the effect of LSTM was considered poor in this study.

Table 7. Classification results of LSTM model.

Model	Batch Size	Learning Rate	Accuracy%	Precision%	Recall	F1-Score
		0.1	50.32	50.10	0.5001	0.5002
	32	0.01	54.29	53.21	0.5321	0.5321
		0.001	54.67	54.60	0.5460	0.5430
		0.1	55.60	44.21	0.4421	0.4421
LSTM	64	0.01	54.30	54.12	0.5420	0.5411
		0.001	56.61	53.43	0.5435	0.5324
		0.1	55.21	44.25	0.6550	0.5220
	128	0.01	56.60	43.21	0.5521	0.4201
		0.001	55.37	50.20	0.5020	0.5020

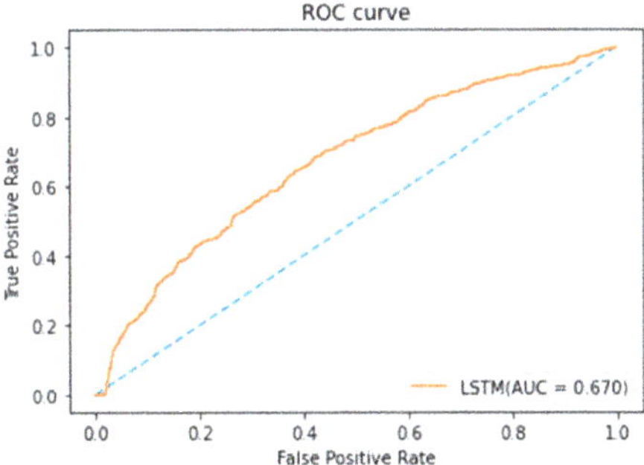

Figure 10. ROC curve of LSTM model.

In this study, the epoch parameter values of the LSTM model were set as 10, and the execution time, loss function, and accuracy of the LSTM model can be observed from the training process data in Table 8. The training time of the LSTM model was only about 2 ms/epoch. The accuracy of the final training set was 56.60%, and the loss function was 0.7562. The accuracy of the test set was 56.61%.

Table 8. Execution time, loss function, and accuracy of LSTM model.

Epoch	Execution Time (ms)	Accuracy (Training) (%)	Loss Function	Accuracy (Validation) (%)	Accuracy (Testing) (%)
1	2	53.32	0.7346	54.89	53.20
2	2	53.63	0.7360	55.32	53.39
3	2	54.29	0.7375	55.36	53.65
4	2	54.42	0.7394	54.22	54.30
5	2	54.68	0.7153	55.89	54.39
6	2	54.56	0.7163	55.90	54.37
7	2	54.04	0.7309	55.91	54.49
8	2	55.60	0.7316	56.01	55.60
9	2	56.01	0.7557	56.43	55.97
10	2	**56.60**	**0.7562**	**56.42**	**56.61**

3.3. Experimental Results of CNN-LSTM

The CNN-LSTM model in this study adopted Keras in Python software for model training [21]. The classification results of the CNN-LSTM model are shown in Table 9. In the CNN-LSTM model, if the parameter value of the batch size was set as 128 and the learning rate was set as 0.01, the CNN-LSTM model could obtain the highest accuracy of 78.57%. In this study, Scikit-Learn [22] in Python software was used to draw the ROC curve of the CNN-LSTM model in Figure 11. It can be seen from Figure 11 that the AUC of the CNN-LSTM model was 0.758 and the classification result of the model was above medium.

Table 9. Classification results of CNN-LSTM model.

Model	Batch Size	Learning Rate	Accuracy%	Precision%	Recall	F1-Score
		0.1	62.49	65.99	0.6666	0.6549
	32	0.01	66.66	64.44	0.6656	0.6333
		0.001	73.20	68.54	0.6756	0.6723
		0.1	70.21	69.45	0.6230	0.7165
CNN-LSTM	64	0.01	69.20	69.44	0.7333	0.7175
		0.001	73.21	67.54	0.6740	0.6740
		0.1	75.30	70.15	0.6563	0.7490
	128	0.01	78.57	70.33	0.6660	0.7500
		0.001	77.33	69.44	0.7475	0.7375

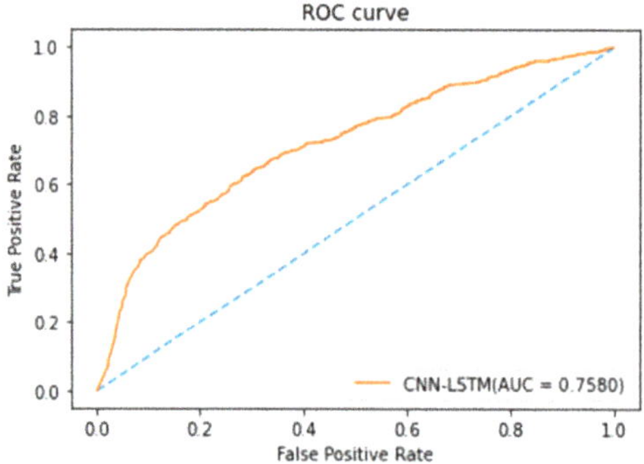

Figure 11. ROC curve of CNN-LSTM model.

In this study, the epoch parameter value of the CNN-LSTM model was set as 10, and the execution time, loss function, and accuracy of the CNN-LSTM model can be observed from the training process data in Table 10. The training time of the CNN-LSTM model was only about 4 to 8 ms/epoch, and the accuracy of the final training set was 84.21%. The loss function was 0.2745, and the test set accuracy was 78.57%.

Table 10. Execution time, loss function, and accuracy of CNN-LSTM model.

Epoch	Execution Time (ms)	Accuracy (Training) (%)	Loss Function	Accuracy (Validation) (%)	Accuracy (Testing) (%)
1	5	42.11	0.9493	50.00	43.50
2	5	57.89	0.8010	66.67	50.65
3	5	63.16	0.6720	66.67	51.27
4	8	73.68	0.5617	66.67	65.90
5	4	84.21	0.3367	83.33	66.37
6	8	84.21	0.3256	83.33	67.47
7	5	84.21	0.3102	83.33	70.30
8	6	84.21	0.3060	83.33	75.98
9	5	84.21	0.2665	83.33	76.35
10	5	**84.21**	**0.2745**	**83.33**	**78.57**

3.4. Experimental Results of CNN-GRU Model

The CNN-GRU model in this study adopted Keras in Python software for model training [21]. The classification results of the CNN-GRU model are shown in Table 11. In the CNN-GRU model, if the parameter value of the batch size was set as 128 and the learning rate was set as 0.001, the highest accuracy of 98.88% of the CNN-GRU model could be obtained. In this study, Scikit-Learn [22] in Python software was used to draw the research results of the ROC curve of the CNN-GRU model in Figure 12. It can be seen that the AUC of the CNN-GRU model was 0.916 and the model classification results were excellent.

Table 11. Classification results of CNN-GRU model.

Model	Batch Size	Learning Rate	Accuracy%	Precision%	Recall	F1-Score
		0.1	92.27	93.21	0.9121	0.9220
	32	0.01	94.52	94.23	0.9422	0.9420
		0.001	95.21	93.20	0.9220	0.9231
		0.1	96.41	95.51	0.9421	0.9412
CNN-GRU	64	0.01	96.70	90.24	0.9026	0.9633
		0.001	96.38	96.31	0.9427	0.9532
		0.1	97.71	96.21	0.9621	0.9621
	128	0.01	98.02	90.47	0.9030	0.9021
		0.001	98.88	91.47	0.9147	0.9147

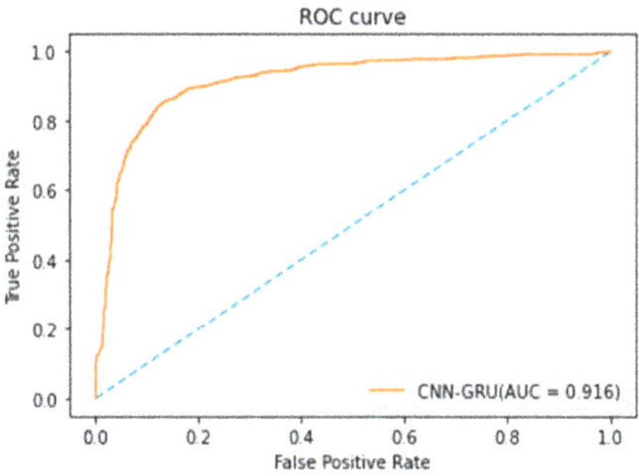

Figure 12. ROC curve of CNN-GRU model.

In this study, the epoch parameter value of the CNN-GRU model was set as 10, and the execution time, loss function, and accuracy of the CNN-GRU model can be observed from the training process data in Table 12. It only took about 2 ms/epoch to train the CNN-GRU model, and the accuracy of the final training set was 98.14%. The loss function was 0.1621, and its test set accuracy was 98.38%.

Table 12. Execution time, loss function, and accuracy of CNN-GRU model.

Epoch	Execution Time (ms)	Accuracy (Training) (%)	Loss Function	Accuracy (Validation) (%)	Accuracy (Testing) (%)
1	2	79.20	0.157	90.77	89.21
2	2	92.27	0.1267	91.08	90.20
3	2	94.52	0.3353	90.97	93.45
4	2	95.21	0.2937	91.16	94.60
5	2	96.41	0.1553	90.77	95.88
6	2	96.70	0.1274	91.36	97.56
7	2	96.83	0.1029	91.20	96.30
8	2	97.71	0.2396	91.40	97.13
9	2	98.02	0.2084	91.63	97.79
10	2	**98.14**	**0.1621**	**91.52**	**98.38**

4. Discussion of Results

According to the experimental results in Section 3, the accuracy values of the CNN model training set and test set were 97.88% and 94.36%, respectively (Table 6). The accuracy of the LSTM model training set and test set was 56.61% (Table 8). The accuracy of the CNN-LSTM model training set was 84.21%, and the accuracy of the test set was 78.57% (Table 10). Finally, the accuracy values of the proposed CNN-GRU model training set and test set were 98.14% and 98.38%, respectively (Table 12). Regardless of the perspective of the training set and test set, the CNN-GRU model had the highest accuracy. In the judgment of the AUC value, the AUC = 0.916 of the CNN-GRU model was also the highest, which was better than the other three models. Various evaluation metrics show that the proposed CNN-GRU model can obtain more accurate judgment results in dysarthria detection.

The results of this study are compared with other methods used in previous studies and summarized in Table 13. Hernandez et al. [23] used a method based on fricative sounds in audio messages and machine learning to detect dysarthria. The average spectral peak in the spectral moment was used to extract the fricatives in the audio as the input features of the SVM model, and the final SVM accuracy was 72%. Narendra et al. [24] trained an SVM with acoustic and glottic features extracted from coded speech utterances and their corresponding dysarthria/health labels and finally achieved an accuracy of 96.38% from the SVM. Narendra et al. [25] developed an end-to-end system that mainly used raw speech signals and raw glottal flow waveforms to detect dysarthria in two deep learning architectures: CNN-MLP and CNN-LSTM. The results showed that the original glottal flow waveform is more suitable for model training than the original speech signal, and the accuracy of CNN-MLP and CNN-LSTM were 87.93% and 77.57%, respectively. Rajeswari et al. [26] enhanced the speech by variational mode decomposition and fed the reconstructed signal to CNN for model training, and the final result achieved 95.95% accuracy. The accuracy of the CNN-GRU model proposed in this study was 98.38%, which is the highest in all studies. However, our approach may take a longer time to execute. After a survey, previous studies have not reported the execution times in their articles. Therefore, an execution time of 2 ms for our approach is appended in Table 13 for further investigation or comparison in the future.

Table 13. Performance comparison.

Author	Classification Method	Dataset	Accuracy (%)	Execution Time
Hernandez et al. (2019) [23]	SVM	UA-Speech	72%	-
Narendra et al. (2019) [24]	SVM	UA-Speech	96.38%	-
Narendra et al. (2020) [10]	CNN-MLP CNN-LSTM	UA-Speech	87.93% 77.57%	-
Rajeswari et al. (2022) [25]	CNN	UA-Speech	95.95%	-
Our Approach	CNN-GRU	UA-Speech	98.38%	2 ms

(-: indicates unknown or uncertainty).

5. Conclusions

Although dysarthria testing can be based on the subjective judgment of doctors, it is also regarded as a costly and time-consuming test, which can easily cause a medical burden. Therefore, if dysarthria testing can be conducted objectively, it can assist doctors in making an immediate judgment. This study used a CNN-GRU classification model for dysarthria detection. The results showed that the proposed CNN-GRU model can achieve the highest accuracy of 98.38%, which is better than the CNN, LSTM, CNN-LSTM models and those of other scholars.

The results can be used as an auxiliary diagnostic procedure for detecting dysarthria in the future. In future studies, it may be possible to take more eigenvalues from audio to analyze the severity level of dysarthria symptoms so that dysarthria detection can be further studied. In addition, others can also use the CNN-GRU model to detect other speech pathologies, such as Parkinson's disease, amyotrophic lateral sclerosis (ALS), and other symptoms of speech detection. The proposed architecture can also be used for image identification, just as Priyanka and Ganesan [26] used different data preprocessing methods combined with machine learning to classify the severity of dementia. Better prediction results may be achieved if the research is conducted through deep learning architecture.

In addition, most of the existing freely available dysarthric speech databases, including [12], contain speech data recorded from a small number of patients [24]. The volume of speech samples recorded in the dataset used in this study is quite large. However, the number of samples included is not immense, and there has been no continuous addition of samples, which makes it challenging to ensure that the results of this study can be adequately transferred to other clinical trials of dysarthria.

Author Contributions: Conceptualization, D.-H.S. and M.-H.S.; Data curation, C.-H.L. and X.-Y.X.; Formal analysis, T.-W.W. and X.-Y.X.; Funding acquisition, D.-H.S.; Investigation, C.-H.L., T.-W.W. and M.-H.S.; Methodology, D.-H.S. and X.-Y.X.; Project administration, D.-H.S.; Resources, C.-H.L.; Software, X.-Y.X.; Validation, C.-H.L.; Visualization, M.-H.S.; Writing—original draft, T.-W.W.; Writing—review and editing, M.-H.S. All authors have read and agreed to the published version of the manuscript.

Funding: This work was partially supported by the Taiwan Ministry of Science and Technology (grant MOST 111-2410-H-224-006). The funder had no role in study design, data collection and analysis, the decision to publish, or the preparation of the manuscript.

Institutional Review Board Statement: Not applicable.

Informed Consent Statement: Not applicable.

Data Availability Statement: Not applicable.

Conflicts of Interest: The authors declare no conflict of interest.

References

1. Gentil, M.; Pollak, P.; Perret, J. Parkinsonian dysarthria. *Rev. Neurol.* **1995**, *151*, 105–112. [PubMed]
2. Rampello, L.; Rampello, L.; Patti, F.; Zappia, M. When the word doesn't come out: A synthetic overview of dysarthria. *J. Neurol. Sci.* **2016**, *369*, 354–360. [CrossRef] [PubMed]

3. Marmor, S.; Horvath, K.J.; Lim, K.O.; Misono, S. Voice problems and depression among adults in the U nited S tates. *Laryngoscope* **2016**, *126*, 1859–1864. [CrossRef] [PubMed]
4. Van Nuffelen, G.; Middag, C.; De Bodt, M.; Martens, J. Speech technology-based assessment of phoneme intelligibility in dysarthria. *Int. J. Lang. Commun. Disord.* **2009**, *44*, 716–730. [CrossRef] [PubMed]
5. Vashkevich, M.; Rushkevich, Y. Classification of ALS patients based on acoustic analysis of sustained vowel phonations. *Biomed. Signal Process. Control* **2020**, *65*, 102350. [CrossRef]
6. Muhammad, G.; Alsulaiman, M.; Ali, Z.; Mesallam, T.A.; Farahat, M.; Malki, K.H.; Al-Nasheri, A.; Bencherif, M.A. Voice pathology detection using interlaced derivative pattern on glottal source excitation. *Biomed. Signal Process. Control* **2017**, *31*, 156–164. [CrossRef]
7. Karan, B.; Sahu, S.S.; Mahto, K. Parkinson disease prediction using intrinsic mode function based features from speech signal. *Biocybern. Biomed. Eng.* **2019**, *40*, 249–264. [CrossRef]
8. Moro-Velazquez, L.; Gómez-García, J.A.; Godino-Llorente, J.I.; Villalba, J.; Orozco-Arroyave, J.R.; Dehak, N. Analysis of speaker recognition methodologies and the influence of kinetic changes to automatically detect Parkinson's Disease. *Appl. Soft Comput.* **2018**, *62*, 649–666. [CrossRef]
9. Albaqshi, H.; Sagheer, A. Dysarthric Speech Recognition using Convolutional Recurrent Neural Networks. *Int. J. Intell. Eng. Syst.* **2020**, *13*, 384–392. [CrossRef]
10. Narendra, N.P.; Alku, P. Glottal source information for pathological voice detection. *IEEE Access* **2020**, *8*, 67745–67755. [CrossRef]
11. Schlauch, R.S.; Anderson, E.S.; Micheyl, C. A demonstration of improved precision of word recognition scores. *J. Speech, Lang. Heart Res.* **2014**, *57*, 543–555. [CrossRef]
12. Kim, H.; Hasegawa-Johnson, M.; Perlman, A.; Gunderson, J.; Huang, T.S.; Watkin, K.; Frame, S. Dysarthric speech database for universal access research. *Interspeech* **2008**, *2008*, 480. [CrossRef]
13. Dumane, P.; Hungund, B.; Chavan, S. Dysarthria Detection Using Convolutional Neural Network. *Techno-Soc.* **2021**, *2020*, 449–457. [CrossRef]
14. Gers, F.; Schmidhuber, E. LSTM recurrent networks learn simple context-free and context-sensitive languages. *IEEE Trans. Neural. Netw.* **2001**, *12*, 1333–1340. [CrossRef] [PubMed]
15. Chaiani, M.; Selouani, S.A.; Boudraa, M.; Yakoub, M.S. Voice disorder classification using speech enhancement and deep learning models. *Biocybern. Biomed. Eng.* **2022**, *42*, 463–480. [CrossRef]
16. Hasannezhad, M.; Ouyang, Z.; Zhu, W.P.; Champagne, B. An integrated CNN-GRU framework for complex ratio mask estimation in speech enhancement. In Proceedings of the 2020 Asia-Pacific Signal and Information Processing Association Annual Summit and Conference (APSIPA ASC), Auckland, New Zealand, 7–10 December 2020; pp. 764–768.
17. Yerima, S.; Alzaylaee, M.; Shajan, A.; Vinod, P. Deep learning techniques for android botnet detection. *Electronics* **2021**, *10*, 519. [CrossRef]
18. Chung, J.; Gulcehre, C.; Cho, K.; Bengio, Y. Empirical evaluation of gated recurrent neural networks on sequence modeling. *arXiv preprint* **2014**, arXiv:1412.3555.
19. Goutte, C.; Gaussier, E. A probabilistic interpretation of precision, recall and F-score, with implication for evaluation. In *European Conference on Information Retrieval*; Springer: Berlin/Heidelberg, Germany, 2005; pp. 345–359.
20. Fawcett, T. An Introduction to ROC analysis. *Pattern Recogn. Lett.* **2006**, *27*, 861–874. [CrossRef]
21. Vasilev, I.; Slater, D.; Spacagna, G.; Roelants, P.; Zocca, V. *Python Deep Learning: Exploring Deep Learning Techniques and Neural Network Architectures with Pytorch, Keras, and TensorFlow*; Packt Publishing Ltd.: Birmingham, UK, 2019.
22. Pedregosa, F.; Varoquaux, G.; Gramfort, A.; Michel, V.; Thirion, B.; Grisel, O.; Duchesnay, E. Scikit-learn: Machine learning in Python. *J. Mach. Learn. Res.* **2011**, *12*, 2825–2830.
23. Hernandez, A.; Chung, M. Dysarthria classification using acoustic properties of fricatives. In Proceedings of Seoul International Conference on Speech Sciences (SICSS) 2019, Seoul, Korea, 15–16 November 2019.
24. Narendra, N.; Alku, P. Dysarthric speech classification from coded telephone speech using glottal features. *Speech Commun.* **2019**, *110*, 47–55. [CrossRef]
25. Rajeswari, R.; Devi, T.; Shalini, S. Dysarthric Speech Recognition Using Variational Mode Decomposition and Convolutional Neural Networks. *Wirel. Pers. Commun.* **2021**, *122*, 293–307. [CrossRef]
26. Priyanka, A.; Ganesan, K. Radiomic features based severity prediction in dementia MR images using hybrid SSA-PSO optimizer and multi-class SVM classifier. *IRBM*, 2022; *in press*.

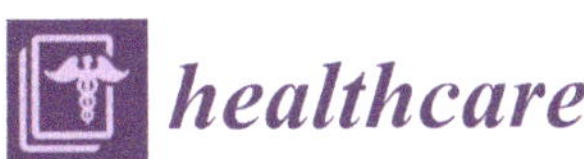

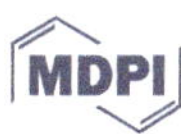

Article

Customized Deep Learning Classifier for Detection of Acute Lymphoblastic Leukemia Using Blood Smear Images

Niranjana Sampathila [1], Krishnaraj Chadaga [2], Neelankit Goswami [1], Rajagopala P. Chadaga [3], Mayur Pandya [2], Srikanth Prabhu [2,*], Muralidhar G. Bairy [1], Swathi S. Katta [4,*], Devadas Bhat [1] and Sudhakara P. Upadya [5]

[1] Department of Biomedical Engineering, Manipal Institute of Technology, Manipal Academy of Higher Education, Manipal 576104, Karnataka, India
[2] Department of Computer Science and Engineering, Manipal Institute of Technology, Manipal Academy of Higher Education, Manipal 576104, Karnataka, India
[3] Department of Mechanical & Industrial Engineering, Manipal Institute of Technology, Manipal Academy of Higher Education, Manipal 576104, Karnataka, India
[4] Manipal Institute of Management, Manipal Academy of Higher Education, Manipal 576104, Karnataka, India
[5] Manipal School of Information Science, Manipal Academy of Higher Education, Manipal 576104, Karnataka, India
* Correspondence: srikanth.prabhu@manipal.edu (S.P.); swathi.ks@manipal.edu (S.S.K.)

Abstract: Acute lymphoblastic leukemia (ALL) is a rare type of blood cancer caused due to the overproduction of lymphocytes by the bone marrow in the human body. It is one of the common types of cancer in children, which has a fair chance of being cured. However, this may even occur in adults, and the chances of a cure are slim if diagnosed at a later stage. To aid in the early detection of this deadly disease, an intelligent method to screen the white blood cells is proposed in this study. The proposed intelligent deep learning algorithm uses the microscopic images of blood smears as the input data. This algorithm is implemented with a convolutional neural network (CNN) to predict the leukemic cells from the healthy blood cells. The custom ALLNET model was trained and tested using the microscopic images available as open-source data. The model training was carried out on Google Collaboratory using the Nvidia Tesla P-100 GPU method. Maximum accuracy of 95.54%, specificity of 95.81%, sensitivity of 95.91%, F1-score of 95.43%, and precision of 96% were obtained by this accurate classifier. The proposed technique may be used during the pre-screening to detect the leukemia cells during complete blood count (CBC) and peripheral blood tests.

Keywords: acute lymphoblastic leukemia (ALL); blood smear; convolutional neural networks; deep learning; white blood cells

Citation: Sampathila, N.; Chadaga, K.; Goswami, N.; Chadaga, R.P.; Pandya, M.; Prabhu, S.; Bairy, M.G.; Katta, S.S.; Bhat, D.; Upadya, S.P. Customized Deep Learning Classifier for Detection of Acute Lymphoblastic Leukemia Using Blood Smear Images. *Healthcare* **2022**, *10*, 1812. https://doi.org/10.3390/healthcare10101812

Academic Editor: Mahmudur Rahman

Received: 18 August 2022
Accepted: 9 September 2022
Published: 20 September 2022

Publisher's Note: MDPI stays neutral with regard to jurisdictional claims in published maps and institutional affiliations.

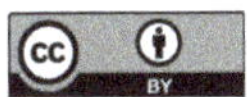

1. Introduction

ALL (acute lymphoblastic leukemia) is a lymphoid blood cell malignancy characterized by the development of immature lymphocytes [1]. These impaired white blood cells harm the entire body and bone marrow, putting the immune system as a whole at risk. It also inhibits the bone marrow's capacity to generate red blood cells and platelets. Moreover, these cancerous cells can enter the bloodstream and cause serious harm to other regions of the human body, including the kidney, liver, brain, heart, and other organs, leading to the development of other deadly cancers. According to worldwide statistics by the World Health Organization (WHO)'s International Agency for Research on Cancer, they reported 437,033 cases of leukemia and 303,006 deaths as of 2022 [2]. The blood, bone marrow, and extramedullary sites all show signs of ALL. This deadly disease is categorized into T-lymphoblastic leukemia (Pre-T), B-lymphoblastic leukemia (Pre-B), and B lymphoblastic leukemia according to the WHO [3]. Mature-B lymphoblastic leukemia starts in the bone marrow and releases an abnormal quantity of white blood cells in the body. These dangerously formed cells are known as "leukemia cells" or "blasts" because they are severely undeveloped. Leukemia is defined by Khullar et al. [4] as an abnormal hyper-proliferation of polymorphonuclear leukocytes which do not produce solid tumor aggregates, i.e., liquid cancer. Acute leukemia cells mature fast and can be lethal if not detected early.

Machine learning plays a crucial part in the battle against various life-threatening diseases [5–7]. It also contributes significantly to educational and clinical studies [8–11]. Machine learning has shown significant potential in medical, engineering, psychology, multi-disciplinary science, earth sciences, analytical practices, healthcare, and other domains. Using blood smear images and CNN, this article provides an early filtering deep learning strategy for correctly identifying ALL. This algorithm can assist clinicians and medical personnel to a great extent. Acute lymphoblastic leukemia is a type of malignant blood cell cancer that affects mostly children and adults above age 65 [12]. Leukocytes, or white blood cells as they are commonly known, make up around one percent of all blood cells. It can be observed in the bone marrow, blood, and extramedullary sites. In this type of leukemia, the immature leukocytes proliferate in the body rapidly, bringing about the need for early detection. Usually, the diagnosis is done based on a bone marrow examination. This method is labor intensive, time-consuming, and might generate inaccurate results. Therefore, there is a need for automation. The peripheral blood smear (PBS) test is one of the methods used for screening for leukemia [13]. A blood samples smear is analyzed under the microscope. To automate the process of recognizing ALL, deep learning is already playing a significant role and will help in reducing manual error as well. Over the past, several strategies have been used to expedite the process of detecting leukemia using artificial intelligence. Automated analysis of PBS introduces a smart healthcare facility by screening a sample for diagnostic purposes [14,15].

The robustness and the performance of CNN inspired our research [16]. Therefore, we developed customized CNN architecture to classify ALL. According to the study, the accuracy and reliability of prediction have improved. In this research, we put forward a method to automate the process of lymphoblast (blast cell) detection in the single-celled image to help in the detection of leukemia. The C_NMC_2019 dataset was used to train the model, and evaluation was done on the same [17]. Deep learning eliminates the process of using hand-crafted features for classification. Instead, the classification is done using a CNN custom architecture. The average accuracy after 6-fold cross-validation on the reliable C_NMC_2019 dataset was 94.95%. A computer-aided diagnosis system can be built on this result, potentially reducing the time and error required for the same.

Over the years, several approaches have been utilized to automate the process of detecting ALL. Many of the methodological procedures resolve the utilization of various machine and deep learning algorithms. Jiang et al. [18] applied Vit-CNN ensemble models to diagnose ALL. An accuracy of 89% was obtained by the models, claims the study. Differentiate enhancement-random sampling (DEES) was used to prevent data imbalance. Leukemia subtypes identification using CNN and microscopic images were researched in [19]. Two image datasets, ASH-Image-Bank and ALL-IDB, were used. The accuracy obtained was 88.25% and 81.74%, respectively. This algorithm was compared with traditional ML algorithms, such as support vector machine, decision tree, and KNN. Ghaderzadeh et al. [20] used CNN to diagnose B-ALL and its further subtypes from peripheral smear images. Ten well-known CNN architectures were used. These models obtained good results with accuracy, specificity, and sensitivity of 99.85%, 99.89%, and 99.82%, respectively. The dataset was obtained from a Kaggle competition. Qiao et al. [21] used a compact CNN model for the preliminary screening of ALL. Two datasets, APL-Cytomorphology-JHH and APL-Cytomorphology-LMU, were used. They yielded a precision of 96.53% and 99.20%, respectively. Promyelocytes were distinguished from normal leukocytes in this study. A hybrid model that used mutual information was used to diagnose ALL [22]. The Deep CNN classifier achieved an accuracy of 98%. The AA-IDB2 database was considered for this study. The rest of the research is described in Table 1.

Table 1. Existing research that diagnoses ALL using deep learning.

Research	Dataset	Algorithm Used	Accuracy	Precision	Recall
[23]	Three hybrid image databases	CNN and SVM	99%	99%	99%
[24]	IDB dataset	AlexNet	96%	-	96.74%
[25]	DNA Sequence images	CNN and other ML models	75%	-	-
[26]	GRTD dataset	VCGNet	96%	93%	93%
[27]	BCCD ALL-IDB2 JTSC CellaVision databases	CNN	97%	80%	94%
[28]	LISC and Dhruv dataset	CNN	97%	80%	94%
[29]	Amreek Clinical Laboratory	CNN	97.75%	-	-

To further support our claim, the remainder of the article has been described in the following manner. The following section describes the workflow and image processing techniques used, and the network is explained. Section 3 presents the results produced by our classifier along with a comparison of the outcomes from other established studies. The conclusion of the article is described in Section 4.

2. Materials and Methods

This section explains the workflow, image processing techniques, and network architecture developed for leukemia classification. Figure 1 describes the workflow followed for this work. After acquiring the dataset, augmentation was carried out to increase the size as well as the robustness. Afterward, the image data was fed to the CNN for automated feature extraction. The network then managed to classify the images as either ALL (blast cell) or HEM (healthy cell).

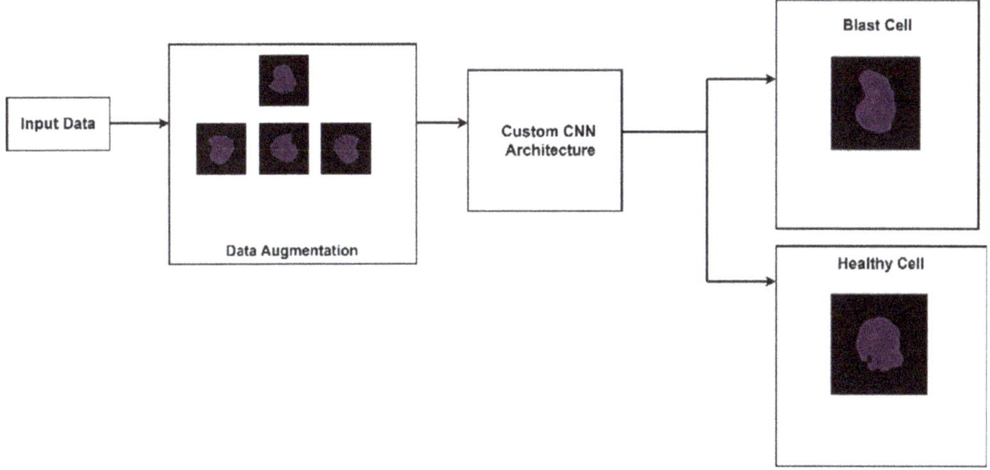

Figure 1. Leukemia screening system.

2.1. Input Data

The dataset used in this research belongs to the "ALL Challenge dataset of ISBI, 2019" [30–33]. The dataset contained cell images of both normal individuals and patients diagnosed with ALL. As shown in Figure 2, the original images acquired from a digital microscope having various components of the blood smear are pictorially depicted. The CNN classification for leukemia is done using segmented white blood cell (WBC) regions. This requires preprocessing and color segmentation. The subsequent process involves finding better segmentation of the region of interest. The HSI color space-based images of blood smears are shown in Figure 3. The white blood cells are seen to have better contrast than the other components of the image. To further localize the white blood cells, we selected the saturated component as it describes the intensity of the color, which is shown in Figure 4. This was then converted to a binary image by performing thresholding, as shown in Figure 5. The thresholding was performed on the gray scale image in such a way that all pixels in the range of (180–255) were converted to white, while all pixels belonging to values below this threshold were converted to black. The segmented image was obtained by finding the product of the original image and the segmented image, which was then used for further processing, as shown in Figure 6.

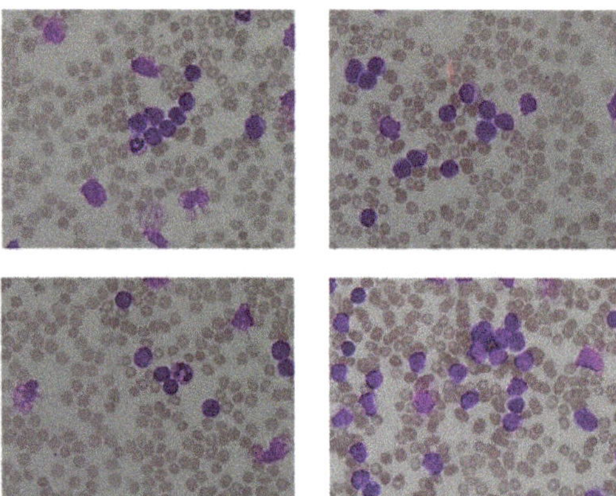

Figure 2. Original images.

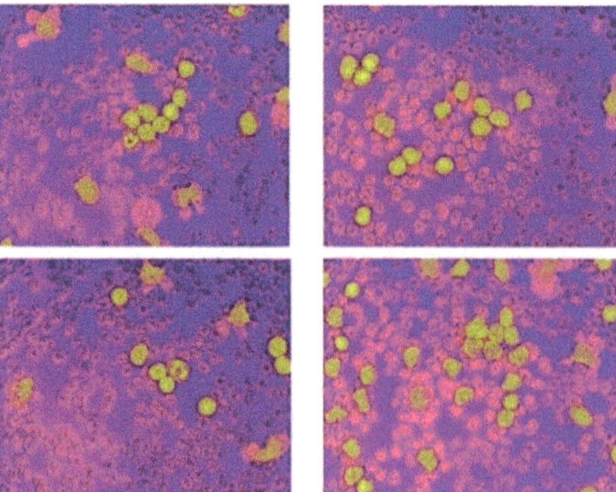

Figure 3. HIS color space.

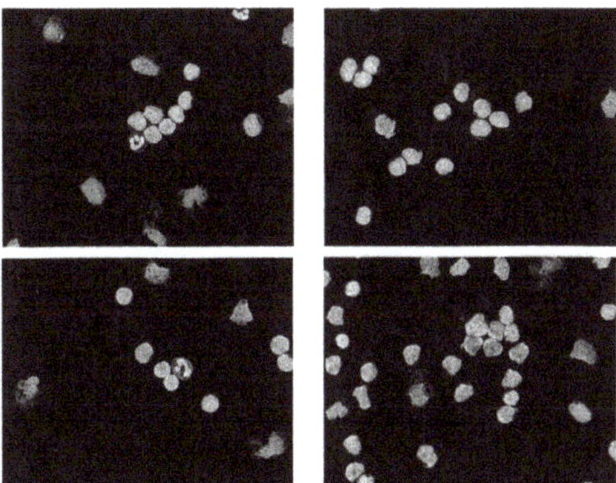

Figure 4. Saturation component.

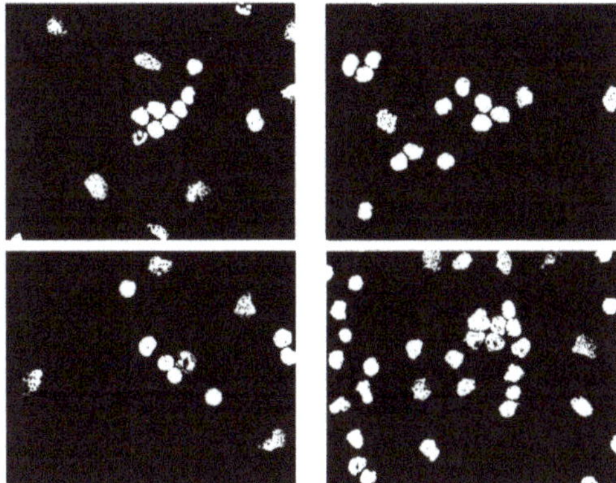

Figure 5. Images after thresholding.

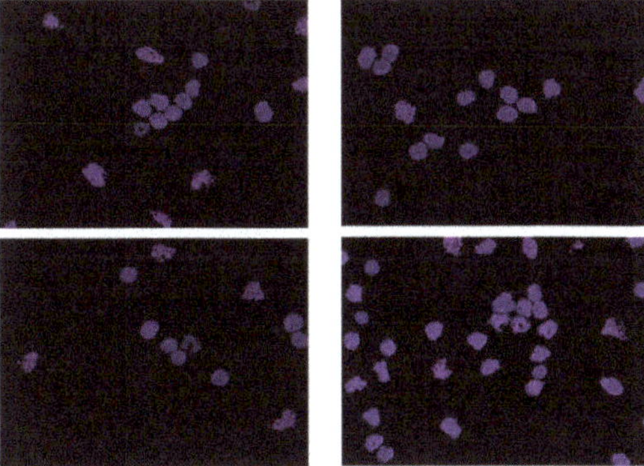

Figure 6. Image after segmentation.

A total of 10,661 images were collected from 73 participants from the C NMC 2019 dataset. There were 7272 images of blast cells and 3389 images of healthy cells in total. The images in this dataset were uniform with a size of $450 \times 450 \times 3$ and had been pre-processed such that only the object of interest (WBC) was included, and everything else was padded with black. Figure 2 gives a glimpse of the kind of image available in the dataset. Figure 7a represents the deadly blast cell, and Figure 7b represents a normal white blood cell. This dataset is reliable since expert oncologists have done the blast/healthy cell classification.

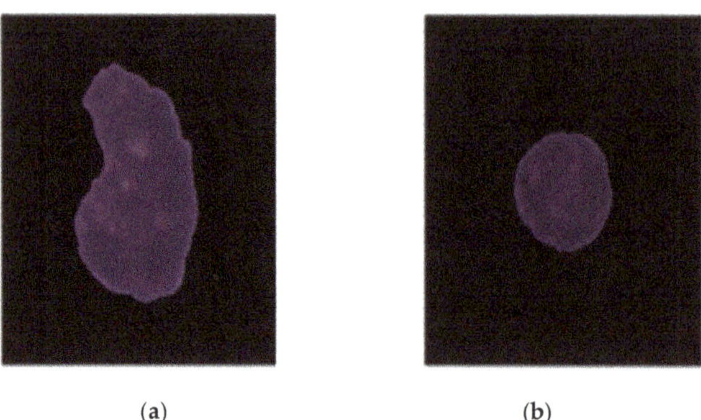

(**a**) (**b**)

Figure 7. Images in the dataset: (**a**) represent blast cells; (**b**) represent healthy cell.

2.2. Data Augmentation

The number of images provided to the neural network plays a pivotal role in the feature extraction procedure. The dataset used had an imbalance of images of the two classes. This would make the classification process biased. So, to remove the bias, the images were subjected to auto orientation and resizing. Augmentation steps involved were: (1) vertical horizontal flipping, (2) clockwise and anti-clockwise rotation, (3) random brightness adjustments (4) random Gaussian blur with the addition of pepper and salt noise to the pixels. The final dataset consisted of 12,000 images, with 6000 images in each class. Figure 8 depicts the images obtained after augmentation.

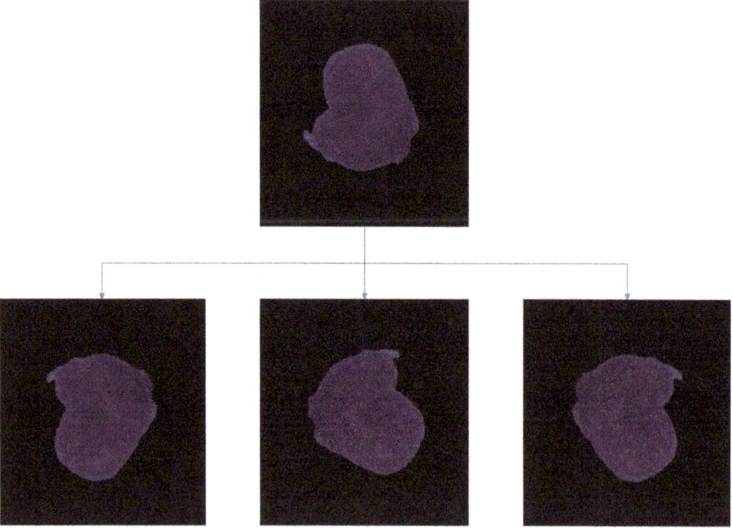

Figure 8. Original image of a blast cell and its augmented versions for the C_NMC_2019 dataset.

2.3. CNN

A CNN has a sequence of layers that transforms an image volume into an output volume through a differential function. The architecture of CNN was inspired by the visual cortex of the brain. The architecture fits the data better because of the reduction in the number of parameters involved and the reusability of weights. There are different types of layers in a convolutional network which includes: convolution (CONV), pooling (Pool), and fully connected (FC).

- **Convolution (CONV) Layers** The convolution layers are the main building blocks of CNN. They comprise a set of independent filters, which are convolved with the input volume to compute an activation map made of neurons. The useful features from the input images are extracted by having multilayered architecture. Each of the filters can be of a different type, and they extract different features, such as vertical lines, horizontal lines, and edges. The CNN layers help in extracting features through convolution. The extracted deep features play a major role in the decision support system.

The 2D convolution is given by Equations (1) and (2), respectively.

$$y[m, n] = x[m, n] \times h[m, n] \tag{1}$$

$$y[m, n] = \sum_{i=-\infty}^{\infty} \sum_{j=-\infty}^{\infty} x[i, j] . h[m - i, n - j] \tag{2}$$

where, $x[m, n]$ = Input
m, n = no. of rows, no. of columns, respectively
i, j = row index and column index
Similarly, the size of the image after convolution is given by Equation (3):

$$Size = \left\lfloor \left(\frac{m + 2p - n}{s} + 1, \ \frac{m + 2p - n}{s} + 1 \right) \right\rfloor \tag{3}$$

where m = number of input features
n = convolution kernel size
p = padding
s = stride

- **Pooling (POOL) Layer** Convolutional neural networks often use pooling layers to decrease the representation size and increase the speed of computation. A pooling layer summarizes the activities of local patches of nodes in the convolutional layers. Pooling can be done in two ways: max pooling and average pooling. In max pooling, the maximum value for each patch of the feature map is stored, while others are discarded. The intuition behind using max pooling is that the maximum value indicates that it has the most impact on that patch of the image. Hence other patches can be discarded. Average pooling follows a similar procedure, except in the place of the maximum value, the average value of the patch is taken, and all other values are discarded.
- **Fully Connected (FC) Layer** The FC input layer takes the output of the previous layers and turns them into a single vector that can be connected to the input layer of the next stage. This layer contains a softmax layer at the end, which predicts the correct label (0, 1). The output layer gives the final probability for each layer. The fully connected part of the CNN determines the most accurate weights by going through its backpropagation. The weights that each node receives are used to determine their respective labels. Since this project is of binary classification, the nodes will be prioritized to either 1 or 0.
- **Batch Normalization** Batch normalization decreases the covariance shift, i.e., the amount by which the hidden unit values shift. If the algorithm is trained to map some input x to some output y, and if the distribution of x changes, the prediction will not work as well, and retraining might be required. Batch normalization allows

the learning of each layer in an independent manner. An advantage of using batch normalization is that learning rates can be set higher as it makes sure that no activation goes high or low. Batch normalization also reduces overfitting as it has regularization effects. To improve the stability of the neural network, batch normalization normalizes the previous activation layers' outputs. This process adds two parameters to each layer, so the normalized output gets multiplied by gamma (standard deviation) and beta (mean). Mathematically, the mini-batch mean is given by Equation (4):

$$\mu_B = \frac{1}{m} \sum_{i=1}^{m} x_i \tag{4}$$

Mini-batch variance is shown in Equation (5):

$$\sigma_B^2 = \frac{1}{m} \sum_{i=1}^{m} (x_i - \mu_B) \tag{5}$$

Normalization is given by Equation (6):

$$\hat{x}_i = \frac{x_i - \mu_B}{\sqrt{\sigma_B^2 + \epsilon}} \tag{6}$$

- **Dropout** Deep neural networks are likely to overfit early on any given dataset. Dropout is a method of regularization that approximates training a large number of neural networks with different architectures in parallel. While training, some dropout layers are randomly ignored. This simulates the effect of a new layer, making the neural network treat it in such a way. In effect, each update is performed with a new outlook on the layer. This method makes the network more robust as additional noise is introduced.
- **Loss function** In the model, the categorical cross-entropy loss function has been implemented. The performance of this binary classification model, i.e., whose output lies between 0 and 1, is measured by the mentioned loss function. Categorical cross-entropy compares the distribution of the predictions with the true distribution, where the probability of the class in consideration is set to 1 and the probability of the other classes is set to 0. Categorical cross-entropy is shown in Equation (7):

$$L(y, \hat{y}) = -\sum_{j=0}^{M} \sum_{i=0}^{N} \left[y_{ij} \times \log\left(\hat{y}_{ij}\right) \right] \tag{7}$$

where y-hat is the predicted expected value and y is the observed value.
- **Optimizer** Optimizers are algorithms used to change the attributes of the neural network such as learning rates and weights to reduce the loss. In the model, adaptive movement estimation (Adam) has been incorporated. Adam is a combination of the root mean square propagation (RMSProp) and adaptive gradient algorithm (AdaGrad). The proposed convolution neural network architecture is shown in Figure 2, which makes use of pooling layers, fully connected layers, convolutional layers, dropout and batch normalization. Features were automatically extracted from the input images by the CNN. Feature extraction is then performed by the convolutional layers and the pooling layers. Four convolutional layers, four max-pooling layers, and 3 fully connected layers were utilized. Batch normalization and Dropout were applied to account for overfitting, vanishing, and exploding of gradients. This model consisted of 95,099,266 parameters in total. The architecture for the designed model can be seen in Figure 9. A more detailed description of the model is described in Table 2.

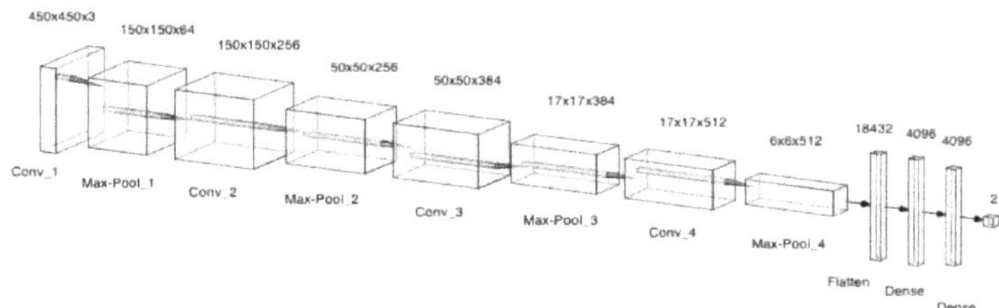

Figure 9. The architecture of CNN (ALLNet).

Table 2. ALLNet Architecture.

Layer (Type)	Layer Shape	Number of Parameters
Conv2D	(450, 450, 3)	1792
Max_Pooling_2D	(150, 150, 64)	-
Conv2D	(150, 150, 256)	147,712
Max_Pooling_2D	(50, 50, 256)	-
Conv2D	(50, 50, 384)	885,120
Batch_Normalization	(50, 50, 384)	1536
Max_Pooling	(17, 17, 384)	-
Dropout	(17, 17, 384)	-
Conv2D	(17, 17, 512)	1,769,984
Batch Normalization	(17, 17, 512)	2048
Max_Pooling	(6, 6, 512)	-
Dropout	(6, 6, 512)	-
Flatten	18,232	-
Dense	4096	75,501,568
Dropout	4096	-
Dense	4096	16,781,312
Dropout	4096	-
Output	2	8194

Total Parameters:—95,099,266, Trainable Parameters:—95,097,474, Non-Trainable Parameters:—1792.

3. Results and Discussion

3.1. Performance Metrics

The performance metrics estimated include *accuracy, precision, recall,* and *F1 score*:

Accuracy: It is the ratio of true positive predictions to the total number of predictions and is given in Equation (8).

$$Accuracy = \frac{True\ positive + True\ Negative}{Total\ samples} \times 100 \tag{8}$$

Precision: It is the ability of the model to return only relevant instances, given by Equation (9).

$$Precision = \frac{True\ Positive\ (TP)}{True\ Positive(TP) + False\ Positive\ (FP)} \times 100 \tag{9}$$

Recall: It is the ability of the model to identify all relevant instances, as shown in Equation (10). It emphasizes false negative results. This is also called the *true positive* rate or sensitivity.

$$Recall = \frac{True\ positive\ (TP)}{True\ positive\ (TP) + False Negative\ (FN)} \times 100 \tag{10}$$

Specificity: It is an important metric to identify false-positive results. It is described in Equation (11)

$$Specificity = \frac{True\ negative\ (TN)}{True\ negative\ (TN) + False\,Positive\ (FP)} \times 100 \tag{11}$$

F1 Score: This is the harmonic mean of precision and recall and is used to indicate a balance between *Precision* and *Recall* given in Equation (12).

$$F1\ Score = 2 \times \frac{Precision \times Recall}{Precision + Recall} \tag{12}$$

3.2. Model Evaluation

The ALL-NET architecture consists of a total of 4 convolution layers alternated with max pooling layers. This setting is followed by a total of 3 fully connected layers. The reason for keeping a max pooling layer after every convolution is to maintain the size of the processed image instance to a minimum. This can create a potential problem; if excessive max pooling is done, then it can lead to potential loss of information or patterns which are not spanning wide or large enough. Further, as observed previously, the data augmentation step has already added noise to the image; such noise can also affect the operation of max pooling. Batch normalization is carried out during every alternate max pooling to make sure that the flowing data is normalized, and every neuron has some input to give. Finally, to avoid any overfitting, we use dropout. These layers will ensure that multiple neurons having similar weight vectors are not unintentionally learning the same pattern in the given image instance. The learning rate was initially set at 1×10^{-3} initially, but it was observed that 1×10^{-5} gave marginally better improvement during the learning phase. The batch size for the training images was set at 16. While the epochs were initially selected to be in the range of 50 to 100. As pointed out in the later sections, it was found that the model was prone to overfitting if the epochs exceeded 70. Further fine tuning was done, and 65 epochs were finally selected as the final parameter value.

After image augmentation, the number of test instances available as blast cell images and healthy cell images was nearly the same as shown in Figure 10, so there was no imbalance present.

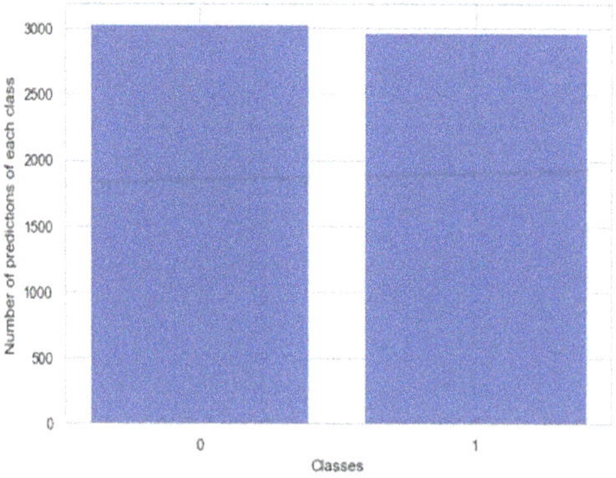

Figure 10. Prediction of classes of the test set images.

The dataset was initially given an 80–20 train test split. The training split was further divided into 5-fold cross-validation. The best performing fold was then utilized for testing on the holdout validation 20% test split. The cross-validation was carried out to overcome any potential overfitting which might occur due to model exposure to one class of images. The proposed model was trained on 12,000 images and tested on 2132 images. Each fold of

5-fold cv was learned by the model for 65 epochs. We performed validation of this model by training and conducting simultaneous test evaluations for five runs. The augmented data was mixed along with the original data to provide a wide range of training samples, this in turn helped the model to generalize better. The accuracy and loss curves are described in Figures 11 and 12, respectively. From Figure 12, it can be noticed how the categorical cross-entropy loss function starts to reduce heavily in the span of 10–30 epochs, referring to Figure 11. The model is performing adequately but stopping the model training at this point would have led to potential underfitting. Epochs after 35 do not provide many variations in the loss, and a steady decrease in the loss function can be observed. This behavior of the ALL-NET was observed in all 5 separate training processes. While increasing the epoch number from 65 would have led to a decrease in the loss even further as well as simultaneous increase in the accuracy, this would have led to overfitting as we will see when the model is evaluated against the holdout test set.

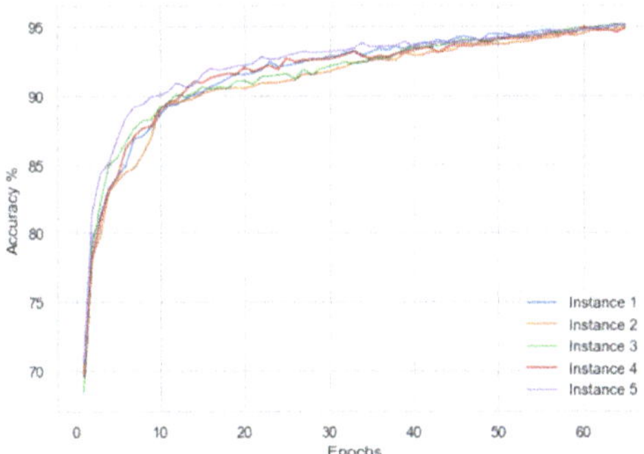

Figure 11. Accuracy for the five instances.

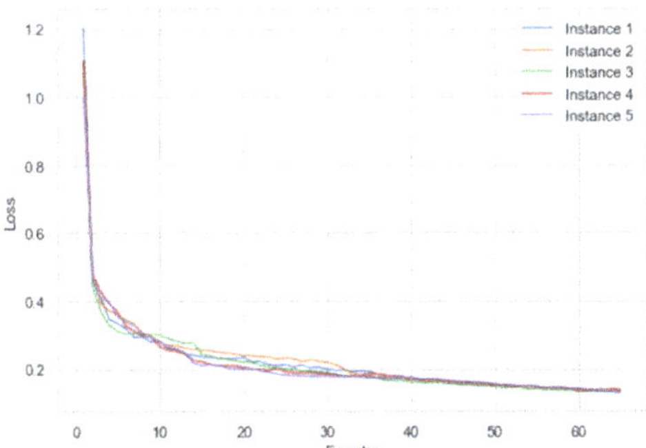

Figure 12. Training loss for the five instances.

During the first instance, the accuracy, specificity, recall, F1-score, and specificity were 94.94%, 94.87%, 94%, 94.96%, and 95.95%, respectively. When the model was run again, the accuracy, specificity, recall, F1-score, and specificity obtained were 94.5%, 95.8%, 93.2%, 93.2% and 96%, respectively. When the model was run the third time, the above metrics obtained were 94.72%, 95.8%, 93.2%, 93.2%, and 96%, respectively. During the fourth iteration, the accuracy, specificity, recall, F1-score, and specificity obtained were 95%, 95.91%, 94%, 94.96 and 95.95%, respectively. In the last instance, the above metrics obtained were 95.45%, 95%, 95.91%, 95.43% and 94.94%, respectively. In Figure 12, the accuracies are plotted against epochs.

A confusion matrix was used to evaluate the number of true predictions. The prediction was done on two possible classes, "ALL", i.e., blast cells and "HEM" i.e., healthy cells.

It was found that from a total of 2132 images, 1454 images were classified as blast cells, and 667 images were classified as healthy cells. During prediction, the model predicted 1996 images, i.e., 94.2% images correctly, and 5.8% images incorrectly. Predictions made per class are seen more clearly in Figure 13, depicting the confusion matrix. These results can be seen in Table 3.

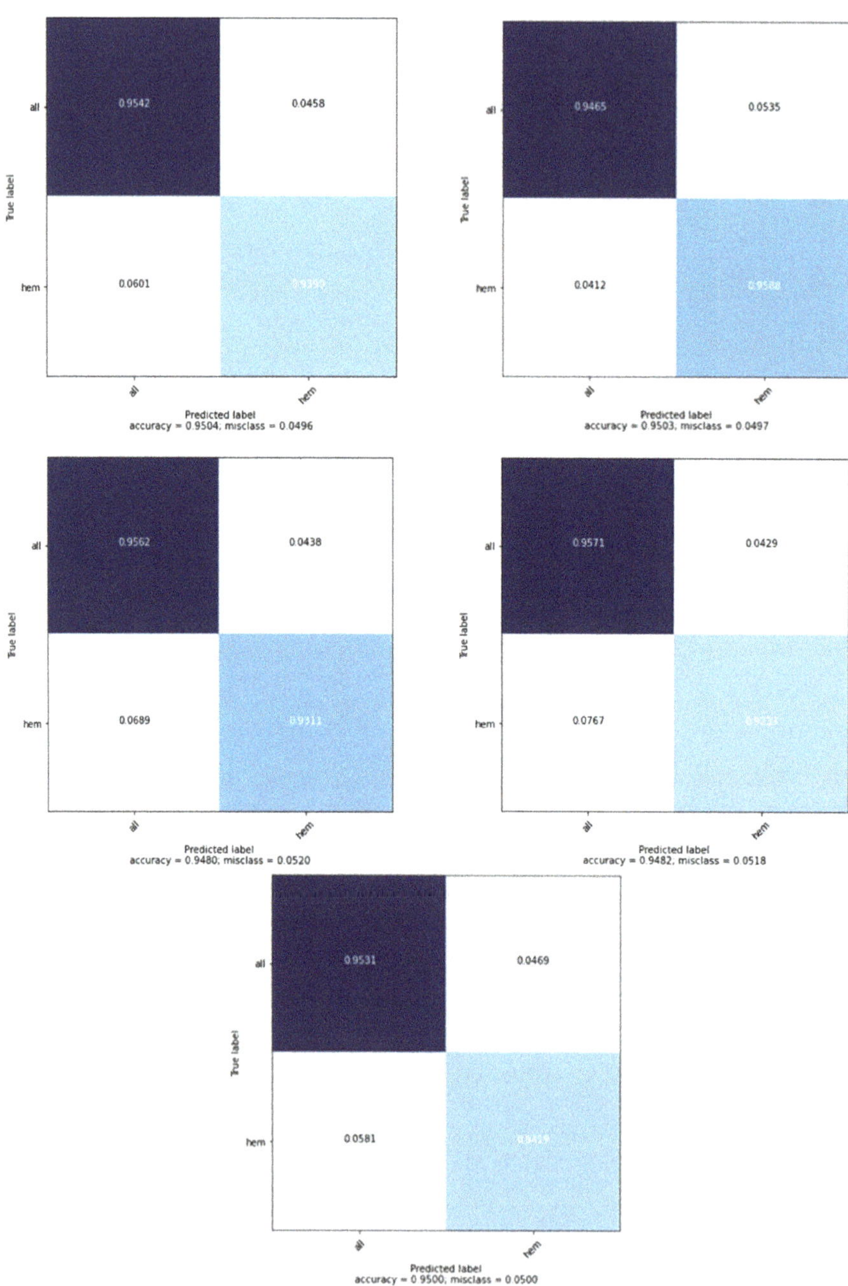

Figure 13. Confusion matrix of 5 separate training instances.

Table 3. Model evaluation results.

Instance	Accuracy (%)	Specificity (%)	Recall (%)	F1-Score (%)	Precision (%)	Matthews Correlation Coefficient (MCC)
Instance 1	94.94	94.87	94	94.96	95.95	89.42
Instance 2	94.5	95.8	93.2	93.2	96	89.53
Instance 3	94.72	95.8	93.2	93.2	96	88.76
Instance 4	95	95.91	94	94.96	95.95	88
Instance 5	95.45	95	95.91	95.43	94.94	89.5

Referring to Table 3, it can be observed that the F1 score obtained by the model in each of the 5 running instances is up to par if not better than the current existing model performances which we shall discuss later. A consistent F1 score of 90 plus in all 5 runs indicates that the balance between the precision and recall is maintained. The balance between precision and recall is quite pertinent for a model such as ALL-NET which can potentially serve as a preliminary screening tool. Our approach of using a simple CNN network for this dataset has given us good results across multiple performance metrics.

Many approaches have been used for classifying leukemia. Of the many, a few approaches with good performance are discussed in Table 4. ALL was diagnosed using Abunadi et al. [34] using an ensemble deep learning approach. The combined model achieved an accuracy of 100%. For the C_NMC_2019 dataset, Yongsheng Pan et al. [35] used a neighborhood correction technique to diagnose this fatal condition at an early stage. An accuracy of 92% was obtained by this algorithm. Khandekar et al. [36] used the YOLOe4 algorithm to diagnose this fatal disease. A maximum recall of 96% was obtained by the deep learning model. Christian et al. [37] have utilized an attention-based neural network to detect ALL. A maximum F1-score of 82% was obtained by this efficient algorithm. Table 4 demonstrates the comparison of prior research with the suggested technique for a similar dataset. The need for preprocessing to tackle this problem may be a slight drawback in this research. The model could be made more robust if it were trained with more data. The intelligent algorithms are promising with the optimized features for screening various problems in digital pathology [38–40]. The improved telehealth framework with the intelligent algorithm will enable the remote diagnosis facility [41–43].

Table 4. Comparison of results on the C_NMC_2019 dataset.

Reference	Method	Salient Features	Performance Measure
[34]	Bagging Ensemble with Deep Learning	Bagging ensembling was utilized	F1-score of 88%
[35]	Neighborhood Correction Algorithm	Fine-tuning a pre-trained residual network, constructing a Fisher vector based on feature maps, and correction using weighted majority.	F1-score of 92%
[37]	CNN	Regional proposal subnetwork.	F1-score of 83%
Proposed	CNN	Improved accuracy	F1-score of 96%

4. Conclusions

A method for early diagnosis of cancer from infinitesimal images of white blood cells using CNN has been proposed in this research. Since the deep learning approaches do not require manual feature engineering, the model performs exceptionally well when compared to traditional image processing techniques. The good performance of blast cell detection is supported by the accurate classification results. Maximum accuracy of 95% was obtained by the custom deep learning ALL-NET classifier. It operates on all data available rather than a portion specified by a feature vector, which is also a benefit. This work can help during the screening, reducing the rate of error, as well as decreasing the computational time. As a result, this research can be used to provide a theoretical framework for a diagnosis support tool for the detection of ALL. The future study includes expanding the dataset with noisy images with very little pre-processing, to address the problem of using actual medical images for prediction. Combining these models with explainabality models provides useful inferences to practitioners. Algorithms such as Yolov4, Resnet, and AlexNet can also be explored since they can perform better on these tasks.

Author Contributions: Conceptualization, N.S. and S.S.K.; formal analysis, K.C. and M.P.; investigation, N.S., K.C. and N.G.; methodology, K.C. and M.P.; project administration, S.S.K.; resources, M.G.B., D.B. and S.P.U.; software, N.G.; supervision, N.S.; visualization, N.S.; writing—original draft, N.S.; writing—review and editing, R.P.C., D.B., S.P.U. and S.P. All authors have read and agreed to the published version of the manuscript.

Funding: This research received no external funding.

Institutional Review Board Statement: Not applicable.

Informed Consent Statement: Not applicable.

Data Availability Statement: Not applicable.

Conflicts of Interest: The authors declare no conflict of interest.

References

1. Cho, S.; Tromburg, C.; Forbes, C.; Tran, A.; Allapitan, E.; Fay-McClymont, T.; Reynolds, K.; Schulte, F. Social adjustment across the lifespan in survivors of pediatric acute lymphoblastic leukemia (ALL): A systematic review. *J. Cancer Surviv.* **2022**, 1–17. [CrossRef] [PubMed]
2. Sheykhhasan, M.; Manoochehri, H.; Dama, P. Use of CAR T-cell for acute lymphoblastic leukemia (ALL) treatment: A review study. *Cancer Gene Ther.* **2022**, *29*, 1080–1096. [CrossRef]
3. Yang, H.; Zhang, H.; Luan, Y.; Liu, T.; Yang, W.; Roberts, K.G.; Qian, M.X.; Zhang, B.; Yang, W.; Perez-Andreu, V.; et al. Noncoding ge-netic variation in GATA3 increases acute lymphoblastic leukemia risk through local and global changes in chromatin con-formation. *Nat. Genet.* **2022**, *54*, 170–179. [CrossRef]
4. Khullar, K.; Plascak, J.J.; Parikh, R.R. Acute lymphoblastic leukemia (ALL) in adults: Disparities in treatment intervention based on access to treatment facility. *Leuk. Lymphoma* **2021**, *63*, 170–178. [CrossRef]
5. Chadaga, K.; Prabhu, S.; Vivekananda, B.K.; Niranjana, S.; Umakanth, S. Battling COVID-19 using machine learning: A review. *Cogent Eng.* **2021**, *8*, 1958666. [CrossRef]
6. Nono Djotsa, A.; Helmer, D.A.; Park, C.; Lynch, K.E.; Sharafkhaneh, A.; Naik, A.D.; Razjouyan, J.; Amos, C.I. Assessing Smoking Status and Risk of SARS-CoV-2 Infection: A Machine Learning Approach among Veterans. *Healthcare* **2022**, *10*, 1244. [CrossRef]
7. Chadaga, K.; Prabhu, S.; Umakanth, S.; Bhat, V.K.; Sampathila, N.; Chadaga, R.P.; Prakasha, K.K. COVID-19 Mortality Prediction among Patients Using Epidemiological Parameters: An Ensemble Machine Learning Approach. *Eng. Sci.* **2021**, *16*, 221–233. [CrossRef]
8. Absar, N.; Das, E.K.; Shoma, S.N.; Khandaker, M.U.; Miraz, M.H.; Faruque, M.R.I.; Tamam, N.; Sulieman, A.; Pathan, R.K. The Efficacy of Machine-Learning-Supported Smart System for Heart Disease Prediction. *Healthcare* **2022**, *10*, 1137. [CrossRef]
9. Chadaga, K.; Prabhu, S.; Bhat, K.V.; Umakanth, S.; Sampathila, N. Medical diagnosis of COVID-19 using blood tests and machine learning. In *Journal of Physics: Conference Series, Proceedings of the 1st International Conference on Artificial Intelligence, Computational Electronics and Communication System (AICECS 2021), Manipal, India, 28–30 October 2021*; IOP Publishing: Bristol, UK, 2022; Volume 2161. [CrossRef]
10. Lukić, I.; Ranković, N.; Savić, N.; Ranković, D.; Popov, Ž.; Vujić, A.; Folić, N. A Novel Approach of Determining the Risks for the Development of Hyperinsulinemia in the Children and Adolescent Population Using Radial Basis Function and Support Vec-tor Machine Learning Algorithm. *Healthcare* **2022**, *10*, 921. [CrossRef]
11. Yamamoto, N.; Sukegawa, S.; Watari, T. Impact of System and Diagnostic Errors on Medical Litigation Outcomes: Machine Learning-Based Prediction Models. *Healthcare* **2022**, *10*, 892. [CrossRef]
12. Li, L.; Han, C.; Yu, X.; Shen, J.; Cao, Y. Targeting AraC-Resistant Acute Myeloid Leukemia by Dual Inhibition of CDK9 and Bcl-2: A Systematic Review and Meta-Analysis. *J. Healthc. Eng.* **2022**, *25*, 2022. [CrossRef] [PubMed]
13. Rastogi, P.; Khanna, K.; Singh, V. LeuFeatx: Deep learning–based feature extractor for the diagnosis of acute leukemia from mi-croscopic images of peripheral blood smear. *Comput. Biol. Med.* **2022**, *19*, 105236. [CrossRef] [PubMed]
14. Alqudah, R.; Suen, C.Y. Intensive Survey on Peripheral Blood Smear Analysis Using Deep Learning. In *Advances in Pattern Recognition and Artificial Intelligence*; World Scientific Publishing: Singapore, 2022; pp. 23–45. [CrossRef]
15. Toret, E.; Demir-Kolsuz, O.; Ozdemir, Z.C.; Bor, O. A Case Report of Congenital Thrombotic Thrombocytopenic Purpura: The Peripheral Blood Smear Lights the Diagnosis. *J. Pediatr. Hematol.* **2022**, *44*, e243–e245. [CrossRef] [PubMed]

16. Roy, A.M. An efficient multi-scale CNN model with intrinsic feature integration for motor imagery EEG subject classification in brain-machine interfaces. *Biomed. Signal Process. Control* **2022**, *74*, 103496. [CrossRef]
17. Anagha, V.; Disha, A.; Aishwarya, B.Y.; Nikkita, R.; Biradar, V.G. Detection of Leukemia Using Convolutional Neural Network. In *Emerging Research in Computing, Information, Communication and Applications*; Springer: Singapore, 2021; pp. 229–242. [CrossRef]
18. Jiang, Z.; Dong, Z.; Wang, L.; Jiang, W. Method for Diagnosis of Acute Lymphoblastic Leukemia Based on ViT-CNN Ensemble Model. *Comput. Intell. Neurosci.* **2021**, *23*, 2021. [CrossRef]
19. Ahmed, N.; Yigit, A.; Isik, Z.; Alpkocak, A. Identification of leukemia subtypes from microscopic images using convolutional neu-ral network. *Diagnostics* **2019**, *9*, 104. [CrossRef]
20. Ghaderzadeh, M.; Aria, M.; Hosseini, A.; Asadi, F.; Bashash, D.; Abolghasemi, H. A fast and efficient CNN model for B-ALL diag-nosis and its subtypes classification using peripheral blood smear images. *Int. J. Intell. Syst.* **2021**, *37*, 5113–5133. [CrossRef]
21. Qiao, Y.; Zhang, Y.; Liu, N.; Chen, P.; Liu, Y. An End-to-End Pipeline for Early Diagnosis of Acute Promyelocytic Leukemia Based on a Compact CNN Model. *Diagnostics* **2021**, *11*, 1237. [CrossRef]
22. Jha, K.K.; Dutta, H.S. Mutual Information based hybrid model and deep learning for Acute Lymphocytic Leukemia detection in single cell blood smear images. *Comput. Methods Programs Biomed.* **2019**, *179*, 104987. [CrossRef]
23. Vogado, L.H.; Veras, R.M.; Araujo, F.H.; Silva, R.R.; Aires, K.R. Leukemia diagnosis in blood slides using transfer learning in CNNs and SVM for classification. *Eng. Appl. Artif. Intell.* **2018**, *72*, 415–422. [CrossRef]
24. Shafique, S.; Tehsin, S. Acute lymphoblastic leukemia detection and classification of its subtypes using pretrained deep convo-lutional neural networks. *Technol. Cancer Res. Treat.* **2018**, *26*, 1533033818802789.
25. He, J.; Pu, X.; Li, M.; Li, C.; Guo, Y. Deep convolutional neural networks for predicting leukemia-related transcription factor bind-ing sites from DNA sequence data. *Chemom. Intell. Lab. Syst.* **2020**, *199*, 103976. [CrossRef]
26. Sahlol, A.T.; Kollmannsberger, P.; Ewees, A.A. Efficient classification of white blood cell leukemia with improved swarm optimi-zation of deep features. *Sci. Rep.* **2020**, *10*, 1–11. [CrossRef]
27. Banik, P.P.; Saha, R.; Kim, K.-D. An Automatic Nucleus Segmentation and CNN Model based Classification Method of White Blood Cell. *Expert Syst. Appl.* **2020**, *149*, 113211. [CrossRef]
28. Naz, I.; Muhammad, N.; Yasmin, M.; Sharif, M.; Shah, J.H.; Fernandes, S.L. Robust Discrimination of Leukocytes Protuberant Types for Early Diagnosis Of Leukemia. *J. Mech. Med. Biol.* **2019**, *19*, 1950055. [CrossRef]
29. Rehman, A.; Abbas, N.; Saba, T.; Rahman, S.I.U.; Mehmood, Z.; Kolivand, H. Classification of acute lymphoblastic leukemia using deep learning. *Microsc. Res. Tech.* **2018**, *81*, 1310–1317. [CrossRef]
30. Gupta, A.; Gupta, R. ALL Challenge Dataset of ISBI 2019 [Data Set]. In *The Cancer Imaging Archive*; National Cancer Institute: Bethesda, ME, USA, 2019. [CrossRef]
31. Gehlot, S.; Gupta, A.; Gupta, R. SDCT-AuxNet: DCT augmented stain deconvolutional CNN with auxiliary classifier for cancer diagnosis. *Med. Image Anal.* **2020**, *61*, 101661. [CrossRef]
32. Goswami, S.; Mehta, S.; Sahrawat, D.; Gupta, A.; Gupta, R. Heterogeneity Loss to Handle Intersub-ject and Intrasubject Variability in Cancer, ICLR workshop on Affordable AI in healthcare. *arXiv* **2020**, arXiv:2003.03295.
33. Clark, K.; Vendt, B.; Smith, K.; Freymann, J.; Kirby, J.; Koppel, P.; Moore, S.; Phillips, S.; Maffitt, D.; Pringle, M.; et al. The Cancer Imaging Archive (TCIA): Maintaining and Operating a Public Information Repository. *J. Digit. Imaging* **2013**, *26*, 1045–1057. [CrossRef]
34. Abunadi, I.; Senan, E.M. Multi-Method Diagnosis of Blood Microscopic Sample for Early Detection of Acute Lymphoblastic Leukemia Based on Deep Learning and Hybrid Techniques. *Sensors* **2022**, *22*, 1629. [CrossRef]
35. Pan, Y.; Liu, M.; Xia, Y.; Shen, D. Neighborhood-Correction Algorithm for Classification of Normal and Malignant Cells. In *ISBI 2019 C-NMC Challenge: Classification in Cancer Cell Imaging*; Springer: Singapore, 2019; pp. 73–82.
36. Khandekar, R.; Shastry, P.; Jaishankar, S.; Faust, O.; Sampathila, N. Automated blast cell detection for Acute Lympho-blastic Leukemia diagnosis. *Biomed. Signal Processing Control* **2021**, *68*, 102690. [CrossRef]
37. Marzahl, C.; Aubreville, M.; Voigt, J.; Maier, A. Classification of Leukemic B-Lymphoblast Cells from Blood Smear Microscopic Images with an Attention-Based Deep Learning Method and Advanced Augmentation Techniques. In *ISBI 2019 C-NMC Challenge: Classification in Cancer Cell Imaging*; Springer: Singapore, 2019; pp. 13–22.
38. Mayrose, H.; Sampathila, N.; Bairy, G.M.; Belurkar, S.; Saravu, K.; Basu, A.; Khan, S. Intelligent algorithm for detection of dengue using mobilenetv2-based deep features with lymphocyte nucleus. *Expert Syst.* **2021**, e12904. [CrossRef]
39. Krishnadas, P.; Sampathila, N. Automated Detection of Malaria implemented by Deep Learning in Pytorch. In Proceedings of the 2021 IEEE International Conference on Electronics, Computing and Communication Technologies (CONECCT), Bangalore, India, 9–11 July 2021; pp. 01–05. [CrossRef]
40. Mayrose, H.; Niranjana, S.; Bairy, G.M.; Edwankar, H.; Belurkar, S.; Saravu, K. Computer Vision Approach for the detection of Thrombocytopenia from Microscopic Blood Smear Images. In Proceedings of the 2021 IEEE International Conference on Electronics, Computing and Communication Technologies (CONECCT), Bangalore, India, 9–11 July 2021; pp. 1–5. [CrossRef]
41. Upadya, P.S.; Sampathila, N.; Hebbar, H.; Pai, B.S. Machine learning approach for classification of maculopapular and vesicular rashes using the textural features of the skin images. *Cogent Eng.* **2022**, *9*, 2009093. [CrossRef]

42. Cornish, T.C.; McClintock, D.S. Whole Slide Imaging and Telepathology. In *Whole Slide Imaging*; Springer: Cham, Switzerland, 2021; pp. 117–152. [CrossRef]
43. Díaz, D.; Corredor, G.; Romero, E.; Cruz-Roa, A. A web-based telepathology framework for collabora-tive work of pathologists to support teaching and research in Latin America. In *Sipaim–Miccai Biomedical Workshop*; Springer: Cham, Switzerland; pp. 105–112.

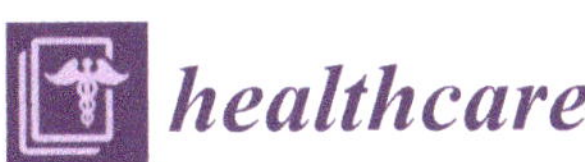
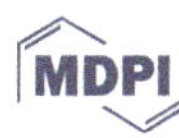

healthcare

Article

Rapid Polyp Classification in Colonoscopy Using Textural and Convolutional Features

Chung-Ming Lo [1,2], Yu-Hsuan Yeh [1], Jui-Hsiang Tang [3], Chun-Chao Chang [3,4,5] and Hsing-Jung Yeh [1,3,4,5,*]

[1] Graduate Institute of Biomedical Informatics, College of Medical Science and Technology,
     Taipei Medical University, Taipei 110301, Taiwan
[2] Graduate Institute of Library, Information and Archival Studies, National Chengchi University,
     Taipei 116011, Taiwan
[3] Division of Gastroenterology and Hepatology, Department of Internal Medicine, School of Medicine,
     College of Medicine, Taipei Medical University, Taipei 110301, Taiwan
[4] Division of Gastroenterology and Hepatology, Department of Internal Medicine,
     Taipei Medical University Hospital, Taipei 110301, Taiwan
[5] Research Center for Digestive Medicine, Taipei Medical University, Taipei 110301, Taiwan
*   Correspondence: yiew@ms10.hinet.net

Abstract: Colorectal cancer is the leading cause of cancer-associated morbidity and mortality worldwide. One of the causes of developing colorectal cancer is untreated colon adenomatous polyps. Clinically, polyps are detected in colonoscopy and the malignancies are determined according to the biopsy. To provide a quick and objective assessment to gastroenterologists, this study proposed a quantitative polyp classification via various image features in colonoscopy. The collected image database was composed of 1991 images including 1053 hyperplastic polyps and 938 adenomatous polyps and adenocarcinomas. From each image, textural features were extracted and combined in machine learning classifiers and machine-generated features were automatically selected in deep convolutional neural networks (DCNN). The DCNNs included AlexNet, Inception-V3, ResNet-101, and DenseNet-201. AlexNet trained from scratch achieved the best performance of 96.4% accuracy which is better than transfer learning and textural features. Using the prediction models, the malignancy level of polyps can be evaluated during a colonoscopy to provide a rapid treatment plan.

Keywords: colorectal cancer; colon polyp; image features; convolutional neural network

Citation: Lo, C.-M.; Yeh, Y.-H.; Tang, J.-H.; Chang, C.-C.; Yeh, H.-J. Rapid Polyp Classification in Colonoscopy Using Textural and Convolutional Features. *Healthcare* **2022**, *10*, 1494. https://doi.org/10.3390/healthcare10081494

Academic Editor: Mahmudur Rahman

Received: 10 July 2022
Accepted: 5 August 2022
Published: 8 August 2022

Publisher's Note: MDPI stays neutral with regard to jurisdictional claims in published maps and institutional affiliations.

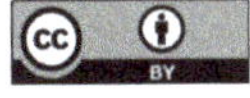

1. Introduction

Colorectal cancer (CRC) is the fourth most common newly diagnosed internal cancer in the United States [1]. In 2020, a total of 147,951 new CRC cases and 52,300 CRC-related deaths were reported [1] including gastrointestinal (GI)-related mortality [2]. The risk factors are drinking, consuming red meat or processed meat, sedentary lifestyle, overweight, smoking, and genetic diseases [3,4]. However, genetic problems are less than five percent associated with colorectal cancer [4,5]. The possible symptoms are blood in the stool, changes in bowel habits, weight loss, anemia, palpable mass, tenesmus, abdominal pain, and fatigue. A CRC often transforms from a benign polyp to a malignant one [6] and can be diagnosed by biopsy-proven tissues obtained from colonoscopy.

Polyp types can be divided into non-neoplastic (hyperplastic polyp) and neoplastic polyps (adenomatous polyps) [7,8]. Hyperplastic polyps are usually <1 cm in diameter and may occur in any part of the colon. They are not considered cancerous unless they are sufficiently large to cause complications, and regular examination is recommended in most cases. Adenomatous polyps including adenomas and sessile serrated adenomas (SSA) are important precursors to the majority of colorectal cancer. Adenomas can be classified into tubular adenomas, tubular villous adenomas, and villous adenomas according to pathological classification. Other rare polyp types are hamartoma, pseudopolyps, carcinoid tumors, and connective tissue polyps. About 70% of colorectal cancers originate from adenomatous polyps. In contrast, 25–30% of colorectal cancer cases originate from sessile serrated polyps [9]. If colon adenomas are removed by colonoscopic polypectomy, patient mortality is reduced by 53% [10]. Consequently, detecting early colon adenomatous polyps is critical. In addition, for patients receiving anticoagulants or antiplatelet drugs such as warfarin and clopidogrel, immediate polypectomy is not recommended [11]. The colonoscopy examination simultaneously provides more information of polyp location and surrounding tissues for further treatment.

With the advancements in image processing and machine learning techniques, computer-aided diagnosis (CAD) systems have been proposed to assist clinical endoscopists to identify different polyp types. In the past literature, CAD has been used by radiologists to detect colon polyps in computed tomography colonoscopy [12–14]. Additionally, the automatized colon polyp segmentation was proposed [15]. Recently, deep convolutional neural networks (DCNN) have been proposed for colon polyp detection [16,17], segmentation [15,18], and classification [19]. The key point of detection task is rapid. The DCNN used in the studies can detect polys in real-time such as YOLO algorithms [16]. To correctly analyze the polyp tissues, segmentation DCNN including Focus U-Net was introduced for a better region extraction. As a CAD used in malignancy evaluation, handcrafted and DCNN features were proposed to classify polyps in endoscopy video-frames [19]. As a widely used artificial intelligence technique, DCNN has been used in the various applications in colonoscopy. For polyp classification, both handcrafted and DCNN features are useful. However, more complete comparisons should be established to realize the differences between features, networks, and training methods.

To explore the classification ability and practice in clinical diagnosis, this study proposes using CAD systems for polyp classification in colorectal endoscopic images using different features, networks, and training methods. As shown in Figure 1, various approaches were implemented to compare the performance differences between machine learning using texture features and deep learning using DCNN features, the performance differences between DCNN models trained from scratch and transfer learning, and the performance differences between various DCNN architectures. The evaluations would provide more practical advice to gastroenterologists about using CAD for polyp classification in colonoscopy.

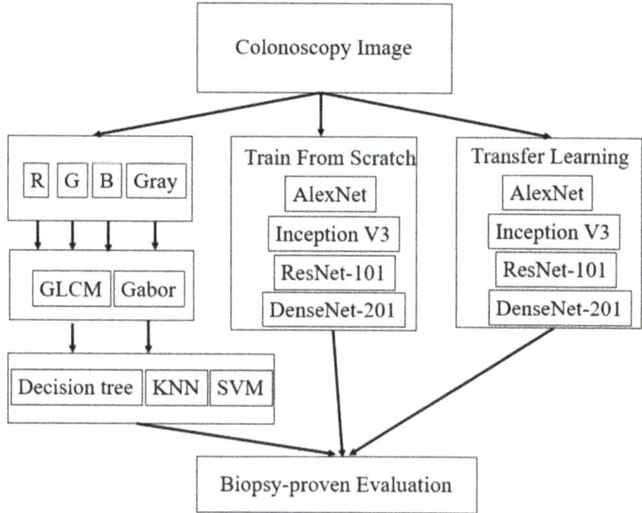

Figure 1. The flowchart of the polyp classification using colonoscopy image features.

2. Materials and Methods

2.1. Colonoscopy Images

This study was approved by the Taipei Medical University-Joint Institutional Review Board (approval no. N201802090c) on 25 February 2020. Between 1 January 2018 and 27 July 2018, 1991 patients underwent colonoscopy. Among these patients, 1053 were biopsy-proven to have hyperplastic polyps, 732 had adenomas, and 206 had adenocarcinomas. The collected colonoscopic images were obtained from colonoscopes (GF-260 and 290, Olympus Corporation, Tokyo, Japan). The format is jpeg with the resolution of 640 × 480. A total of 24 bits were used for a pixel, that is, the bit depth is 8 for red (R), green (G), and blue (B) individually. In the experiment, patient information was removed and the image part completely presenting the lesion area was cropped to be the image database (Figure 2). Colon polyps usually have a round or oval shape under the colonoscopy.

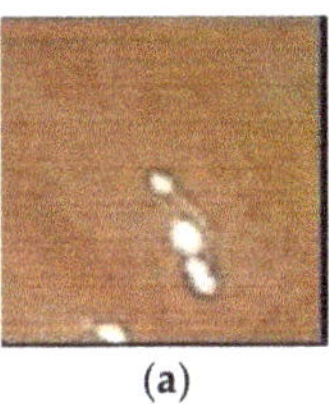 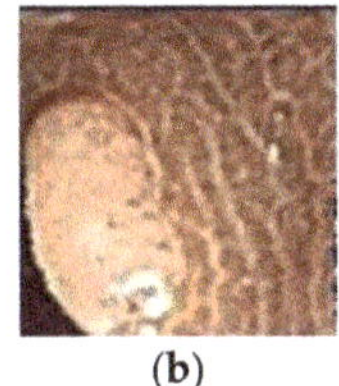 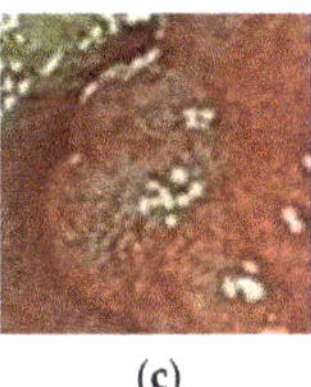

(**a**)   (**b**)   (**c**)

Figure 2. Different polys in endoscopy: (**a**) hyperplastic polyps; (**b**) adenoma; (**c**) adenocarcinoma.

2.2. Textural Features

Quantitative image analysis is widely used for medical images [20,21]. Some image features used to interpret lesions can be observed by human eyes such as color and shape. Other types of image features, such as texture features, are subtle and denote correlations between adjacent pixel values. From the visual observations by gastroenterologists, the lesions including hyperplastic polyps, adenomas, and adenocarcinomas as shown in Figure 1 are mass-like which is related to shape properties. However, the light reflection and color differences would cause the lesion segmentation to fail. That is, shape features are hardly well-extracted from poor segmentations. Alternatively, texture features have been proposed in many CAD systems. The pattern differences between various lesion types can provide meaningful diagnostic information including the light reflection appeared in endoscopy. To present the color difference among different types, the texture features can be extracted from different color channels individually. Thus, texture features including gray-level co-occurrence matrix (GLCM) [13] and Gabor features [22,23] were proposed in this study for polyp classification.

GLCM extracts the spatial correlations between pixels as the texture features. First, the co-occurrence matrices $p = [p\,(i, j\,|\,d, \theta)]$ are generated to show the frequencies of each pixel (a gray value i) and its neighboring pixels (a gray value j) between a distance d and the direction θ. In the experiment, one pixel distance and four directions: $0°, 45°, 90°$, and $135°$ were calculated and averaged. From the matrices, the statistical analysis was performed to generate various GLCM features including energy, mean, entropy, variance, correlation, homogeneity, dissimilarity, angular second moment, and contrast [24]. These features present the value distributions of tissue patterns. Energy is the sum of the squares of the element values in GLCM. If all values in the matrix are equal, the energy value is small; conversely, if some of the values are large and others are small, the energy value is large. A large energy value indicates a more uniform and regularly changing texture pattern. Entropy expresses the randomness of the texture. It is a measure of the amount of information that the image has, such as uniformity or complexity. When all pixels in the matrix are almost equal, entropy is relatively large. Contrast reflects the distribution of values in the matrix. The greater the grayscale difference, the greater the contrast and the greater this value. Correlation reflects the similarity among pixels in the matrix in a row or column. Homogeneity can also be called variance, which reflects the homogeneity of the image texture. If the image texture is uniform between different areas and changes slowly, homogencity will be greater, and if the image texture is nonuniform, homogeneity will be smaller.

Gabor wavelets generated another kind of texture feature used in the experiment which was performed after Fourier transform. The Gabor features with various scales and rotations were then created. A total of forty Gabor filters in five scales and eight orientations are shown in Figure 3. In the Gabor, the sinusoid frequency and the orientation of the normal to the parallel stripes are used [25]. Gabor filter is used for extracting texture patterns such as what kind of specific frequency appeared in the pixels. The Gabor filter has real and imaginary parts that are orthogonal to each other. The two can form a complex number or be used alone. After filtering the real part, the image will be smooth, and filtering the imaginary part is used to detect edges [22]. Texture features are extracted from gray-scale pixels. Thus, from the original color image, three color channels were separated into three images. Additionally, a transformed gray-scale image was generated. As shown in Figure 4, four images were used for the feature extraction.

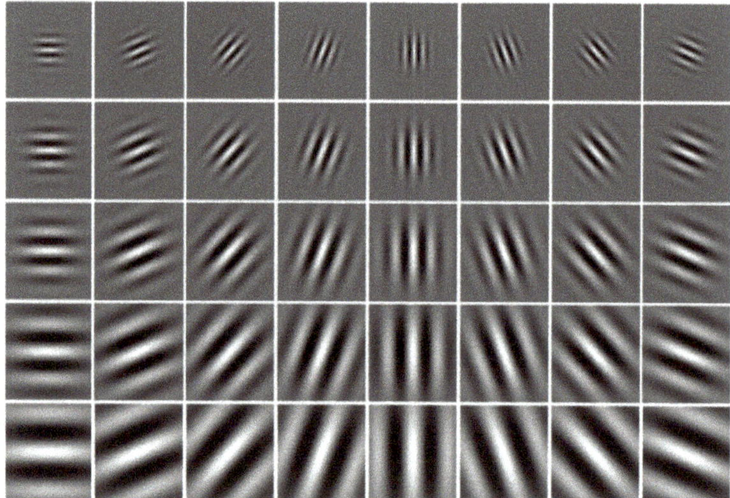

Figure 3. The 40 Gaussian filters in the Gabor filter.

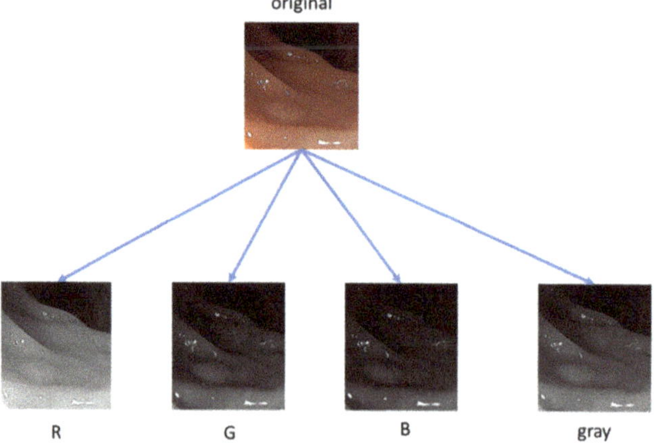

Figure 4. Conversions from a RGB image to four R, G, B, and grayscale images.

The use of GLCM and Gabor textures refer to the complete domain information, that is, Gabor collected texture features from frequency domain and GLCM collected texture features from spatial domain. After feature extraction, these image features were combined in various classifiers to establish polyp classification models. A total of 21 classifiers from MATLAB Classification Learner App (MathWorks Inc., Natick, MA, USA) were used, including decision tree, logistic regression, k-nearest neighbors, ensemble learning, and support vector machine (SVM). A 10-fold cross-validation was also performed during model evaluation. Principal component analysis was also performed as the feature selection to deal with the numerous features. The analysis reduces the feature dimension but minimizes information loss at the same time [26].

2.3. DCNN Features

DCNN is a deep learning technique that uses multiple layers in artificial neural networks [27–29]. Image features can be automatically extracted through linear or nonlinear transformation in multiple processing layers [30]. DCNN does not require the quantification of features through artificially designed metrics [31]. The essential architecture is composed of convolution layers, pooling layers, fully connective layers, and activation (nonlinearity) layers. The success of DCNN is based on the statistical analysis used to generate feature rules for the following classification. Therefore, a large number of input images is necessary. However, in the medical field, image data are not easily obtained such as natural images. To solve this problem, transfer learning was introduced to use features obtained from a pretrained model [32]. This is also called knowledge transfer, which means acquiring the knowledge of how to perform pattern recognition in natural images and using it in medical image classification. At present, the most widely known image database for transfer learning is ImageNet. In its implementation, the last few layers were removed from the pretrained model and were replaced with new layers. Then, the polyp images were fed to train parameters of new layers. An illustration is shown in Figure 5.

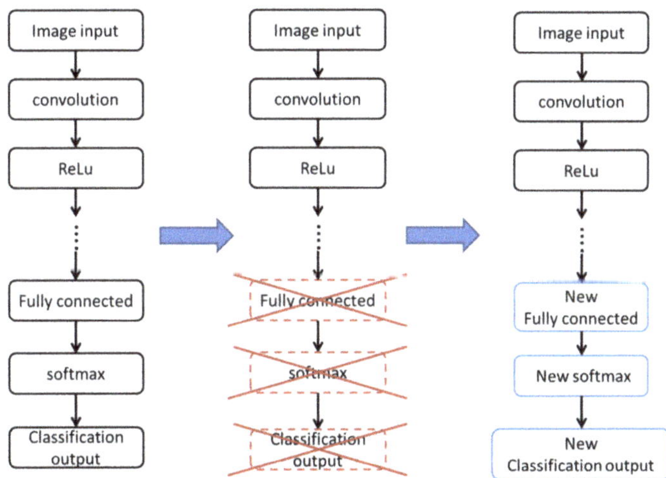

Figure 5. Illustration of transferred convolutional neural network.

In the experiment, two ways were used to train a DCNN model. A DCNN trained from scratch means all the parameters for feature extraction and classification are learned from the target image database, i.e., the colonoscopy in this study. Another way to train a model is transferring parameters from a pre-trained big dataset such as ImageNet. However, ImageNet does not have too many colonoscopy images and may not be as helpful as expected. Thus, the comparisons are shown in this study to emphasize the differences. Moreover, the performances of different DCNN architectures were compared including

AlexNet [33], Inception-V3 [34], ResNet-101 [35], and DenseNet-201 [36]. In the model training, the training and test datasets were randomly selected. Each network was trained 10 times, and the averaged accuracy values were regarded as the final result.

3. Results

In the experiment, input images were firstly divided into R, G, B, and grayscale images. After extracting GLCM and Gabor features, 21 classifiers were used. That is, the results contained 4 image types × 2 feature types × 21 classifiers = 168 prediction models with 10-fold cross-validation. The highest accuracy of 75.6% was obtained using GLCM from B images (Table 1), and the area under receiver operating characteristic curve was 0.82.

Table 1. The top five accuracies using the texture features and different classifiers.

Model Type	Accuracy	Feature
Ensemble Bagged Trees	75.6%	GLCM_B
Coarse KNN	75.0%	GLCM_B
Ensemble Booted Trees	73.9%	GLCM_G
Ensemble RUSBooted Trees	73.5%	Gabor_B
Quadratic SVM	72.8%	GLCM_B

B = blue channel; G = green channel.

Using DCNN features, the performances of four types of DCNN with and without transfer learning were also explored, including AlexNet, Inception-V3, Resnet-101, and DenseNet-201. The parameters used in the training are learning rate = 0.001 and mini batch size = 64 to gradually achieve the local minimum with affordable image number. Epoch as the training iteration is set 30 for train from scratch and 3~15 for transfer learning. The determination is based on when to achieve the training convergence.

In Table 2, without transfer learning, the networks achieved the accuracies of 96.4%, 82.4%, 80.6%, and 87.4%, respectively. All of them have accuracy higher than 80% and the best one is 96.4%. Considering transfer learning in Table 3, the accuracies were 81.3%, 78.2%, 85.3%, and 87.7%. Inception-V3 only had 78.2% but still better than conventional texture features. The best one is 87.7% which is no better than AlexNet trained from scratch.

Table 2. The performances of various convolutional neural networks trained from scratch.

Train from Scratch	Accuracy	Sensitivity	Specificity
Alex	96.4%	95.7%	97.2%
Inception-V3	82.4%	78.7%	85.9%
ResNet-101	80.6%	87.2%	74.5%
DenseNet-201	87.4%	86.2%	87.7%

Table 3. The performances of various convolutional neural networks using transfer learning.

Transfer Learning	Accuracy	Sensitivity	Specificity
Alex	81.3%	90.4%	72.6%
Inception-V3	78.2%	67.0%	87.7%
ResNet-101	85.3%	81.9%	87.7%
DenseNet-201	87.7%	83.0%	91.5%

4. Discussion

CAD has been used for polyp detection under computed tomography [13]. Based on the success, this study explored extracting image features from colonoscopy image for polyp type classification. Recent literature proposed using texture features only or using DCNN features only in the classification of colon polyps [29,37]. The implementation of texture features is time-consuming, while it relatively costs less than DCNN. Nevertheless, texture features are easier to be explained. In the training of DCNN, a large image dataset and computational power are required. Although it may generate a higher accuracy, not all the medical intuitions can afford the computation power. With respect to achieving a higher accuracy, DCNN trained from scratch and transfer learning were implemented. According to the result, AlexNet trained from scratch can achieve the best performance of 96.4% accuracy. Transfer learning may not improve the performance with respect to the different networks used for the colonoscopy images. Some performances were increased or decreased or similar. Nevertheless, the worst one had 78.2% accuracy which was still higher than the best texture features, i.e., 75.6%.

Compared to a recent study using handcrafted and DCNN features for polyp classification [19], Ay, Betul et al. obtained 96.3% to 98.3% accuracies from different combinations of features and classifiers using video-frames of 80 participants. Although the number of 80 patients is much smaller than the 1991 patients used in this study, DCNN features performed better than handcrafted features in both studies. The accuracies higher than 96% would show the classification abilities of DCNN in polyp classification.

In clinical use, training from scratch may take more time compared to transfer learning. However, the accuracy difference is substantial such as 15.1% between AlexNet trained from scratch and transfer learning. It seems necessary to train an optimal model for a specific target task to obtain a good performance. Another way to improve the performance would be combining various features such as texture features or intensity features and various DCNN features in machine learning classifiers. This relates to more techniques about feature combination and feature selection. Whether the model can be applied to other datasets generated in different settings would be the next experiment. Then, we can estimate if a customized model is needed for different datasets and training methods. Meanwhile, a split validation would be performed to obtain more comparable results [38]. So far, the result shows that the prediction model can help gastroenterologists determine the polyp types during a colonoscopy.

It is helpful for gastrologists to predict the possible pathological results of polyps. With the prediction model based on the image features, gastrologist can have an early estimation of tissue malignancy. Some treatment plans can be arranged in advance without having to wait a few weeks. Using an image-based estimation model on other modalities is also helpful, including abnormal detections in capsule endoscopy which would be a time-consuming task for gastrologist. More trial or experiments will be executed after the preparation of data collection.

Compared with the general population, inflammatory bowel disease has a higher incidence of colorectal polyps [39] and colon cancer [40,41]. The proposed method may be used to predict the severity of intestinal mucosal pathological outcomes of inflammatory bowel disease in the future.

5. Conclusions

This study proposed the CAD system for the classification of polyp types using colonoscopy. Various features, networks, and training methods were implemented in the experiment. GLCM texture features in the B channel had the accuracy of 75.6%, while AlexNet trained from scratch obtained the accuracy of 96.4%. Based on the performance comparisons, DCNN can achieve a substantial performance and training from scratch is a promising way to build a model if the image data are good enough. The evaluations would provide more practical advice to gastroenterologists about using CAD for polyp classification during a colonoscopy. More CAD systems for intestinal tumors or inflammatory bowel diseases such as Crohn's disease and ulcerative colitis would be possible in the future.

Author Contributions: Conceptualization, C.-M.L.; Data curation, C.-M.L.; Methodology, Y.-H.Y. and C.-M.L.; Validation, C.-M.L.; Writing—original draft, C.-M.L. and Y.-H.Y.; Writing—review and editing, H.-J.Y.; Investigation, H.-J.Y.; Visualization, H.-J.Y.; Software, Y.-H.Y.; Resources, J.-H.T. and C.-C.C. All authors have read and agreed to the published version of the manuscript.

Funding: This research received no external funding.

Institutional Review Board Statement: The study was conducted in accordance with the Declaration of Helsinki, and approved by the Joint Institutional Review Board of Taipei Medical University (protocol code is N201802090c and date of approval is 25 February 2020).

Acknowledgments: The authors would like to thank the Division of Gastroenterology and Hepatology, Department of Internal Medicine, Taipei Medical University Hospital for financially supporting this research.

Conflicts of Interest: The authors declare no conflict of interest.

References

1. Siegel, R.L.; Miller, K.D.; Jemal, A. Cancer statistics, 2020. *CA Cancer J. Clin.* **2020**, *70*, 7–30. [CrossRef]
2. Siegel, R.L.; Fedewa, S.A.; Anderson, W.F.; Miller, K.D.; Ma, J.; Rosenberg, P.S.; Jemal, A. Colorectal Cancer Incidence Patterns in the United States, 1974–2013. *J. Natl. Cancer Inst.* **2017**, *109*, djw322. [CrossRef] [PubMed]
3. WHO. *World Cancer Report*; World Health Organization Press: Geneva, Switzerland, 2014; Chapter 5.5.
4. Institute, N.C. *Colorectal Cancer Prevention (PDQ®)—Health Professional Version*; North Carolina Institute: Chapel Hill, NC, USA, 2014.
5. Hiramatsu, K.; Sakata, H.; Horita, Y.; Orita, N.; Kida, A.; Mizukami, A.; Miyazawa, M.; Hirai, S.; Shimatani, A.; Matsuda, K.; et al. Mesenteric phlebosclerosis associated with long-term oral intake of geniposide, an ingredient of herbal medicine. *Aliment. Pharmacol. Ther.* **2012**, *36*, 575–586. [CrossRef] [PubMed]
6. Carethers, J.M.; Jung, B.H. Genetics and Genetic Biomarkers in Sporadic Colorectal Cancer. *Gastroenterology* **2015**, *149*, 1177–1190. [CrossRef] [PubMed]
7. Byrne, M.F.; Chapados, N.; Soudan, F.; Oertel, C.; Linares Pérez, M.; Kelly, R.; Iqbal, N.; Chandelier, F.; Rex, D.K. Real-time differentiation of adenomatous and hyperplastic diminutive colorectal polyps during analysis of unaltered videos of standard colonoscopy using a deep learning model. *Gut* **2019**, *68*, 94–100. [CrossRef] [PubMed]
8. Corley, D.A.; Jensen, C.D.; Marks, A.R.; Zhao, W.K.; Lee, J.K.; Doubeni, C.A.; Zauber, A.G.; de Boer, J.; Fireman, B.H.; Schottinger, J.E.; et al. Adenoma detection rate and risk of colorectal cancer and death. *N. Engl. J. Med.* **2014**, *370*, 1298–1306. [CrossRef]
9. Mann, R.; Gajendran, M.; Umapathy, C.; Perisetti, A.; Goyal, H.; Saligram, S.; Echavarria, J. Endoscopic Management of Complex Colorectal Polyps: Current Insights and Future Trends. *Front. Med.* **2022**, *8*, 728704. [CrossRef] [PubMed]
10. Zauber, A.G.; Winawer, S.J.; O'Brien, M.J.; Lansdorp-Vogelaar, I.; van Ballegooijen, M.; Hankey, B.F.; Shi, W.; Bond, J.H.; Schapiro, M.; Panish, J.F.; et al. Colonoscopic polypectomy and long-term prevention of colorectal-cancer deaths. *N. Engl. J. Med.* **2012**, *366*, 687–696. [CrossRef]
11. Shalman, D.; Gerson, L.B. Systematic review with meta-analysis: The risk of gastrointestinal haemorrhage post-polypectomy in patients receiving anti-platelet, anti-coagulant and/or thienopyridine medications. *Aliment. Pharmacol. Ther.* **2015**, *42*, 949–956. [CrossRef]
12. Yoshida, H.; Nappi, J.; MacEneaney, P.; Rubin, D.T.; Dachman, A.H. Computer-aided diagnosis scheme for detection of polyps at CT colonography. *Radiographics* **2002**, *22*, 963–979. [CrossRef]
13. Tan, J.; Gao, Y.; Cao, W.; Pomeroy, M.; Zhang, S.; Huo, Y.; Li, L.; Liang, Z. GLCM-CNN: Gray Level Co-occurrence Matrix based CNN Model for Polyp Diagnosis. In Proceedings of the 2019 IEEE EMBS International Conference on Biomedical & Health Informatics (BHI), Chicago, IL, USA, 19–22 May 2019; pp. 1–4.
14. Lee, J.-G.; Hyo Kim, J.; Hyung Kim, S.; Sun Park, H.; Ihn Choi, B. A straightforward approach to computer-aided polyp detection using a polyp-specific volumetric feature in CT colonography. *Comput. Biol. Med.* **2011**, *41*, 790–801. [CrossRef]
15. Sánchez-González, A.; García-Zapirain, B.; Sierra-Sosa, D.; Elmaghraby, A. Automatized colon polyp segmentation via contour region analysis. *Comput. Biol. Med.* **2018**, *100*, 152–164. [CrossRef]
16. Pacal, I.; Karaman, A.; Karaboga, D.; Akay, B.; Basturk, A.; Nalbantoglu, U.; Coskun, S. An efficient real-time colonic polyp detection with YOLO algorithms trained by using negative samples and large datasets. *Comput. Biol. Med.* **2022**, *141*, 105031. [CrossRef]
17. Pacal, I.; Karaboga, D. A robust real-time deep learning based automatic polyp detection system. *Comput. Biol. Med.* **2021**, *134*, 104519. [CrossRef]
18. Hu, K.; Zhao, L.; Feng, S.; Zhang, S.; Zhou, Q.; Gao, X.; Guo, Y. Colorectal polyp region extraction using saliency detection network with neutrosophic enhancement. *Comput. Biol. Med.* **2022**, *147*, 105760. [CrossRef]
19. Ay, B.; Turker, C.; Emre, E.; Ay, K.; Aydin, G. Automated classification of nasal polyps in endoscopy video-frames using handcrafted and CNN features. *Comput. Biol. Med.* **2022**, *147*, 105725. [CrossRef]

20. Cai, W.-L.; Hong, G.-B. Quantitative image analysis for evaluation of tumor response in clinical oncology. *Chronic Dis. Transl. Med.* **2018**, *4*, 18–28. [CrossRef]

21. Yang, Q.; Li, L.; Zhang, J.; Shao, G.; Zheng, B. A new quantitative image analysis method for improving breast cancer diagnosis using DCE-MRI examinations. *Med. Phys.* **2015**, *42*, 103–109. [CrossRef]

22. Moreno, P.; Bernardino, A.; Santos-Victor, J. Gabor Parameter Selection for Local Feature Detection. In *Iberian Conference on Pattern Recognition and Image Analysis*; Springer: Berlin/Heidelberg, Germany, 2005; pp. 11–19.

23. Buciu, I.; Gacsadi, A. Gabor wavelet based features for medical image analysis and classification. In Proceedings of the 2009 2nd International Symposium on Applied Sciences in Biomedical and Communication Technologies, Bratislava, Slovakia, 24–27 November 2009; pp. 1–4.

24. Chaddad, A.; Desrosiers, C.; Bouridane, A.; Toews, M.; Hassan, L.; Tanougast, C. Multi Texture Analysis of Colorectal Cancer Continuum Using Multispectral Imagery. *PLoS ONE* **2016**, *11*, e0149893. [CrossRef]

25. Haghighat, M.; Zonouz, S.; Abdel-Mottaleb, M. CloudID: Trustworthy cloud-based and cross-enterprise biometric identification. *Expert Syst. Appl.* **2015**, *42*, 7905–7916. [CrossRef]

26. Jolliffe, I. Principal Component Analysis. In *Encyclopedia of Statistics in Behavioral Science*; John Wiley & Sons, Inc.: Hoboken, NJ, USA, 2005. [CrossRef]

27. Gales, M.a.S.Y. The application of hidden Markov models in speech recognition. *Found. Trends Signal Process.* **2008**, *1*, 195–304. [CrossRef]

28. Bengio, Y.; Courville, A.; Vincent, P. Representation learning: A review and new perspectives. *IEEE Trans. Pattern Anal. Mach. Intell.* **2013**, *35*, 1798–1828. [CrossRef] [PubMed]

29. Schmidhuber, J. Deep learning in neural networks: An overview. *Neural Netw.* **2015**, *61*, 85–117. [CrossRef]

30. Boyd, S.; Parikh, N.; Chu, E.; Peleato, B.; Eckstein, J. Distributed optimization and statistical learning via the alternating direction method of multipliers. *Found. Trends Mach. Learn.* **2011**, *3*, 1–122. [CrossRef]

31. Han, S.; Pool, J.; Tran, J.; Dally, W. Learning both weights and connections for efficient neural network. In *Advances in Neural Information Processing Systems*; Morgan Kaufmann Publishers Inc.: San Francisco, CA, USA, 2015.

32. Pan, S.J.; Yang, Q. A Survey on Transfer Learning. *IEEE Trans. Knowl. Data Eng.* **2010**, *22*, 1345–1359. [CrossRef]

33. Yuan, Z.-W.; Zhang, J. *Feature Extraction and Image Retrieval Based on AlexNet*; SPIE: Bellingham, WA, USA, 2016; Volume 10033.

34. Szegedy, C.; Liu, W.; Jia, Y.; Sermanet, P.; Reed, S.; Anguelov, D.; Erhan, D.; Vanhoucke, V.; Rabinovich, A. Going deeper with convolutions. In Proceedings of the IEEE Conference on Computer Vision and Pattern Recognition, Boston, MA, USA, 7–12 June 2015.

35. Zhai, Y.; Fu, J.; Lu, Y.; Li, H. Feature Selective Networks for Object Detection. In Proceedings of the IEEE Conference on Computer Vision and Pattern Recognition, Honolulu, HI, USA, 21–26 July 2017.

36. Huang, G.; Liu, S.; Van der Maaten, L.; Weinberger, K.Q. Condensenet: An efficient densenet using learned group convolutions. In Proceedings of the IEEE Conference on Computer Vision and Pattern Recognition, Salt Lake City, UT, USA, 18–23 June 2018; pp. 2752–2761.

37. Pogorelov, K.; Ostroukhova, O.; Jeppsson, M.; Espeland, H.; Griwodz, C.; Lange, T.d.; Johansen, D.; Riegler, M.; Halvorsen, P. Deep Learning and Hand-Crafted Feature Based Approaches for Polyp Detection in Medical Videos. In Proceedings of the 2018 IEEE 31st International Symposium on Computer-Based Medical Systems (CBMS), Karlstad, Sweden, 18–21 June 2018; pp. 381–386.

38. Liu, X.; Faes, L.; Kale, A.U.; Wagner, S.K.; Fu, D.J.; Bruynseels, A.; Mahendiran, T.; Moraes, G.; Shamdas, M.; Kern, C.; et al. A comparison of deep learning performance against health-care professionals in detecting diseases from medical imaging: A systematic review and meta-analysis. *Lancet Digit. Health* **2019**, *1*, e271–e297. [CrossRef]

39. Hsu, Y.-C.; Wu, T.-C.; Lo, Y.-C.; Wang, L.-S. Gastrointestinal complications and extraintestinal manifestations of inflammatory bowel disease in Taiwan: A population-based study. *J. Chin. Med. Assoc.* **2017**, *80*, 56–62. [CrossRef]

40. Torres, J.; Mehandru, S.; Colombel, J.-F.; Peyrin-Biroulet, L. Crohn's disease. *Lancet* **2017**, *389*, 1741–1755. [CrossRef]

41. Beaugerie, L.; Itzkowitz, S.H. Cancers Complicating Inflammatory Bowel Disease. *N. Engl. J. Med.* **2015**, *372*, 1441–1452. [CrossRef]

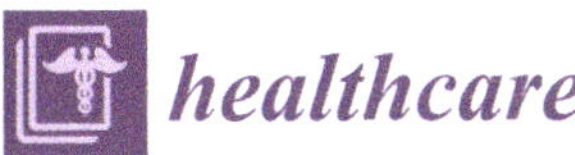

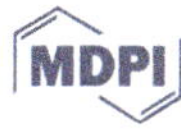

Article

Osteoporosis Pre-Screening Using Ensemble Machine Learning in Postmenopausal Korean Women

Youngihn Kwon [1,†], Juyeon Lee [2,†], Joo Hee Park [2], Yoo Mee Kim [3], Se Hwa Kim [3], Young Jun Won [3,*] and Hyung-Yong Kim [2,*]

1   Insilicogen, Inc., Yongin-si 16954, Korea; yikwon@insilicogen.com
2   AIDX, Inc., Yongin-si 16954, Korea; jylee@aidx.kr (J.L.); jheepark@aidx.kr (J.H.P.)
3   Department of Internal Medicine, International St. Mary's Hospital, Catholic Kwandong University College of Medicine, Incheon 22711, Korea; ymkim@ish.ac.kr (Y.M.K.); endojune@ish.ac.kr (S.H.K.)
*   Correspondence: yjwon@ish.ac.kr (Y.J.W.); hygkim@aidx.kr (H.-Y.K.)
†   These authors contributed equally to this work.

Abstract: As osteoporosis is a degenerative disease related to postmenopausal aging, early diagnosis is vital. This study used data from the Korea National Health and Nutrition Examination Surveys to predict a patient's risk of osteoporosis using machine learning algorithms. Data from 1431 postmenopausal women aged 40–69 years were used, including 20 features affecting osteoporosis, chosen by feature importance and recursive feature elimination. Random Forest (RF), AdaBoost, and Gradient Boosting (GBM) machine learning algorithms were each used to train three models: A, checkup features; B, survey features; and C, both checkup and survey features, respectively. Of the three models, Model C generated the best outcomes with an accuracy of 0.832 for RF, 0.849 for AdaBoost, and 0.829 for GBM. Its area under the receiver operating characteristic curve (AUROC) was 0.919 for RF, 0.921 for AdaBoost, and 0.908 for GBM. By utilizing multiple feature selection methods, the ensemble models of this study achieved excellent results with an AUROC score of 0.921 with AdaBoost, which is 0.1–0.2 higher than those of the best performing models from recent studies. Our model can be further improved as a practical medical tool for the early diagnosis of osteoporosis after menopause.

Keywords: machine learning; feature selection; osteoporosis; postmenopausal women; pre-screening; risk assessment

Citation: Kwon, Y.; Lee, J.; Park, J.H.; Kim, Y.M.; Kim, S.H.; Won, Y.J.; Kim, H.-Y. Osteoporosis Pre-Screening Using Ensemble Machine Learning in Postmenopausal Korean Women. *Healthcare* **2022**, *10*, 1107. https://doi.org/10.3390/healthcare10061107

Academic Editor: Mahmudur Rahman

Received: 12 May 2022
Accepted: 11 June 2022
Published: 14 June 2022

Publisher's Note: MDPI stays neutral with regard to jurisdictional claims in published maps and institutional affiliations.

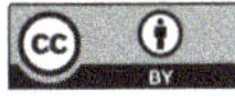

1. Introduction

Osteoporosis is a representative disease that accompanies aging and is closely related to skeletal fractures and deaths [1]. Therefore, a methodology for early diagnosis and prevention has been proposed. Osteoporosis is diagnosed by measuring bone mineral density (BMD) using dual-energy X-ray absorptiometry (DXA) equipment [2]. However, the associated costs are expensive [3]. Hence, with the accelerating growth of aged populations, the financial burdens of individuals and governments are increasing dramatically [4,5]. Notably, a pre-screening diagnosis method that leverages data from surveys and checkups to evaluate osteoporosis risk in advance would greatly benefit prevention and treatment while reducing economic and financial burdens on society. For these reasons, pre-screening diagnosis methods have been actively studied. Thus, many conventional methods of predicting osteoporosis risk are used, including the Osteoporosis Self-Assessment Tool for Asians [6], the osteoporosis risk assessment instrument [7], simple calculated osteoporosis risk estimation [8], and the osteoporosis index of risk [9,10], because these methods rely on only two or three features to predict osteoporosis simply. However, because enormous amounts of medical data are collected nowadays, it is necessary to apply complicated statistical methods to utilize data in advance for better results [3].

Machine learning is an artificial intelligence technique for learning patterns and predicting outcomes based on input data [11]. Machine learning is especially effective at identifying trends and making predictions from multi-dimensional data and has already been applied to osteoporosis diagnosis. For example, E et al. [12] attempted to improve the low accuracy of osteoporosis prevalence predictions using machine learning, and Kim et al. [13] applied machine learning techniques to pre-screen osteoporosis in postmenopausal women in Korea.

Feature selection is important for machine learning efficiency and accuracy [14]. In most machine learning osteoporosis diagnosis methods, selected features known to influence osteoporosis are used to train machine learning models from prepared datasets [12,13,15,16]. This study instead applies a method of selecting features optimized for machine learning from high-dimensional data, rather than by filtering features in advance based on expert knowledge. The performance of this method turns out to be better than those of extant feature selection methods.

The Korea National Health and Nutrition Examination Survey (KNHANES) is a nationwide survey of Korean residents that collects general health and nutrition data, including those of bone densitometry. Lee and Lee [15], Shim et al. [16], and Yoo et al. [17] studied machine learning models that predict osteoporosis based on the features related to osteoporosis, achieving area under the receiver operating characteristic (AUC) curve performances of 0.710, 0.743, and 0.827, respectively. Based on this, the current study trains and evaluates a machine learning model that predicts osteoporosis in postmenopausal women using raw data from the KNHANES (2008–2011).

2. Materials and Methods

2.1. Data Collection

The KNHANES database was established to identify the health and nutritional statuses of Korean citizens following the 1998 enactment of Article 16 of the National Health Promotion Act. Hence, the survey has been conducted yearly with raw data released online. KNHANES include data from common participant information, health behavior surveys, health examinations, and nutrition surveys [18]. The current study uses raw data from the V-4 (2008–2009) and V-5 (2010–2011) surveys, when osteoporosis tests were performed using DXA equipment [19]. The current study's use of KNHANES data received ethical approval from the Institutional Review Board of the Korea Centers for Disease Control and Prevention (IRB Num. IS19EISI0063). Data were downloaded from the KNHANES website (https://knhanes.kdca.go.kr/knhanes/main.do (accessed on 7 October 2020)).

2.2. Study Participants

Among the 21,303 participants, four exclusion criteria were applied to meet the purpose of this study. First, those who were not tested for osteoporosis were excluded. Second, osteopenia patients were excluded because the purpose of this study is to determine whether patients have osteoporosis or normal as binary classification. Third, men were excluded, as the focus of the study is postmenopausal women. Furthermore, patients who had experienced both menopause and a hysterectomy were included as they have a high chance of contracting osteoporosis, based on previous studies [20]. Fourth, only participants aged 40–69 years were included as most over 70 have already suffered osteoporosis. Considering all four criteria, 1431 participants remained.

2.3. Bone Mineral Density and T-Score

Osteoporosis is normally diagnosed using BMD tests via DXA, which measures the inorganic content in bone to determine the risk of fracture and identify the prevalence of osteoporosis. BMDs of the lumbar spine and femur are usually measured, but those of the wrist, finger, or heel may be substituted [21].

In KNHANES V-4 and V-5, BMD was measured in three areas: lumbar spine, femur neck, and the whole femur. The individually measured BMDs were used to diagnose osteoporosis after calculating T-scores and comparing them to the BMDs of healthy adults, according to a recommendation by the World Health Organization. The largest BMD dataset from Asia Japan (DISCOVERY-W; fan-beam densitometer, Hologic, Inc., USA) was used as the healthy adult group [22].

$$\text{T-score} = (\text{BMD} - \text{group's BMD mean}) * \text{group's BMD stddev}, \tag{1}$$

T-scores calculated using the above equation were classified: a T-score of -1 or higher was classified as normal, -1 to -2.5 was classified as osteopenia, and less than -2.5 was classified as osteoporosis [23]. Based on above criteria, T-scores were classified into three different classes, and only two classes (normal and osteoporosis) as a dependent variable were used to train binary classification model.

2.4. Experimental Design

Figure 1 displays a flowchart explaining the study design. Prior to analysis, participants were selected considering the criteria explained in Section 2.2, and data preprocessing was conducted afterward (see Section 2.5). Machine learning algorithms were applied to predict the occurrence of osteoporosis based on 20 features having high classification influence, chosen via discussions with medical specialists and feature importance scoring from trained machine learning algorithms. The features consisted of 10 biochemical screening results (Model A) and 10 survey results (Model B). When combined, Model C is obtained.

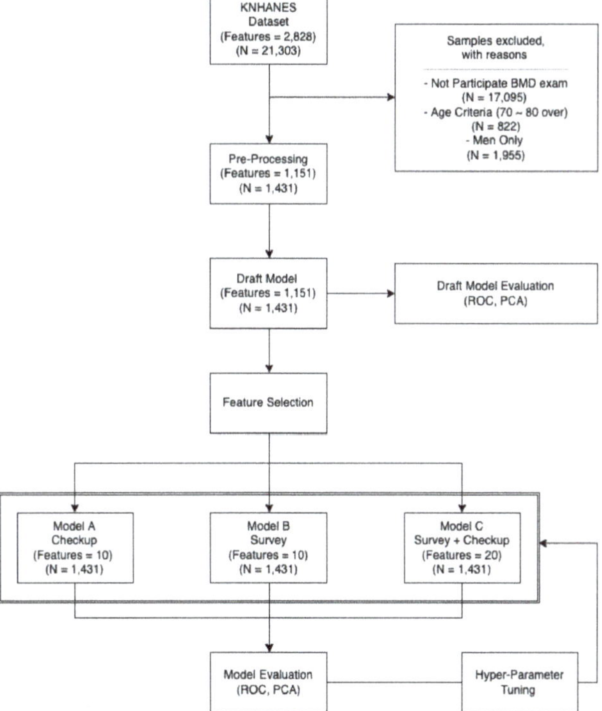

Figure 1. Study procedure. Model A—trained Model based on checkup features. Model B—trained Model based on survey features. Model C—trained Model based on total (checkup + survey) features.

2.5. Data Preprocessing

Data preprocessing was performed using Python V.3.8 using the pandas, numpy, and scikit-learn libraries. Outliers and non-responses were converted into missing values

("N/A") based on the KNHANES data guidelines, and multinominal data were analyzed using the one-hot encoding method. Feature engineering was used to integrate features with overlapping meanings by year, and all data were conditions with standard scaling prior to training.

2.6. Feature Selection

As shown in Figure 1, feature selection was performed based on feature importance and recursive feature elimination (RFE), following data processing. Feature importance refers a measure of the individual contribution of the corresponding feature for a particular classifier, regardless of the shape or direction of the feature effect [24]. The higher the feature importance, the greater the influence on algorithmic decision-making. RFE is a backward feature selection technique that removes features with low importance, considering the size of the input feature set. The machine learning model was trained on all features initially, and unimportant features were then eliminated from the set.

2.7. Machine Learning Algorithms

A total of eight different machine learning models (KNN, Decision Tree, LDA, QDA, SVC, Random Forest, AdaBoost, and Gradient Boosting Machine) were trained and evaluated based on the KNHANES data during study. Among them, three machine learning models (Random Forest, AdaBoost, and Gradient Boosting Machine) were selected with the highest performance. In this study, three ensemble machine learning algorithms were used to analyze KNHANES data: Random Forest (RF), AdaBoost, and Gradient Boosting Machine (GBM). Ensemble learning connects several weak learning algorithms to obtain stronger results, which is effective in solving classification and regression problems. RF generates a strong decision tree by combining the outputs of several randomly generated ones [25]. AdaBoost is a classification-based model that synthesizes a classifier strengthened through weight modification by combining many weak classifiers. GBM sequentially generates trees in a manner that mitigates the errors of previous trees using gradient boosting classifiers [26].

2.8. Model Training

The k-fold cross-validation method was used for machine learning training and verification k times by allocating verification data differently for each iteration after dividing the dataset into k folds [27]. In this study, the training and testing datasets were divided 80:20 for learning and performance measurement, and k was set to five. This study repeated this cross-validation method 10 times, followed by an accuracy comparative analysis of 50 total learned models. During training, hyperparameters were optimized using the grid-search approach, a tuning technique that computes the optimal combination of hyperparameters by verifying the performance of all possible combinations using cross-validation [28].

2.9. Model Evaluation

Two indicators are normally required to evaluate machine learning performance. The first is the area under the curve (AUC) score from the receiver operating characteristic curve, which is curve-plotting sensitivity vs. one minus specificity. In statistic fields, the accuracy of the machine learning model will improve as the AUC approaches one [29].

Principal component analysis (PCA) is a multivariate analysis method that finds the main components represented by a linear combination of variables by identifying the variation–covariant relationships between large quantitative variables. PCA was used in the present study to visualize the clusters of target patients using two-dimensional reduced principal component variables.

2.10. Statistical Analysis

As the dependent variable of this study is the T-score, point-biserial correlation and phi correlation analyses were performed to calculate correlations instead of using the

Pearson coefficient. Point-biserial correlation measures the correlation when one variable is a binary variable and the other is continuous [30]. The phi correlation analysis determines the degree of correlation between two variables when both independent and dependent variables are binary [31].

3. Results

3.1. Draft Model Building

Training with 1151 features (original data), the AdaBoost model showed the best performance in terms of the AUC (0.91), followed by the GBM (0.90) and RF (0.86). See Figure 2A. Additionally, the osteoporosis per se (dependent variable) was not clearly classified into two separate groups (normal and osteoporosis) based on only two main features (PC1 and PC2), whereas the PCA was performed on 1151 features (Figure 2B).

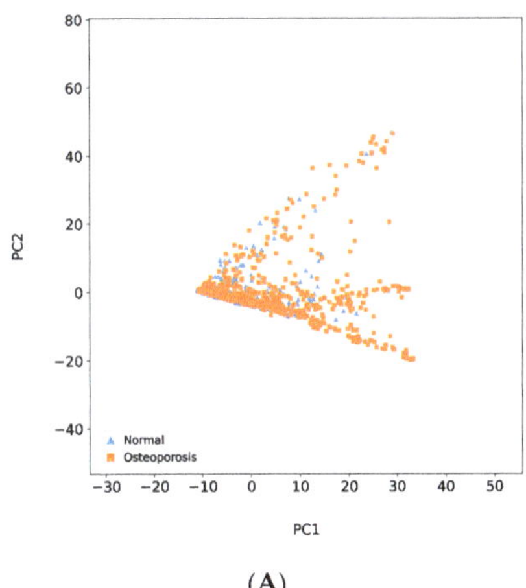

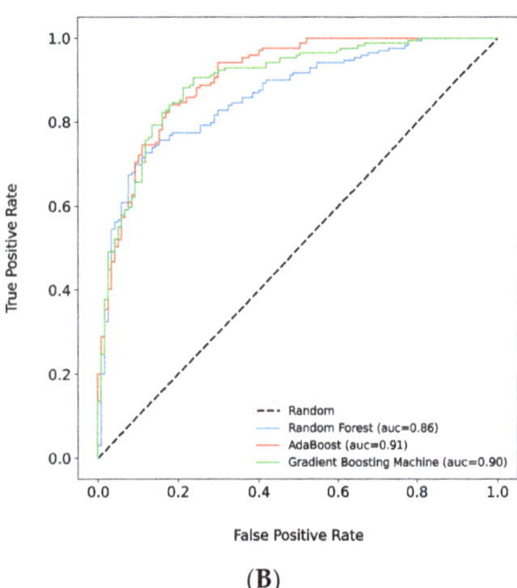

(A) (B)

Figure 2. Draft Model Performance. (**A**): The result of principal component analysis plot based on 1151 features. GBM—Gradient Boosting Machine. (**B**): Receiver operating characteristic (ROC) curve for three different best models (Random Forest, AdaBoost, and Gradient Boosting Machine) based on total features (the number of features = 1151).

3.2. Feature Selection and Statistical Analysis

Survey data are questions that the patient can directly respond to and are related to people's life patterns. Checkup data are collected with the biochemical screening result of participants. Table 1 shows the descriptive statistics of the 20 features selected for importance, and Table 2 presents a list of 20 variables selected by referring to the feature importance as well as one-to-one correlation coefficients between each variable and DX_OST (dependent variable). As a result of the point-biserial correlation analysis, the age variable had the highest correlation at 0.540 in the positive direction, followed by age of menarche (0.24) and use of estrogen (0.17). Among the survey data, education level had the greatest negative correlation at −0.34. Serum alkaline phosphatase level was the highest at 0.233 for screening questions with a positive correlation. From the screening questions, weight (HE_wt) scored the highest negative correlation (−0.43) with the DX_OST, followed by height (HE_ht) at −0.37.

Table 1. Descriptive statistics of normal and osteoporosis subjects in the study.

Variables	Characteristics	Normal (*n* = 610)	Osteoporosis (*n* = 821)
Age	Age (years)	55.15 (49.46, 60.84)	62.34 (56.92, 67.77)
LW_mp_a	Age of menopause (years)	49.53 (45.07, 53.99)	48.86 (43.93, 53.78)
LW_ms_a	Age of menarche (years)	15.22 (13.37, 17.07)	16.21 (14.16, 18.26)
BP8	Average sleeping time for a day (hours)	6.6 (5.25, 7.96)	6.5 (4.93, 8.08)
BD2	Beginning age of drinking (years)	23.42 (7.69, 39.16)	22.07 (2.02, 42.12)
HE_fev1fvc	Expired lung vol. for 1	0.8 (0.75, 0.86)	0.79 (0.72, 0.86)
HE_HDL_st2	HDL cholesterol	49.58 (38.28, 60.87)	48.35 (37.58, 59.11)
HE_ht	Height (cm)	156.71 (151.59, 161.82)	152.65 (147.57, 157.72)
DX_Q_ht	Highest height of the young (cm)	158.88 (154.2, 163.56)	156.26 (151.22, 161.3)
HE_insulin	Insulin	10.7 (2.73, 18.66)	10.07 (4.5, 15.64)
LQ_VAS	Quality of life scale (index)	72.96 (54.39, 91.53)	68.32 (47.18, 89.46)
HE_ALP	Serum alkaline phosphatase (IU/L)	231.77 (165.21, 298.33)	267.75 (188.13, 347.37)
HE_sbp2	Systolic blood pressure (mmHg)	124.67 (106.22, 143.12)	127.36 (109.16, 145.56)
HE_crea	Serum Creatinine (mg/dL)	0.72 (0.62, 0.82)	0.7 (0.52, 0.89)
HE_vitD	Vitamin D (ng/mL)	18.58 (11.98, 25.18)	18.49 (11.38, 25.61)
HE_wt	Weight (kg)	62.03 (53.58, 70.48)	54.52 (47.07, 61.98)
HE_wc	Waist Circumference (cm)	83.71 (74.44, 92.98)	80.62 (71.98, 89.26)
BE5_1	Muscle exercise per week (%) *		
1	Never	80	88.94
2	One day a week	3.97	1.84
3	Two days a week	4.13	2.21
4	Three days a week	4.63	2.83
5	Four days a week	2.15	1.6
6	More than five days a week	5.12	2.58
edu	Education Level (%) *		
1	Primary or less	37.25	72.52
2	Middle	23.18	12.52
3	High	28.64	12.15
4	College or more	10.93	2.82
LW_wh	Use of estrogen (%) *		
0	No	25.96	12.93
1	Yes	74.04	87.07

* indicates categorical variables, and the number of each characteristic under categorical variables refers to percentage.

Table 2. The results of univariate correlation analysis with the list of 20 independent variables and dependent variable.

Data Type	Variables	Characteristics	Correlation
Checkup	HE_wt	Weight (kg)	−0.426 (−0.467, −0.383)
	HE_ht	Height (cm)	−0.367 (−0.411, −0.321)
	HE_wc	Waist Circumference (cm)	−0.170 (−0.219, −0.119)
	HE_fev1fvc	Expired lung vol. for 1 s	−0.115 (−0.172, −0.056)
	HE_HDL_st2	HDL cholesterol (mg/dL)	−0.055 (−0.108, −0.002)
	HE_insulin	Insulin (μIU/mL)	−0.046 (−0.103, 0.010)
	HE_Crea	Serum Creatinine (mg/dL)	−0.045 (−0.098, 0.008)
	HE_vitD	Vitamin D (ng/mL)	−0.006 (−0.059, 0.047)
	HE_sbp2	Systolic blood pressure (mmHg)	0.073 (0.021, 0.124)
	HE_ALP	Serum alkaline phosphatase (IU/L)	0.233 (0.183, 0.283)
Survey	Edu	Education Level	−0.345 (−0.390, −0.298)
	DX_Q_ht	Highest height of the young (cm)	−0.261 (−0.317, −0.203)
	LQ_VAS	Quality of life scale (index)	−0.112 (−0.163, −0.060)
	BE5_1	muscle exercise per week (days)	−0.107 (−0.158, −0.055)
	LW_mp_a	Age of menopause (years)	−0.070 (−0.123, −0.016)
	BD2	Beginning age of drinking (hours)	−0.037 (−0.088, 0.015)
	BP8	Average sleeping time for a day (years)	−0.034 (−0.085, 0.018)
	LW_wh	Use of estrogen	0.17
	LW_ms_a	Age of menarche (years)	0.243 (0.192, 0.292)
	Age	Age (years)	0.540 (0.503, 0.576)

Parentheses under the correlation column indicate a 95% confidence interval.

3.3. Models (A, B, and C) Performance

The three machine learning models were each trained using Models A, B, and C, and grid search and five-fold cross-validation techniques were used to determine the optimized hyperparameters for the best performance. The performance of Model C (Figure 3) had a high average AUC of 0.88. Models A and B had AUCs exceeding 0.80 and 0.83, respectively.

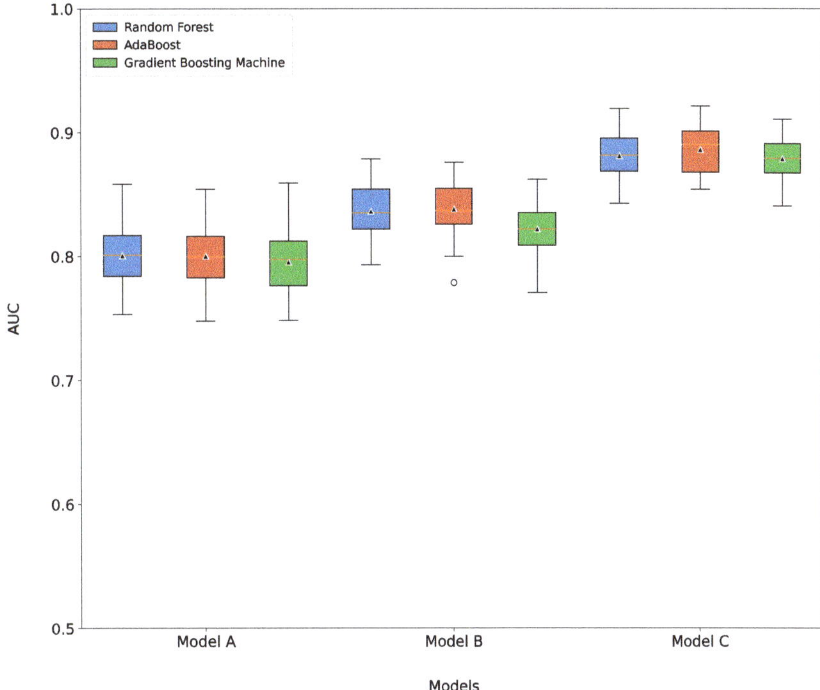

Figure 3. The box plot for AUROC score of three different prediction models among three different data types. Model A—trained model based on checkup features. Model B—trained model based on survey features. Model C—trained model based on total (survey + checkup) features.

Figure 4 and Table S2 show the performance of Model C, and using the same process, the results of the best model performances of Models A and B can be viewed in the supplementary section (Figures S2 and S3). Figure 4A shows the result of the ROC curves for RF, AdaBoost, and GBM. The AUCs of the RF and AdaBoost algorithms were both 0.92, and the GBM showed no significant difference at 0.91. Referring to Supplementary Table S2, the performance indicators of accuracy, precision, and recall resulted in low variations among algorithms and were stable. Figure 4B shows the results of the two-dimensional PCA for the 20 selected features. Osteoporosis and normal clusters were not completely separated, but two clusters of PC1 could be distinguished between zero and one along the *x*-axis.

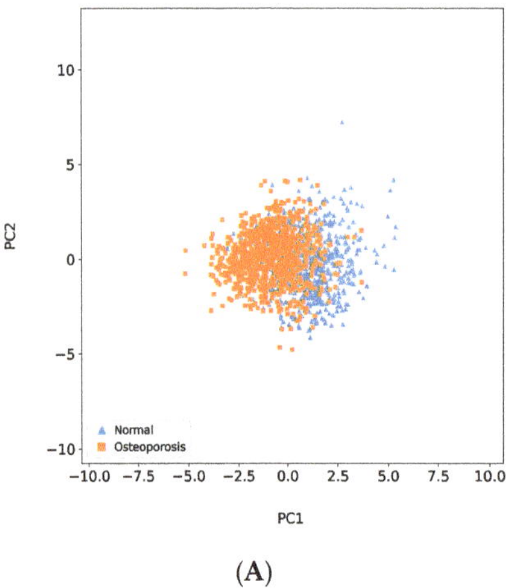

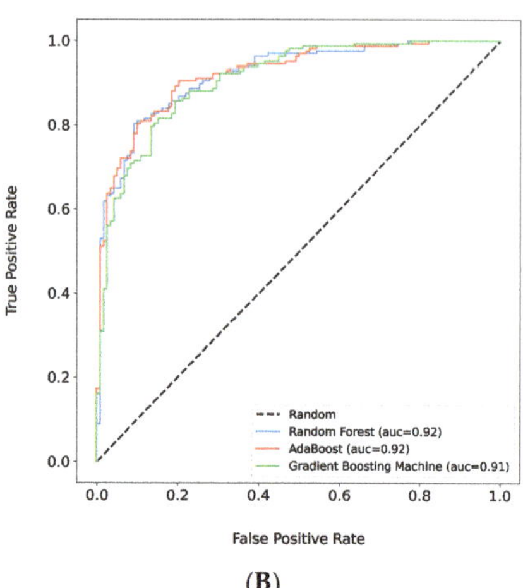

(A)

(B)

Figure 4. Best Model (Model C) Performance. (**A**): The result of 2D principal component analysis plot based on selected 20 features. (**B**): Receiver operating characteristic (ROC) curve of three different best models (Random Forest, AdaBoost, and Gradient Boosting Machine) based on 20 selected features (total).

4. Discussion

In this study, a PCA was performed prior to feature selection and afterward to confirm the relationships between osteoporosis and the selected features. According to the PCA plot (Figure 2B) of the draft model, the normal and osteoporosis groups could not be clearly distinguished based on the two principal components. However, the results of Model C (Figure 4B) implied that the clusters were distinguishable on the right side (normal) and the left side (osteoporosis) based on the specific value at the x-axis (between zero and one). There was no significant difference between the AUC of the draft model and Model C. For Model C, the variation in the AUCs among the three machine learning algorithms was small. Thus, training machine learning models with a small number of features is more effective than using all features in terms of model efficiency and stability.

Checkup data would be used to predict the occurrence of osteoporosis with an 80% accuracy when applying Model A and survey data would be used to predict the occurrence of osteoporosis with an 85% accuracy if Model B was applied. Finally, if both checkup and survey data were available, Model C would be appropriate to predict the occurrence of osteoporosis with an 88% accuracy. To sum up, each model would be used practically depending on the type of data collected.

Prior studies selected features that potentially affected osteoporosis based on knowledge of the medical domain. However, in this study, the feature selection step was performed using medical domain knowledge alongside feature importance and RFE techniques. Instead of collecting commonly known significant features, a large dataset was used to describe the participants in as much detail as possible. A manual data preprocessing step was also necessary to improve training and prediction accuracy. For example, the beginning age of drinking is meaningful only within the group that already had experience in drinking. Therefore, in this case, a feature engineering technique was used to convert the variable into a new one combining drinking experience and the beginning age of drinking. Using this feature selection method with preprocessing, the machine learning models of this study had better results, with AUCs of 0.919 (RF), 0.921 (AdaBoost), and 0.908 (GBM). These scores are approximately 0.1–0.2 higher than the scores of the best model performance from previous studies. Although this study did not fully consider the clinical knowledge, the unique feature selection method and data preprocessing step had a positive influence on model performance via the selection of more suitable features and the merging of various raw data into more meaningful data. In particular, the features selected in this study could be classified into two different groups (i.e., checkup and survey), each of which results in an AUC score of at least 0.80. Therefore, the trained machine learning model from this study may serve as an osteoporosis assistant diagnostic program that predicts the occurrence of osteoporosis and determines the necessity of more thorough examinations.

There were several limitations in this study. First, the raw data from the KNHANES were gathered from cross-sectional observational studies performed at limited points in time across a limited sample population. Second, as participant selection was restricted to women between 40 and 69 years old, it may be difficult to generalize the results of this study to all populations in Korea.

The results of this study can be used as an auxiliary diagnosis program for osteoporosis in the future. In a further study, the models will verify if clinical data with the same features collected from medical institutions can be generalized. Furthermore, as medical image data and deep learning technology can be used for osteoporosis diagnosis, combined with the results of this study, it might be used as a more objective and accurate osteoporosis auxiliary diagnostic tool [32,33].

5. Conclusions

This study generated a prediction model for classifying the osteoporosis using three machine learning algorithms based on 20 features obtained through the feature selection step. The model (Model C) including both checkup and survey features, had an AUROC value (0.92) based on 20 features. Additionally, the model (Model A) with only checkup features, scored an AUROC value (0.81), and the model (Model B) with only survey features, attained an AUROC value (0.85). The trained osteoporosis prediction models when each dataset is available are expected to be useful as an auxiliary diagnostic tool for women after menopause.

Supplementary Materials: The following supporting information can be downloaded at: https://www.mdpi.com/article/10.3390/healthcare10061107/s1, Figure S1: Machine Learning Curve for each best models using Grid search method; Figure S2: ROC Curve for three different best models based on 10 selected Checkup features; Figure S3: ROC Curve for three different best models based on 10 selected Survey features; Figure S4: Feature importance bar graph for 20 features measured by three different ensemble machine learning models; Table S1: The number of normal and osteoporosis patients distributed in women; Table S2: Summary of the Model C's Performances on the test set ($n = 287$).

Author Contributions: Conceptualization, Y.K., J.L., S.H.K., H.-Y.K. and Y.J.W.; methodology, Y.K., J.L., Y.M.K. and H.-Y.K.; software, Y.K., J.L., J.H.P. and H.-Y.K.; validation, Y.K., J.L. and S.H.K.; formal analysis, Y.K., J.L., J.H.P. and H.-Y.K.; investigation, Y.K., J.L., Y.M.K., H.-Y.K. and Y.J.W.; resources, Y.M.K., S.H.K. and Y.J.W.; data curation, Y.K., J.L., J.H.P., Y.M.K., S.H.K. and H.-Y.K.; writing—original draft preparation, Y.K. and J.L.; writing—review and editing, Y.K., J.L., H.-Y.K. and Y.J.W.; visualization, Y.K., J.L. and J.H.P.; supervision, H.-Y.K. and Y.J.W.; project administration, H.-Y.K. and Y.J.W.; funding acquisition, Y.J.W. All authors have read and agreed to the published version of the manuscript.

Funding: This research received no external funding.

Institutional Review Board Statement: This study was approved by the Catholic Kwandong University College of Medicine. The KNHANES received ethical approval from the Institutional Review Board of the Korea Centers for Disease Control and Prevention.

Informed Consent Statement: Informed consent was obtained from all subjects involved in the study.

Data Availability Statement: The data presented in this study are available to download at https://knhanes.kdca.go.kr/knhanes/main.do (accessed on 7 October 2020) for research purposes. It is necessary to obtain IRB registration of the KNHANES dataset for publishing the study.

Acknowledgments: The IRB registration of the KNHANES dataset was supported by the YUHAN Corporation in Seoul, South Korea (IRB Num. IS19EISI0063).

Conflicts of Interest: The authors declare no conflict of interest.

References

1. Bernabei, R. Screening, Diagnosis and Treatment of Osteoporosis: A Brief Review. *Clin. Cases Miner. Bone Metab.* **2014**, *11*, 201. [CrossRef] [PubMed]
2. Jeremiah, M.P.; Unwin, B.K.; Greenawald, M.H. Diagnosis and Management of Osteoporosis. *Am. Fam. Physician* **2015**, *92*, 10.
3. Nayak, S.; Roberts, M.S.; Greenspan, S.L. Cost-Effectiveness of Different Screening Strategies for Osteoporosis in Postmenopausal Women. *Ann. Intern. Med.* **2011**, *155*, 751. [CrossRef] [PubMed]
4. Trajanoska, K.; Rivadeneira, F. The Genetic Architecture of Osteoporosis and Fracture Risk. *Bone* **2019**, *126*, 2–10. [CrossRef] [PubMed]
5. Barron, R.L.; Oster, G.; Grauer, A.; Crittenden, D.B.; Weycker, D. Determinants of Imminent Fracture Risk in Postmenopausal Women with Osteoporosis. *Osteoporos. Int. J. Establ. Result Coop. Eur. Found. Osteoporos. Natl. Osteoporos. Found. USA* **2020**, *31*, 2103–2111. [CrossRef]
6. Koh, L.K.; Sedrine, W.B.; Torralba, T.P.; Kung, A.; Fujiwara, S.; Chan, S.P.; Huang, Q.R.; Rajatanavin, R.; Tsai, K.S.; Park, H.M.; et al. A Simple Tool to Identify Asian Women at Increased Risk of Osteoporosis. *Osteoporos. Int. J. Establ. Result Coop. Eur. Found. Osteoporos. Natl. Osteoporos. Found. USA* **2001**, *12*, 699–705. [CrossRef]
7. Cadarette, S.M.; Jaglal, S.B.; Kreiger, N.; McIsaac, W.J.; Darlington, G.A.; Tu, J.V. Development and Validation of the Osteoporosis Risk Assessment Instrument to Facilitate Selection of Women for Bone Densitometry. *CMAJ Can. Med. Assoc. J. J. Assoc. Medicale Can.* **2000**, *162*, 1289–1294.
8. Lydick, E.; Cook, K.; Turpin, J.; Melton, M.; Stine, R.; Byrnes, C. Development and Validation of a Simple Questionnaire to Facilitate Identification of Women Likely to Have Low Bone Density. *Am. J. Manag. Care* **1998**, *4*, 37–48.
9. Sedrine, W.B.; Chevallier, T.; Zegels, B.; Kvasz, A.; Micheletti, M.-C.; Gelas, B.; Reginster, J.-Y. Development and Assessment of the Osteoporosis Index of Risk (OSIRIS) to Facilitate Selection of Women for Bone Densitometry. *Gynecol. Endocrinol.* **2002**, *16*, 245–250. [CrossRef]
10. Rud, B.; Hilden, J.; Hyldstrup, L.; Hróbjartsson, A. The Osteoporosis Self-Assessment Tool versus Alternative Tests for Selecting Postmenopausal Women for Bone Mineral Density Assessment: A Comparative Systematic Review of Accuracy. *Osteoporos. Int.* **2009**, *20*, 599–607. [CrossRef]
11. Roth, J.A.; Battegay, M.; Juchler, F.; Vogt, J.E.; Widmer, A.F. Introduction to Machine Learning in Digital Healthcare Epidemiology. *Infect. Control Hosp. Epidemiol.* **2018**, *39*, 1457–1462. [CrossRef] [PubMed]
12. Erjiang, E.; Wang, T.; Yang, L.; Dempsey, M.; Brennan, A.; Yu, M.; Chan, W.P.; Whelan, B.; Silke, C.; O'Sullivan, M.; et al. Machine Learning Can Improve Clinical Detection of Low BMD: The DXA-HIP Study. *J. Clin. Densitom. Off. J. Int. Soc. Clin. Densitom.* **2021**, *24*, 527–537. [CrossRef]
13. Kim, S.K.; Yoo, T.K.; Kim, D.W. Osteoporosis Risk Prediction Using Machine Learning and Conventional Methods. In Proceedings of the 2013 35th Annual International Conference of the IEEE Engineering in Medicine and Biology Society (EMBC), Osaka, Japan, 3–7 July 2013; IEEE: Osaka, Japan, 2013; pp. 188–191. [CrossRef]
14. Kira, K.; Rendell, L.A. A Practical Approach to Feature Selection. In *Machine Learning Proceedings 1992*; Elsevier: Amsterdam, The Netherlands, 1992; pp. 249–256. [CrossRef]
15. Lee, I.-J.; Lee, J. Predictive of Osteoporosis by Tree-based Machine Learning Model in Post-menopause Woman. *J. Radiol. Sci. Technol.* **2020**, *43*, 495–502. [CrossRef]
16. Shim, J.-G.; Kim, D.W.; Ryu, K.-H.; Cho, E.-A.; Ahn, J.-H.; Kim, J.-I.; Lee, S.H. Application of Machine Learning Approaches for Osteoporosis Risk Prediction in Postmenopausal Women. *Arch. Osteoporos.* **2020**, *15*, 169. [CrossRef]
17. Yoo, T.K.; Kim, S.K.; Kim, D.W.; Choi, J.Y.; Lee, W.H.; Oh, E.; Park, E.-C. Osteoporosis Risk Prediction for Bone Mineral Density Assessment of Postmenopausal Women Using Machine Learning. *Yonsei Med. J.* **2013**, *54*, 1321. [CrossRef]
18. Choi, Y.J.; Oh, H.J.; Kim, D.J.; Lee, Y.; Chung, Y.-S. The Prevalence of Osteoporosis in Korean Adults Aged 50 Years or Older and the Higher Diagnosis Rates in Women Who Were Beneficiaries of a National Screening Program: The Korea National Health and Nutrition Examination Survey 2008–2009. *J. Bone Miner. Res.* **2012**, *27*, 1879–1886. [CrossRef]
19. Kweon, S.; Kim, Y.; Jang, M.-J.; Kim, Y.; Kim, K.; Choi, S.; Chun, C.; Khang, Y.-H.; Oh, K. Data Resource Profile: The Korea National Health and Nutrition Examination Survey (KNHANES). *Int. J. Epidemiol.* **2014**, *43*, 69–77. [CrossRef]
20. Yeh, Y.-T.; Li, P.-C.; Wu, K.-C.; Yang, Y.-C.; Chen, W.; Yip, H.-T.; Wang, J.-H.; Lin, S.-Z.; Ding, D.-C. Hysterectomies Are Associated with an Increased Risk of Osteoporosis and Bone Fracture: A Population-Based Cohort Study. *PLoS ONE* **2020**, *15*, e0243037. [CrossRef]
21. Blake, G.M.; Fogelman, I. The Role of DXA Bone Density Scans in the Diagnosis and Treatment of Osteoporosis. *Postgrad. Med. J.* **2007**, *83*, 509–517. [CrossRef]
22. Kim, M.S.; Koo, J.O. Comparative Analysis of Food Habits and Bone Density Risk Factors between Normal and Risk Women Living in the Seoul Area. *Korean J. Community Nutr.* **2008**, *13*, 125–133.
23. Kanis, J.A.; Kanis, J.A. Assessment of Fracture Risk and Its Application to Screening for Postmenopausal Osteoporosis: Synopsis of a WHO Report. *Osteoporos. Int.* **1994**, *4*, 368–381. [CrossRef] [PubMed]
24. Saarela, M.; Jauhiainen, S. Comparison of Feature Importance Measures as Explanations for Classification Models. *SN Appl. Sci.* **2021**, *3*, 272. [CrossRef]

25. Breiman, L. Random forests. *Mach. Learn.* **2001**, *45*, 5–32. [CrossRef]
26. Mason, L.; Baxter, J.; Bartlett, P.L.; Frean, M.R. Boosting Algorithms as Gradient Descent. In *Advances in Neural Information Processing Systems*; The MIT Press: Cambridge, MA, USA, 1999; pp. 512–518.
27. Berrar, D. Cross-Validation. In *Encyclopedia of Bioinformatics and Computational Biology*; Elsevier: Amsterdam, The Netherlands, 2019; pp. 542–545. [CrossRef]
28. Liashchynskyi, P. Grid Search, Random Search, Genetic Algorithm: A Big Comparison for NAS. *arXiv* **2019**, arXiv:1912.06059.
29. Zou, K.H.; O'Malley, A.J.; Mauri, L. Receiver-Operating Characteristic Analysis for Evaluating Diagnostic Tests and Predictive Models. *Circulation* **2007**, *115*, 654–657. [CrossRef]
30. Kornbrot, D. Point Biserial Correlation. In *Encyclopedia of Statistics in Behavioral Science*; Everitt, B.S., Howell, D.C., Eds.; John Wiley & Sons, Ltd.: Chichester, UK, 2005; p. bsa485. [CrossRef]
31. Chedzoy, O.B. Phi-Coefficient. In *Encyclopedia of Statistical Sciences*; Kotz, S., Read, C.B., Balakrishnan, N., Vidakovic, B., Johnson, N.L., Eds.; John Wiley & Sons, Inc.: Hoboken, NJ, USA, 2006; p. ess1960.pub2. [CrossRef]
32. Tiulpin, A.; Klein, S.; Bierma-Zeinstra, S.M.A.; Thevenot, J.; Rahtu, E.; Van Meurs, J.; Oei, E.H.G.; Saarakkala, S. Multimodal Machine Learning-Based Knee Osteoarthritis Progression Prediction from Plain Radiographs and Clinical Data. *Sci. Rep.* **2019**, *9*, 20038. [CrossRef]
33. Yamamoto, N.; Sukegawa, S.; Kitamura, A.; Goto, R.; Noda, T.; Nakano, K.; Takabatake, K.; Kawai, H.; Nagatsuka, H.; Kawasaki, K.; et al. Deep Learning for Osteoporosis Classification Using Hip Radiographs and Patient Clinical Covariates. *Biomolecules* **2020**, *10*, 1534. [CrossRef]

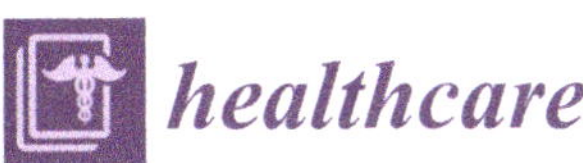

Review

Artificial Intelligence Applied to Pancreatic Imaging: A Narrative Review

Maria Elena Laino [1,*], Angela Ammirabile [2,3,*], Ludovica Lofino [2,3], Lorenzo Mannelli [4], Francesco Fiz [5,6], Marco Francone [2,3], Arturo Chiti [2,7], Luca Saba [8], Matteo Agostino Orlandi [9] and Victor Savevski [1]

[1] Artificial Intelligence Center, IRCCS Humanitas Research Hospital, Via Manzoni 56, Rozzano, 20089 Milan, Italy
[2] Department of Biomedical Sciences, Humanitas University, Via Rita Levi Montalcini 4, Pieve Emanuele, 20072 Milan, Italy
[3] Department of Diagnostic and Interventional Radiology, IRCCS Humanitas Research Hospital, Via Manzoni 56, Rozzano, 20089 Milan, Italy
[4] Department of Radiology, SDN, 80131 Napoli, Italy
[5] Nuclear Medicine Unit, Department of Diagnostic Imaging, E.O. Ospedali Galliera, 56321 Genoa, Italy
[6] Department of Nuclear Medicine and Clinical Molecular Imaging, University Hospital, 72074 Tübingen, Germany
[7] Department of Nuclear Medicine, IRCCS Humanitas Research Hospital, Via Manzoni 56, Rozzano, 20089 Milan, Italy
[8] Department of Radiology, University of Cagliari, 09124 Cagliari, Italy
[9] Department of Radiology, ASST Lodi, Ospedale Maggiore di Lodi, 26900 Lodi, Italy
* Correspondence: mariaelena.laino@humanitas.it (M.E.L.); angela.ammirabile@humanitas.it (A.A.)

Citation: Laino, M.E.; Ammirabile, A.; Lofino, L.; Mannelli, L.; Fiz, F.; Francone, M.; Chiti, A.; Saba, L.; Orlandi, M.A.; Savevski, V. Artificial Intelligence Applied to Pancreatic Imaging: A Narrative Review. *Healthcare* **2022**, *10*, 1511. https://doi.org/10.3390/healthcare10081511

Academic Editor: Mahmudur Rahman

Received: 20 June 2022
Accepted: 8 August 2022
Published: 11 August 2022

Publisher's Note: MDPI stays neutral with regard to jurisdictional claims in published maps and institutional affiliations.

Abstract: The diagnosis, evaluation, and treatment planning of pancreatic pathologies usually require the combined use of different imaging modalities, mainly, computed tomography (CT), magnetic resonance imaging (MRI), and positron emission tomography (PET). Artificial intelligence (AI) has the potential to transform the clinical practice of medical imaging and has been applied to various radiological techniques for different purposes, such as segmentation, lesion detection, characterization, risk stratification, or prediction of response to treatments. The aim of the present narrative review is to assess the available literature on the role of AI applied to pancreatic imaging. Up to now, the use of computer-aided diagnosis (CAD) and radiomics in pancreatic imaging has proven to be useful for both non-oncological and oncological purposes and represents a promising tool for personalized approaches to patients. Although great developments have occurred in recent years, it is important to address the obstacles that still need to be overcome before these technologies can be implemented into our clinical routine, mainly considering the heterogeneity among studies.

Keywords: artificial intelligence; radiomics; pancreatic imaging; MRI; CT; PET

1. Introduction

Pancreatic imaging is one of the body imaging domains that has witnessed increasing interest from researchers due to challenging differential diagnosis and high morbidity. Both computed tomography (CT) and magnetic resonance imaging (MRI) have been widely used as essential tools in the early diagnosis and staging of pancreatic disease [1]. The diagnosis of pancreatic pathologies usually requires the combined use of different morphological and functional imaging modalities, mainly, CT, MRI, and positron emission tomography (PET). Native CT and contrast-enhanced CT (CECT) are widely used for the diagnosis of pancreatic pathologies but also for presurgical evaluation, as they help to determine tumor size, evaluate vascular involvement, and identify disease spread. MRI is useful for characterizing both cystic lesions and solid tumors as it allows noninvasive evaluation of the pancreatic ducts, pancreatic parenchyma, adjacent soft tissues, and vascular network [2,3].

PET utilizes many radiopharmaceuticals to characterize biological features of tumors such as metabolic intensity and receptor expression [4,5].

Artificial intelligence (AI) has the potential to transform the clinical practice of medical imaging due to its ability to discriminate subtle image features. For this reason, it has recently emerged as a noninvasive tool for a better characterization of lesions, thus helping to achieve a more "personalized" approach [5,6].

Computer-aided diagnosis (CAD) and radiomics have been applied to various radiological techniques for different purposes, such as segmentation, detection, and characterization of lesions, risk stratification, and prediction of response to treatments [7,8].

However, their potential applications in pancreatic imaging are still under investigation, both for non-oncological and oncological purposes.

The aim of the present review is to critically assess the available literature on the role of AI and radiomics applied to pancreatic imaging.

2. Materials and Methods

We performed a search of PubMed, Scopus, Embase, Web of Science, and Cochrane library databases for articles relevant to the application of AI and radiomics in pancreatic imaging. On the PubMed database, we used the following MeSH headings: "artificial intelligence", "Machine Learning", "Deep Learning", "neural networks, computer". The search algorithm was constructed using specific strings for each library, as reported in Supplementary Material File S1.

We included original research papers based on human subjects, written and published (including those distributed as "online first") in the English language up to July 2021 that focused on CT, MRI, or PET as imaging techniques.

After screening for duplicates and eligibility, we further refined the selection of manuscripts according to our subjective assessment of their relevance and novelty. The detailed description of the study inclusion process is reported in Figure 1.

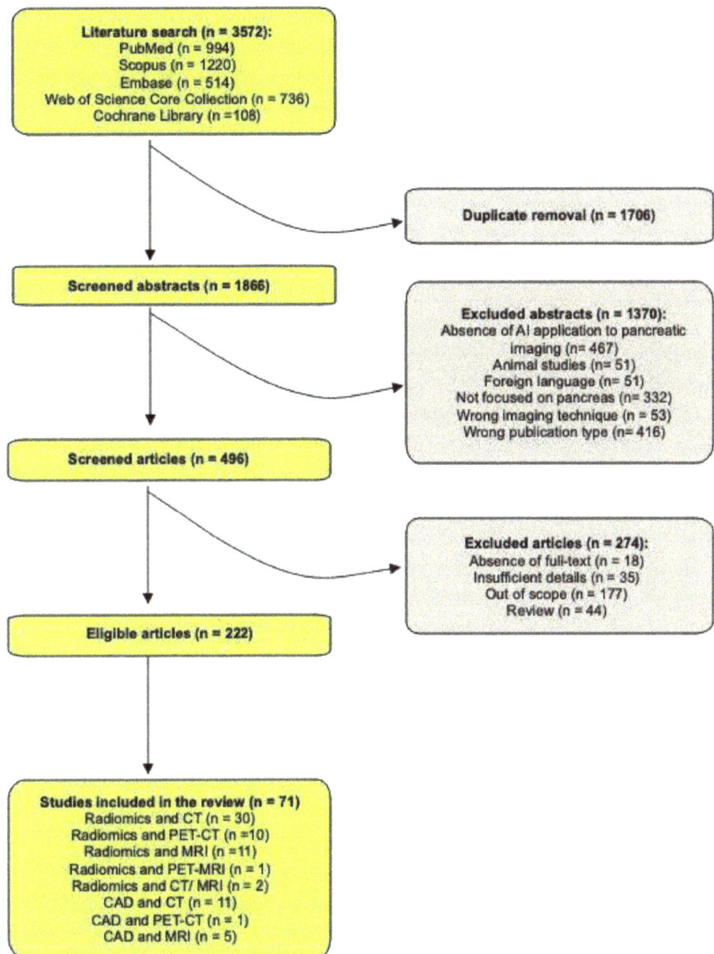

Figure 1. Flowchart of the study inclusion process.

3. Insights on Radiomics Applied to Pancreatic Imaging

In recent years, researchers have investigated the field of radiomics to try and improve patient care [7]. This is even more compelling when dealing with pancreatic imaging, as both clinicians and surgeons have been relying on imaging to improve work-up and prognosis in a field where mortality and morbidity are still very high [2,3] (Figure 2).

3.1. Radiomics and CT

CT represents, by far, the most diffused multislice diagnostic method, with an estimated 400 million examinations per year worldwide. This availability of data has made large-scale radiomics studies possible. In pancreatic imaging, CT features both an excellent spatial and temporal resolution, allowing for a precise assessment of small structures as well as enabling the evaluation of multiple contrast phases. These characteristics have made it possible for CT to be used in a variety of oncological and non-oncological settings [9–37].

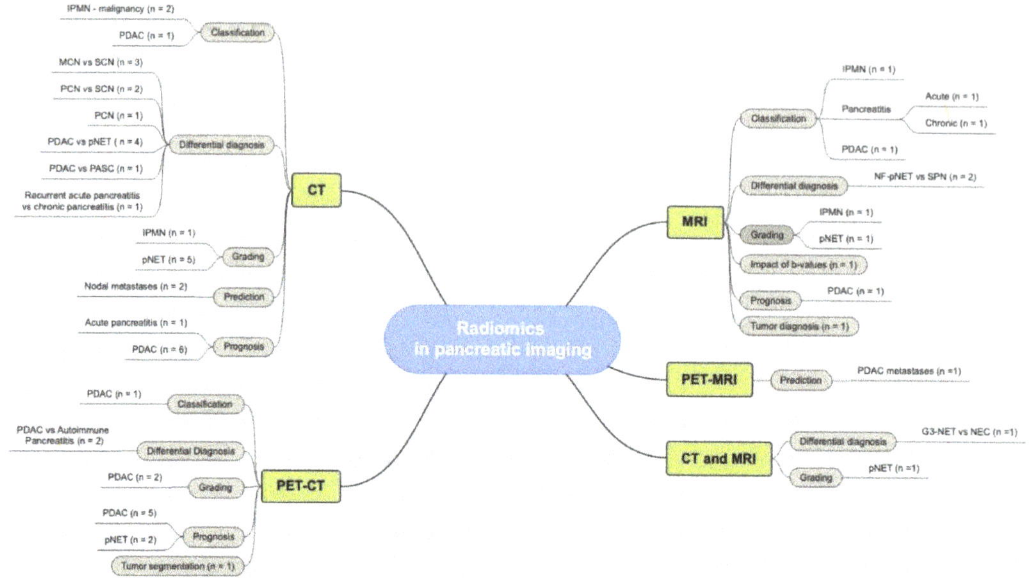

Figure 2. Summary of radiomics applications in pancreatic imaging.

3.1.1. Oncological Applications

Differentiating various lesions (from benign to different levels of malignancy) is the foundation of patient care assessment and many authors have been extensively studying this field. One of the most frequent differential diagnoses a radiologist can come across is differentiating cystic lesions. While some authors have tried to create an algorithm that ties together clinical and radiological features with radiomics signatures [11,13,14], others focus solely on radiomics and its validity in differentiating different cystic neoplasms [9,10,12]

When investigating pancreatic lesions, pancreatic neuroendocrine tumors (pNETs) have a peculiar enhancement pattern that differentiates them from other tumors. Nevertheless, when coming across very small or heterogeneous lesions, it is still quite challenging to understand whether it is a pNET or a pancreatic ductal adenocarcinoma (PDAC); hence, the majority of research is found in this field. We found that most authors focus on differentiating a PDAC from pNET [19–21,23], whereas others investigated radiomics use to predict the histological grade of a pNET [22,25–27].

On the other hand, when it comes to adenocarcinoma, the core investigation is about prognosis prediction. Recent studies show how radiomics features could be related with mortality, whether based on tumor analysis [32–34] or node involvement [35,36].

Cystic Lesions

Cystic findings within the pancreatic parenchyma represent a diagnostic challenge since it might be hard to tell apart pure benign lesions from the ones with transformation potential. However, the combined evaluation of macroscopic morphological features and texture analysis has afforded a great improvement in the diagnostic performance when it comes to the characterization of cystic lesions [9].

Yang et al. [9] evaluated the consistency of textural features between different slice thicknesses extracted from CT images of 2 mm- and 5 mm-thick slices and found a good correlation among the extracted features. They included 25 patients with mucinous cystic neoplasms (MCNs) and 53 patients with serous cystic neoplasms (SCNs) using a preliminary model based on texture extracted from CECT images selected via LASSO regression and random forest classifiers. In the validation group, they achieved an accuracy of 74% in the 2 mm slice-thickness group and 83% in the 5 mm slice-thickness group. This study highlighted the ability of radiomics in reducing misdiagnosis and avoiding overtreatment. In a similar study, the same authors assessed the potential of CT texture analysis in discriminating pancreatic serous cystadenoma from mucinous cystadenoma and improving the diagnostic performance by combining morphological characteristics and textural features. They used a combination of morphological characteristics of CT images and textural features that achieved an impressive AUC of 0.893 [10].

Shen et al. [11] analyzed the potential of CECT in the discrimination of the different subtypes of pancreatic cystic neoplasms (PCNs), considering that only SCNs have a lower malignant potential and need only periodic follow-up. Using a Boruta algorithm, five radiomics features (Histogram_Entropy, Histogram_Skeweness, LLL_GLSZM_GLV, Histogram_Uniformity, HHL_Histogram_Kurtosis) and four clinical factors (serum carbohydrate antigen 19-9, sex, age, and serum carcinoembryonic antigen) were significantly different across SCNs, MCNs and intraductal papillary mucinous neoplasms (IPMNs). Among the three machine learning (ML) algorithms, the random forest classifier achieved an accuracy of 79.59% in the validation cohort.

In a different study, Wei et al. [12] also used radiomics as a way to avoid overtreatment of benign lesions, as they used it as a diagnostic model to differentiate SCNs from other PCNs. Their results showed that texture features, including intensity T-range, wavelet intensity T-median, and wavelet neighborhood gray-tone difference matrix (NGTDM) busyness, and five guideline-based features (sex, location, moment difference, mean rectangular fitting factor, and size) were the most statistically significant in identifying SCNs. The model achieved an accuracy of ~76% in the cross-validation cohort and ~83% in an independent validation cohort.

Xie et al. [13] applied radiomics to differentiate atypical serous cystadenomas (ASCNs) and MCNs and compared radiomics and radiological analysis. They trained an ML model with radiomics features and then demonstrated that adding radiological features such as lesion location, shape, cyst wall, and wall enhancement into this model could significantly improve its performance. Similarly, Tobaly et al. [14] developed a radiomics model mostly based on high-order CT radiomics features, which showed high diagnostic performance in differentiating benign from malignant IPMNs. Their results showed that 85 radiomics features were significantly different between patients with benign and malignant IPMNs, reaching an AUC of 0.84.

Recently, Chen et al. [15] also developed and validated a CT-based radiomics nomogram for differentiating SCNs from mucin-producing PCNs in a preoperative setting. They included a total of 89 patients (31 SCNs, 30 IPMNs, and 28 MCNs) who underwent preoperative CT. The authors used a comprehensive nomogram incorporating clinical features and a fusion radiomics signature. The fusion radiomics signature used was obtained by the combination of the radiomics features extracted in the plain, late arterial, and venous phases. This nomogram obtained an AUC of 0.960 in the training cohort and 0.817 in the validation cohort.

Other studies focused on the prediction of the malignant potential of the IPMN whose management is challenging, owing to the low reliability of conventional imaging techniques in the identification of suspicious lesions. Hanania et al. [16] correlated the histopathological grade of an IPMN with a cross-validated panel of 10 radiomics markers within the cyst contours, reaching an AUC of 0.96 at a sensitivity of 97% and specificity of 88%. Permuth et al. [17] tested a combined model of radiomics features and miRNA genomic classifier (MGC) data, considered as potential biomarkers of pancreatic tumorigenesis, to achieve an AUC of 0.95, higher than those of the single variables (AUC of 0.77 for radiomics features and AUC of 0.83 for MGC data). Attiyeh et al. [18] focused only on a branch-duct IPMN (BD-IPMN) on a preoperative CT scan to create a combined model of quantitative and clinical features. It reached an AUC of 0.79, outperforming the single models (AUC of 0.67 for radiomics and AUC of 0.76 for clinical parameters), and the quantitative mural nodularity feature demonstrated a significant role in the prediction of high-risk disease.

pNET

For pNETs, the use of radiomics and CT has been studied for differentiating and classifying pancreatic tumors. He et al. [19] developed three models to differentiate non-functional pNETs and PDACs. Their model combined a radiomics signature and clinical-radiological features, reaching an AUC of 0.960 and 0.884 in the primary and validation cohort, respectively.

In relation to pNETs, Li et al. [20] examined the use of volumetric CT texture analysis in differentiating atypical pNETs from PDACs. The authors retrospectively analyzed 127 patients with 50 PDACs and 77 pNETs. They found that the fifth percentile and fifth+skewness were optimal parameters for alone and combined diagnosis with an AUC of 0.811 and 0.792, respectively, compared to the mean CT value (AUC = 0.678).

In another study by Yu et al. [21], radiomics was used to differentiate non-hypervascular pNETs from PDACs in 120 patients. Specifically, the authors compared the performances of significant features on conventional imaging techniques (maximum diameter on axial section, margins, calcification, tumor vascularity, and heterogeneity) and texture analysis both in the arterial phase and portal vein phase, achieving an AUC of 0.780, 0.855, and 0.929, respectively, on logistic regression.

Canellas et al. [22] also assessed whether CT texture and CT features are predictive of pNETs. Preoperative contrast-enhanced CT images of 101 patients with pNETs were assessed. The images were evaluated for tumor location, tumor size, tumor pattern, predominantly solid or cystic composition, presence of calcification, presence of heterogeneous enhancement on contrast-enhanced images, presence of pancreatic duct dilatation, presence of pancreatic atrophy, presence of vascular involvement by the tumor, and presence of lymphadenopathy. Their results showed that a size larger than 2.0 cm is useful for predicting aggressive tumors (grades 2 and 3). The only texture parameter predictive of tumor grade was entropy with a spatial scale filter 2 (AUC of 0.65).

Reinert et al. [23] also assessed the role of CT texture analysis for differentiation of PDACs from pNETs in the portal venous phase, comparing this data with visual assessment and tumor-to-pancreas attenuation ratios obtained by placing large hand-drawn ROIs in ^{18}F-FDG PET/CT, 68Ga-DOMITATE-PET/CT, dual-phase CT (including an arterial phase), and contrast-enhanced MRI of the pancreas. They obtained highly significant ($p < 0.005$) discriminatory textural features between PDACs and pNETs, and their model correctly classified PDACs or pNETs in 75.8% of patients. Specifically, 42/53 patients were predicted correctly as PDACs (sensitivity 79.2%) and 12/42 patients were predicted correctly as pNETs (sensitivity 71.4%).

Multiple studies have evaluated the possibility of predicting the histological grade of a pNET with CT-based texture analysis [24]. Some authors focused on the distinction between grade 1 and grade 2/3 pNETs, according to the different degrees of surgical resection needed (parenchyma-sparing vs. radical) and reported the performance of the tested nomogram (radiomics + clinical features) with an AUC of 0.894-0.902, which was higher than those of the single variables [25]. Moreover, Liang et al. [26] described a significant association between the Ki67 level and the rate of nuclear mitosis as an expression of cell proliferation, and a significant difference in overall survival between the G1 and G2/3 groups, predicted by the nomogram, as further confirmation of its prognostic value. As opposed to the previous studies, Guo et al. [27] tested radiomics features to distinguish pNETs with grade 1/2 or grade 3 with histopathological analysis, because the latter usually need chemotherapy or radiotherapy in addition to surgery. They found that, among conventional imaging features, arterial and portal enhancement ratios have the best sensitivity (86–94%) and specificity (92–100%), whereas among radiomics imaging features, mean gray-level intensity, entropy, and uniformity demonstrated good sensitivity (73–91%) and specificity (85–100%); when incorporating all these features together, the resulting AUC was $\geq$0.90.

Adenocarcinoma

For adenocarcinoma, radiomics and CT have been studied for differential diagnosis and survival prediction. Ren et al. [28] used CT and radiomics to assess their predictive ability in the differential diagnosis between pancreatic adenosquamous carcinoma (PASC) and PDAC. For this purpose, 81 patients with PDAC and 31 patients with PASC who underwent preoperative CECT were included. The authors selected seven radiomics features from late arterial phase images and three from the portal venous phase out of 792 radiomics features by using the random forest method extracted from the late arterial phase and portal venous phase. They validated their radiomics signature by using the 10-times leave-group-out cross-validation (LGOCV) method. Their signature showed promising results as a noninvasive method in the differential diagnosis between PASC and PDAC with 94.5% accuracy, 98.3% sensitivity, 90.1% specificity, 91.9% positive predictive value (PPV), and 97.8% negative predictive value (NPV).

Radiomics could be a supportive tool for the distinction of molecular phenotypes of PDAC that have different behaviors in terms of response to treatment and survival. A random forest (RF) ML algorithm by Kaissis et al. [29] was tested to distinguish between quasi-mesenchymal (QM − KRT81+) and non-quasi-mesenchymal (non-QM − HNF1a+) subtypes from radiomics features, reaching an AUC of 0.93, a sensitivity of 0.84, and a specificity of 0.92. Moreover, differences were reported in the median OS for identified QM and non-QM tumors at 16.1 and 20.9 months, respectively (HR 1.59).

Considering the poor outcome of PDAC, multiple studies have tested the application of radiomics in prognosis prediction, especially in patients that underwent curative surgery at risk for postoperative recurrence [30,31]. According to Xie et al. [32], a CT-based Rad-score with five features resulted in an independent prognostic factor for disease-free survival (DFS, HR 2.556) and overall survival (OS, HR 3.741) and patients with a higher Rad-score demonstrated a significantly poorer prognosis. No significant correlation was found between Rad-score and tumor recurrence. The combination of texture parameters with clinical data (differentiation grade, CA19-9, and TNM stage) into a radiomics nomogram could be a good survival estimator, also outperforming the clinical model and the TNM staging, with a C-index of 0.697 in the DFS analysis and 0.726 in the OS analysis.

Other authors focused on specific radiomics features, especially related to tumor heterogeneity and its prognostic role. Kim et al. [33] evaluated the differences in gray-level non-uniformity (GLN) as a texture parameter, and also created a Kaplan–Meier survival curve. After ROI placement on arterial CT images, significantly higher GLN values were found in tumors compared to normal pancreatic tissue and in cases with T3 diseases or poorly differentiated tumors. After multivariate analysis, a high GLN135 value, i.e., increased tissue heterogeneity, was statistically associated with a poor prognosis, and consequently, with short recurrence-free survival. Moreover, the presence of a non-uniform texture reflected an increased biological aggressiveness of the tumor, considering the nodal stage and the tumor differentiation. Authors further highlighted the prognostic role of texture analysis through the identification of histopathological features of the tumor, correlating the lower uniformity of pixel values and the higher level of hypoxia markers. Eilaghi et al. [34] described that uniformity, entropy, and correlation are significantly different in healthy and diseased parenchyma, but they are not associated with survival. On the contrary, the dissimilarity and inverse difference normalized were significantly related to OS, both with an AUC of 0.716, overcoming tumor intensity and tumor size.

The presence of nodal metastases is another indicator of poor prognosis after surgery that, according to Fang et al. [35], could be predicted with a texture analysis of a preoperative CT scan. In their cohort of 155 operable patients (73 with and 82 patients without nodal involvement), 10 texture features were significantly different in the two groups. The SumAverage, i.e., the measure of overall image brightness, resulted in being the most common co-occurrence matrix-based feature on portal venous images that indicated the overall density of the CT image, either at 1.25 mm or 5 mm. Differently, Li et al. [36]

developed a combined prediction nomogram, based on the pathological grade, CT-based node status and a radiomics signature of 15 features that yielded an AUC of 0.912.

3.1.2. Non-Oncological Applications

As for non-oncological application, there is still little evidence about CT radiomics and its implications with pancreatitis. While some authors have looked into the prediction of recurrence [37], others tried to evaluate whether a radiomics model could differentiate between acute and chronic pancreatitis [38].

Pancreatitis

Radiomics has been also tested in the support of non-oncological diagnosis, mainly in the identification of recurrent acute pancreatitis (AcP). Chen et al. [37] evaluated texture features on CT images at the first AcP episode to build a radiomics model of 10 features. This radiomics predictive model reached an AUC of 0.929, an accuracy of 89%, a sensitivity of 83.8%, and a specificity of 97.7%, outperforming the clinical model (an AUC of 0.671, an accuracy of 61%, a sensitivity of 60.5% and a specificity of 62.2%). Mashayekhi et al. [38] also included functional abdominal pain and chronic pancreatitis (CP) in the differential diagnosis with recurrent AcP. Their radiomics model included 11 features, 10 of which belonged to the gray-level co-occurrence matrix (GLCM) category and demonstrated high performance in the distinction of recurrent AP from nonspecific abdominal pain with AUC values of 0.77–0.95 and from CP with AUC values of 0.73–0.92. Then, an overall predictive accuracy of 82.1 % was found for the three diagnoses with an IsoSVM classifier, and recurrent AcP had the lowest rate of misclassification (5% vs. 21% for abdominal pain and 25% for CP).

Table 1 provides a summary of the papers included in the review, focused on the application of radiomics in CT images.

3.2. Radiomics and PET-CT

3.2.1. Oncological Applications

Some PET-based radiomics studies have also been proposed [3,4,39–46]. PET images help in the characterization of biological features of tumors, which are usually associated with their sensitivity and/or aggressiveness [4]. Moreover, [^{18}F]F-fluorodeoxyglucose (FDG) positron emission tomography/computed tomography (PET/CT) combines functional information and anatomic information [3].

Tumor delineation is one of the factors that may affect radiomics features. PET images are considered to be difficult to delineate as edge contours of uptake regions are not sharp and clear. Belli et al. [4] investigated the impact of delineation variability on PET radiomics features. For this purpose, they included 25 pancreatic cancer patients previously treated with FDG PET/CT. The authors found that PET_edge was sufficiently robust against manual delineation, which suggests the possibility of replacing manual with semiautomatic delineation of pancreatic tumors. In a different study, Zhang et al. [39] concluded that the quantified radiomics model is significantly superior to both human doctors and clinical factor-based prediction models in terms of accuracy and specificity for the differentiation of autoimmune pancreatitis and PDAC in F-FDG PET/CT images. According to their results, the combination of the SVM-RFE feature selection strategy and linear SVM classifier had the highest diagnostic performance, with an AUC of 0.93.

Table 1. Applications of radiomics in pancreatic CT images.

Author	Year	Radiomics Analysis	Task	N Pts	Data Split	Ref Standard	CT Phase	Results
Yang	2019	LIFEx software	Differential diagnosis (MCN vs. SCN)	78 (25 MCNs, 53 SCNs)	RW (TS:DS = 4:1)	Histopathology	AP, PVP	Radiomics features, 2 mm: AUC 0.66, Acc 74%, Sen 86%, Spe 71% Radiomics features, 5 mm: AUC 0.75, Acc 83%, Sen 85%, Spe 83%
Yang (1)	2019	LIFEx software	Differential diagnosis (MCN vs. SCN)	91 (32 MCNs, 59 SCNs)	SW	Histopathology	PAP	Textural features: AUC 0.777 Textural features + morphological characteristics: AUC 0.893
Xie	2019	In-house algorithm (MATLAB R2017a)	Differential diagnosis (MCN vs. SCN)	57 (31 MCNs, 26 SCNs)	SW	Radiologist	AP, PVP, DP	Radiomics model: AUC 0.989, Acc 94.7%, Sen 93.6%, Spe 96.2% Combined model (radiomics + radiological features): AUC 0.994, Acc 98.2%, Sen 96.8%, Spe 100%
Chen	2021	Analysis Kit Software (v 3.0.0.R)	Differential diagnosis (PCN vs. SCN)	89 (31 SCNs, 30 IPMNs, 28 MCNs)	RW (63 TS, 26 VS)	Radiologist	NECT, AP, PVP	Radiomics signature NECT + AP + PVP: AUC 0.817
Wei	2019	NS	Differential diagnosis (PCN vs. SCN)	260 (102 SCNs, 158 non-SCNs)	SW (200 TS, 60 VS)	Radiologist	AP, PVP	Radiomics method: AUC 0.837, Sen 66.7%, Spe 81.8%
Shen	2020	ANN, RF, SVM (MATLAB 2017b)	Differential diagnosis (PCN)	164 (76 SCAs, 40 MCNs, 48 IPMNs)	SW (115 TS, 41 VS)	Histopathology	AP	Radiomics model (nine features) Acc 71.43% (SVM, ANN), 79.59% (RF)
He	2019	Pyradiomics	Differential diagnosis (PDAC vs. pNET)	147 (80 PDACs, 67 pNETs)	SW (100 TS, 47 VS)	Radiologist	PAP, PVP	Radiomics signature: AUC 0.873, Acc 76.6%, Sen 92.3%, Spe 70.6% Integrated model (radiomics + clinical features): AUC 0.884, Acc 80.4%, Sen 80.0%, Spe 80.8%
Li	2018	FireVoxel Software	Differential diagnosis (PDAC vs. pNET)	75 (50 PDACs, 25 pNETs)	SW	Radiologist	AP, PVP	Combined fifth + skewness as the best parameters: AUC 0.887, Sen 90%, Spe 80%
Reinert	2020	Pyradiomics	Differential diagnosis (PDAC vs. pNET)	95 (53 PDACs, 42 pNETs)	SW	Radiologist	PVP	Significant discriminatory features: first-order features, i.e., median, total energy, energy, 10th percentile, 90th percentile, minimum, maximum; second-order feature, i.e., gray-level co-occurrence matrix informational measure of correlation (Sen 79%, Spe 71%)

Table 1. *Cont.*

Author	Year	Radiomics Analysis	Task	N Pts	Data Split	Ref Standard	CT Phase	Results
Yu	2020	Analysis Kit Software	Differential diagnosis (PDAC vs. pNET)	120 (80 PDACs, 40 pNETs)	RW	Radiologist	AP, PVP	AP texture model: AUC 0.855 PVP texture model: AUC 0.929
Ren	2020	Analysis Kit Software (v 3.0.0.R)	Differential diagnosis (PDAC vs. PASC)	112 (81 PDACs, 31 PASCs)	RW (TS:DS = 2:1)	Histopathology	PAP, PVP	Acc 94.5%, Sen 98.3%, Spe 90.1%, PPV 91.9%, NPV 97.8%
Tobaly	2020	Pyradiomics (v 2.2.0)	IPMN grading	408 (181 benign, 227 malignant)	SW (296 TS, 112 VS)	Histopathology	PAP, PVP	Benign vs. malignant IPMN radiomics model: AUC 0.71, Acc 64%, Sen 69%, Spe 57% Radiomics + surgical indication: AUC 0.75, Acc 67%, Sen 69%, Spe 65%
Hanania	2016	IBEX	Prediction of IPMN malignancy	53 (34 high-grade, 19 low-grade)	SW(TS:DS = 7:3)	Histopathology	AP	Radiomics panel (10 features): AUC 0.96, Sen 97%, Spe 88%
Permuth	2016	In-house algorithm (Definiens Platform)	Prediction of IPMN malignancy	38 (20 benign, 18 malignant)	SW(TS:DS = 9:1)	Histopathology	AP, PVP	Radiomics signature (14 features): AUC 0.77, Sen 83%, Spe 74% Integrated model 1 (radiomics + genomic data): AUC 0.92, Sen 83%, Spe 89% Integrated model 2 (radiomics + standard imaging + genomic data): AUC 0.93, Sen 89%, Spe 89%
Canellas	2018	TexRAD (v 3.1)	pNET grading	101 (63 grade 1, 35 grade 2, 3 grade 3)	SW	Histopathology	PVP	Entropy as an independent predictor: OR 3.7, AUC 0.65, values > 4.65 with differences in DFS (G1 vs. G2/G3)
Gu	2019	Pyradiomics (v 1.3.0)	pNET grading (G1 vs. G2/G3)	138 (57 grade 1, 69 grade 2, 12 grade 3)	RW (104 TS, 34 VS)	Histopathology	AP, PVP	Nomogram (radiomics features + clinical risk factor tumor margin): AUC 0.902
Guo	2019	MATLAB R2014a	pNET grading (G1/G2 vs. G3)	37 (13 grade 1, 11 grade 2, 13 grade 3)	RW	Histopathology	NECT, AP, PVP	Texture features AUC 0.93, Sen 91.7%, Spe 84.6% Size/margin + texture features AUC 0.958, Sen 91.6%, Spe 87.5%
Liang	2019	In-house algorithm (MATLAB R2016a)	pNET grading (G1 vs. G2/G3)	137 (70 grade 1, 67 grade 2/3)	RW (86 TS, 51 VS)	Histopathology	AP	Nomogram (eight radiomics features + clinical stage): AUC 0.891

Table 1. *Cont.*

Author	Year	Radiomics Analysis	Task	N Pts	Data Split	Ref Standard	CT Phase	Results
D'Onofrio	2019	MaZda Software (v 4.6)	pNET grading	100 (31 grade 1, 52 grade 2, 17 grade 3)	RW	Radiologist	AP, PVP	Kurtosis is different among three G groups: AUC 0.924, Sen 82%, Spe 85% for G3 diagnosis Entropy different between G1 and G3 and G2 and G3 groups: AUC 0.732, Sen 82%, Spe 64% for G3 diagnosis
Kaissis	2020	Pyradiomics	PDAC classification	207 (45 QM, 136 non-QM, 26 unclassifiable)	SW (181 TS, 26 VS)	Histopathology	PVP	AUC 0.93, Sen 0.84, Spe 0.92
Attiyeh	2018	MATLAB R2015a	PDAC prognosis	161	SW (113 TS, 48 VS)	Radiologist	PVP	Model A, preoperative CA19-9 and image features: c-index 0.69 Model B, preoperative CA19-9, Brennan score (postresection pathological variables), and image features: c-index 0.74
Khalvati	2019	Pyradiomics	PDAC prognosis	98	SW (30 TS, 68 VS)	Radiologist	PAP, PVP	Radiomics signature: HR 1.35 (Reader 2), 1.56 (Reader 1)
Yun	2018	NS	PDAC prognosis	88 (70 recurrence, 18 non-recurrence)	SW	Radiologist	PAP, PVP	Correlation of recurrence with texture features Average: AUC 0.736, standard deviation: AUC 0.709, contrast: AUC 0.692, correlation: AUC 0.698 Survival analysis nodal metastasis: HR 2.0375, average: HR 0.5599, standard deviation HR 0.5745
Xie	2020	NS	PDAC prognosis	220	SW (147 TS, 73 VS)	NS	PAP	Rad-score: low-RS correlated with better prognosis (AUC 0.715), HR 2.556 for DFS, HR 3.741 for OS
Kim	2019	NS	PDAC prognosis	116	SW	Radiologist	AP	GLN135: higher levels correlated with shorter DFS (HR 6.030)
Eilaghi	2017	MATLAB R2015a	PDAC prognosis	30	SW	Radiologist	PAP, PVP	Prediction of OS Tumor dissimilarity: AUC 0.716 Inverse difference normalized: AUC 0.716
Fang	2020	MaZda Software (v 4.6)	Prediction of LN metastasis	155 (73 nodal matastases, 82 without nodal metastases)	RW	Histopathology	AP, PVP	Ten texture features with significance in ROC analysis: biggest AUC 0.630 for wavelet-based feature WavEnLH_s-2

Table 1. *Cont.*

Author	Year	Radiomics Analysis	Task	N Pts	Data Split	Ref Standard	CT Phase	Results
Li	2020	Pyradiomics	Prediction of LN metastasis	159 (59 nodal matastases, 100 without nodal metastases)	SW (118 TS, 41 VS)	Histopathology	AP, PVP	Radiomics signature (15 features): AUC 0.912
Chen	2019	IBEX	AcP prognosis	389 (181 recurrent AcP)	RW (271 TS, 118 VS)	Radiologist	AP, PVP	Recurrence prediction: AUC 0.929, Acc 89.0%
Mashayekhi	2020	In-house algorithm (MATLAB)	Differential diagnosis (recurrent AcP vs. CP)	56 (20 recurrent AcP, 19 functional abdominal pain, 17 CP)	SW	Radiologist	PVP	Acc 82.1%; recurrent AP: AUC 0.88, Sen 95%, Spe 78%; CP: AUC 0.90, Sen 71%, Spe 95%

Acc—accuracy, ANN—artificial neural network, AP—arterial phase, AcP—acute pancreatitis, AUC—area under the curve, CECT—contrast-enhanced computed tomography, CNN —convolutional neural network, CP—chronic pancreatitis, CT—computed tomography, DFS—disease-free survival, DP—delayed phase, HR—hazard ratio, IPMN—intraductal papillary mucinous neoplasm, MCN—mucinous cystic neoplasm, NECT—non-enhanced computed tomography, NS—not specified, OR—odds ratio, OS—overall Survival, PAP—pancreatic phase, PASC—pancreatic adenosquamous carcinoma, PDAC—pancreatic ductal adenocarcinoma, PCN—pancreatic cystic neoplasm, pNET—pancreatic neuroendocrine tumor, PVP—portal venous phase, RF—random forest, RW—recorc-wise, SCA—serous cystic adenoma, SCN—serous cystic neoplasm, SVM—support vector machine, Sen—sensitivity, Spe—specificity, SW—subject-wise, TS—training set, VS—validation set.

pNET

Other studies have assessed the potentiality of radiomics analysis extracted by [68Ga]Ga-DOTATOC PET/CT [40,41]. Mapelli et al. [40] found that specific texture features derived from preoperative [68Ga]Ga-DOTATOC and 18F-FDG PET/CT could noninvasively predict specific tumor characteristics and outcomes of patients with NETs. Meanwhile, Liberini et al. [41] carried out a pilot study on two NET patients. Their preliminary results suggested the use of RFs and TLSREwb-50 and SRETVwb-50 as parameters to evaluate the response to peptide receptor radionuclide therapy (PRRT) in their patients.

Adenocarcinoma

Lim et al. [42] investigated FDG PET/CT images of 48 patients with PDAC. Their results showed that genetic alterations of KRAS (correlated with reduced low-intensity textural signatures) and SMAD4 (correlated with reduced high-intensity textural signatures) had significant associations with FDG PET-based radiomics features in PDAC.

Moreover, Xing et al. [3] developed and validated a model based on radiomics features derived from [18F]F-fluorodeoxyglucose PET/CT images to preoperatively predict the pathological grade of PDACs. Their model, based on a twelve-feature-combined radiomics signature, could stratify PDAC patients into grade 1 and grade 2/3 groups with an AUC of 0.994 in the training set and 0.921 in the validation set.

Other studies focused on the identification of prognostic features in FDG PET/CT images in patients treated with stereotactic body radiation therapy. Cui et al. [43] included 139 patients with locally advanced pancreatic cancer that underwent the PET/CT study for the planning of the radiation treatment, and they identified a prognostic signature of seven features, including texture feature, shape complexity, and SUV intensity distribution. Through multivariate analysis, the proposed model was significantly associated with overall survival with a hazard ratio of 3.72 and outperformed conventional imaging parameters, i.e., gross tumor volume and maximum standardized uptake value (SUVmax). Yue et al. [44] identified five significant prognostic variables with multivariate Cox analysis (age, node stage, variations of homogeneity, variance, and cluster tendency) that are able to predict therapy response using both pre- and post-treatment FDG PET/CT. Specifically, they evaluated the texture variation between the two examinations as an index of locoregional metabolic response: a lower texture variation (<15%) was found in the high-risk group with a shorter mean overall survival (17.7 months).

Liu et al. [45] developed a radiomics-based prediction model using dual-time PET/CT imaging for the noninvasive classification of PDAC and autoimmune pancreatitis (AIP) lesions. In their series, they included 112 patients (48 patients with AIP and 64 patients with PDAC). Their model was developed from a combination of the SVM-RFE and linear SVM with the required quantitative features. The multimodal and multidimensional features obtained an average AUC of 0.9668, an accuracy of 89.91%, a sensitivity of 85.31%, and a specificity of 96.04%.

Toyama et al. [46] evaluated the prognostic value of FDG PET radiomics and found that the gray-level zone length matrix (GLZLM) gray-level non-uniformity (GLNU) PET parameter was the most relevant factor for predicting 1-year survival, followed by total lesion glycolysis (TLG). The combination of GLZLM, GLNU, and TLG stratified patients into three groups according to the risk of poor prognosis.

Table 2 provides a summary of the papers included in the review, focused on the application of radiomics in PET-CT images.

Table 2. Applications of radiomics in pancreatic PET-CT images.

Author	Year	Radiomics Analysis	Task	N Pts	Data Split	Reference Standard	Radiotracer	CT Phase	Results
Liu	2021	SVM (MATLAB R2018a)	Differential diagnosis (PDAC vs. autoimmune pancreatitis)	112 (64 PDACs, 48 autoimmune pancreatitis)	RW	Radiologist	FDG	NECT	AUC 0.9668, Acc 89.91%, Sen 85.31%, Spe 96.04%
Zhang	2019	SVM (MATLAB R2017a)	Differential diagnosis (PDAC vs. autoimmune pancreatitis)	111 (66 PDACs, 45 autoimmune pancreatitis)	RW	Radiologist	FDG	NECT	AUC 0.93, Acc 85%, Sen 86%, Spe 84%
Lim	2020	MIM (v 6.4)	PDAC classification	48	SW	Radiologist	FDG	NECT	KRAS gene mutation: significant association with long-run emphasis (AUC 0.806), zone emphasis (AUC 0.794), large-zone emphasis (AUC 0.829); SMAD4 gene mutation: significant association with standardized uptake value skewness (AUC 0.727), long-run emphasis (AUC 0.692), high-intensity textural features such as run emphasis (AUC 0.775), short-run emphasis (AUC 0.736), zone emphasis (AUC 0.750), and short-zone emphasis (AUC 0.725)
Xing	2021	Pyradiomics	PDAC grading	149	RW (99 TS, 50 VS)	Nuclear medicine physician	FDG	NECT	Prediction model (12 features): AUC 0.921 for G1 vs. G2/3
Mapelli	2020	Chang-Gung Image Texture Analysis software package (v 1.3)	pNET prognosis	61	RW	NS	DOTADOC, FDG	NECT	DOTATOC PET: SZV, entropy, intensity variability, and SRD were predictive of tumor dimension; FDG PET: intensity variability, SZV, homogeneity, SUVmax, and MTV were predictive for tumor dimension
Liberini	2020	LIFEx software (v 5.10)	pNET prognosis	2	SW	NS	DOTADOC	NECT	A significant difference of 28 radiomics features in pre- and post-treatment studies

Table 2. *Cont.*

Author	Year	Radiomics Analysis	Task	N Pts	Data Split	Reference Standard	Radiotracer	CT Phase	Results
Toyama	2020	LIFEx software	PDAC prognosis	161	SW	Histopathology	FDG	NECT	GLZLM GLNU as an independent predictor factor for poor prognosis (HR 2.0)
Cui	2016	MITK software (v 3.1.0.A)	PDAC prognosis	139	SW (90 TS, 49 VS)	NS	FDG	NECT	Prognostic signature (seven features): HR 3.72
Yue	2017	3D kernel-based approach	PDAC prognosis	26	SW	NS	FDG	NECT	Low-risk group: higher texture variation (>30%) and longer mean OS (29.3 months); high-risk group: lower texture variation (<15%) and shorter mean OS (17.7 months)
Belli	2018	CGITA software (v 1.4)	Tumor segmentation	25	SW	Radiologist	FDG	NECT	DSC 0.73

Acc—accuracy, AUC—area under the curve, CT—computed tomography, DOTADOC—DOTA-Tyr-octreotide, FDG—fluorodeoxyglucose, HR—hazard ratio, NECT—non-enhanced computed tomography, NS—not specified, OS—overall survival, PET—positron emission tomography, pNET—pancreatic neuroendocrine tumor, PDAC—pancreatic ductal adenocarcinoma, RW—record-wise, Sen—sensitivity, Spe—specificity, SW—subject-wise, TS—training set, VS—validation set.

3.3. Radiomics and MRI

3.3.1. Oncological Applications

MRIs offer several advantages in the diagnosis of pancreatic tumors, such as contrast resolution and a better examination of the pancreaticobiliary system [47].

When evaluating cystic lesions with MRI, one of the daily challenges of a radiologist is examining IPMNs and expressing the likelihood of malignant degeneration. On this note, some authors investigated the use of MR radiomics signatures to predict the risk of malignancy of IPMNs through texture analysis alone [48] or combining both clinical characteristics and radiological characteristics [49].

As previously stated, the radiomics of pNETs has been studied thoroughly for their immediate clinical implications. When it comes to MRI findings, some authors [50] have investigated radiomics models that could predict the histopathologic grade of pNETs. On the other hand, other authors have focused mainly on differentiating pNETs from SPNs, either with T1WI and postcontrast phases [51] or with the use of DWI sequences together with other standard phases [52].

As for adenocarcinoma, most studies about the radiomics of MRI rely on ADC metrics either to differentiate normal parenchyma from pancreatic neoplasm [53] or for outcome prediction and overall survival [54].

Cystic Lesions

Jeon et al. [48] studied the utility of MR findings and texture analysis for predicting the malignant potential of pancreatic IPMNs. The authors found seven significant predictors of malignancy: effective diameter, surface area, sphericity, compactness, entropy, and gray-level co-occurrence matrix entropy ($p < 0.05$). They calculated the diagnostic performance by using Cohen's κ for predicting malignant IPMNs, which was 0.80 (good agreement). Recently, Cui et al. [49] assessed the use of a nomogram combining clinical characteristics and radiomics features, including histograms, texture parameters, the RLM (run-length matrix), and the GLCM (gray-level co-occurrence matrix), for the diagnosis of high-grade branching-type IPMNs in 202 patients from three medical centers. Their radiomics signature obtained AUC values of 0.836 in the training cohort, 0.811 in the first external validation cohort, and 0.822 in the second external validation cohort, whereas using the radiomics nomogram, the high-grade disease-associated AUC values were 0.903 (training cohort), 0.884 (external validation cohort 1), and 0.876 (external validation cohort 2). Their radiomics nomogram model could effectively distinguish high-grade patients with IPMN preoperatively, resulting in better treatment methods and tailored therapy in patients with IPMN.

pNET

Regarding pNETs, Guo et al. [50] proved that MRI findings, including tumor margin, texture, local invasion or metastases, tumor enhancement, and diffusion restriction, as well as texture parameters, can aid in the prediction of pNET grading. For this purpose, they evaluated the performance of MRI findings and texture parameters for the prediction of the histopathologic grade of a pNET with 3-T magnetic resonance. They included 31 G1, 29 G2, and 17 G3 patients. G2/G3 tumors showed higher frequencies of an ill-defined margin, a predominantly solid tumor type, local invasion or metastases, hypoenhancement in the arterial phase, and restriction diffusion. The AUCs of six predicting models on T2WI and DWI ranged from 0.703 to 0.989. Song et al. [51] assessed the value of radiomics parameters derived from MRI in the differentiation of hypovascular nonfunctional pancreatic neuroendocrine tumors (hypo-NF-pNETs) and solid pseudopapillary neoplasms of the pancreas (SPNs) by including fifty-seven SPN patients and twenty-two hypo-NF-pNET patients. They extracted radiomics features from the T1WI, arterial, portal, and delayed phases of MR images. The radiomics signature of the arterial phase was picked to build a clinic-radiomics nomogram. The nomogram, composed of the age and radiomics signature of the arterial phase, showed sufficient performance for discriminating SPNs and hypo-NF-pNETs with AUC values of 0.965 and 0.920 in the training and validation cohorts, respectively. Similarly, Li et al. [52] tested preoperative MRI-based texture analysis to differentiate NF-pNETs (201 patients) and SPNs (101 patients). Nonlinear discriminant analysis (NDA) had a lower value of misclassification rate, especially with DWI sequences (7.92%) than radiologists (34.65%), and the postcontrast DCE-T1WI+fs sequence appeared to provide more information for the distinction with mean and percentile as the most discriminative features.

Adenocarcinoma

In adenocarcinoma, MR and radiomics have shown great results in differentiating normal pancreatic parenchyma from pancreatic neoplasm. In 2019, Taffel et al. [53] evaluated whole-lesion 3D histogram apparent diffusion coefficient (ADC) metrics for the assessment of pancreatic malignancy. For this purpose, forty-two patients with pancreatic malignancies (36 PDACs, 6 PanNETs) had undergone abdominal MRI with diffusion-weighted imaging before endoscopic ultrasound biopsy or surgical resection. The volumetric ADC histogram metrics showed to be effective as a noninvasive biomarker of pancreatic malignancy with an AUC = 0.787–0.792.

The identification of the specific PDAC subtypes could have an important prognostic role in a different rate of treatment response and changes in the overall survival. PDAC has a high heterogeneity on a genetic, proteomic, and transcriptomic level that cannot be appreciated on conventional imaging techniques. Kaissis et al. [54] developed an ML model for the extraction of radiomics features from the diffusion-weighted imaging (DWI)-derived ADC maps for a prognostic evaluation of the tumor. Their algorithm achieved high performances in the outcome prediction with 87% sensitivity, 80% specificity, and 90% AUC in the distinction of above- versus below-median overall survival and the main indicative imaging features belonged to the heterogeneity-related group. Moreover, according to the histopathological classification, almost all the patients with a quasi-mesenchymal tumor subtype (8/9) demonstrated a below-median overall survival. The same research group performed a similar study, focusing on molecular PDAC subtypes and response to chemotherapy. Specifically, KRT81+ patients had a significantly lower median overall survival than KRT81- patients (7.0 vs. 22.6 months, HR 4.03) and a better response to gemcitabine-based chemotherapy over FOLFIRINOX (10.14 vs. 3.8 months median overall survival, HR 2.33). On the contrary, FOLFIRINOX was more effective in KRT81- patients than the gemcitabine-based treatment (30.8 vs. 13.4 months median overall survival, HR 2.41) [55].

3.3.2. Non-Oncological Applications

In 2016, Becker et al. [56] demonstrated that b-values significantly affect texture analysis on DWI images. To this purpose, echo-planar DWI sequences at 16 b-values ranging between 0 and 1000 s/mm2 were acquired at 3-T in 8 healthy male volunteers. According to the authors, several texture features vary systematically in healthy tissues at different b-values, which needs to be taken into account if DWI data with different b-values are analyzed.

Pancreatitis

Radiomics models have been applied to the study of pancreatitis whose diagnosis is mainly based on morphological changes in the pancreas using conventional imaging techniques [57,58]. In the very early phases of acute pancreatitis, those pancreatic abnormalities are not easy to evaluate and could lead to underestimating the incidence of the disease. Starting from this idea, Lin et al. [57] developed a radiomics model using contrast-enhanced MRI (CE-MRI), specifically on the portal venous phase images, for the prediction of the AcP severity also in the early stages of the disease. Their model had an AUC of 0.848 in the training cohort and outperformed the conventional scoring systems, i.e., the MR severity index (MRSI; AUC 0.719), Acute Physiology and Chronic Health Evaluation (APACHE II; 0.725), and bedside index for severity in AcP (BISAP; AUC 0.708).

In 2020, Frokjaer et al. [58] assessed the texture analysis in MRI examinations from 77 patients with CP and 22 controls and obtained a 97% sensitivity, 100% specificity, and 98% accuracy in the classification of chronic pancreatitis vs. healthy controls.

Table 3 provides a summary of the papers included in the review, focused on the application of radiomics in MRI images.

3.4. Radiomics and PET-MRI
Oncological Applications

A study by Gao et al. [59] assessed the use of PET-MRI and radiomics for oncologic treatment prediction outcomes. Specifically, they focused on the imaging biomarkers of glucose metabolic activity and DWI derived from pretreatment integrated ^{18}F-fluorodeoxyglucose PET-MRI imaging as potential predictive factors of metastasis in patients with PDAC. The AUC was 0.939, 0.894, 0.924, and 0.909 for PET-GLRLM_LRHGE, ADC-GLRLM_LRHGE, ADCGLRLM_GLNU, and ADC-GLRLM_RLNU, respectively, whereas the logistic regression model with proposed features obtained an AUC of 1.000.

Table 4 provides a summary of the papers included in the review, focused on the application of radiomics in PET-MRI images.

3.5. Radiomics in Combined CT and MRI Studies
Oncological Applications

Other studies included radiomics applied to both CT and MRI. In 2019, Azoulay et al. [60] compared morphological imaging features and CT texture histogram parameters between grade 3 pancreatic neuroendocrine tumors (G3-pNETs) and neuroendocrine carcinomas (NECs). For this purpose, they included patients with pathologically proven G3-pNETs and NECs who had CT and MRI examinations between 2006–2017 and were retrospectively included. Two radiologists reviewed both CT and MRI for tumor size, enhancement patterns, hemorrhagic content, liver metastases, and lymphadenopathies, and a texture histogram analysis of tumors was performed on arterial and portal phase CT images. The authors found that pancreatic NECs are larger, more frequently hypoattenuating, and more heterogeneous with hemorrhagic content than G3-pNETs on CT and MRI with an AUC of 0.694, 78% sensitivity, and 58% specificity. Recently, Ohki et al. [61] used ADC values in the differential diagnosis of malignant pancreatic disease. They found that texture analysis may aid in differentiating between G1 and G2–3-pNETs.

Table 5 provides a summary of the papers included in the review, focused on the application of radiomics in CT and MRI images.

Table 3. Applications of radiomics in pancreatic MRI images.

Author	Year	Radiomics Analysis	Task	N Pts	Data Split	Reference Standard	MRI Phase	Results
Song	2021	Pyradiomics	Differential diagnosis (NF-pNET vs. SPN)	79 (22 NF-pNETs, 57 SPNs)	RW (TS:DS = 7:3)	Histopathology	T2WI, DWI, T1WI, CE-T1WI	Precontrast T1WI: AUC 0.853 AP: AUC 0.907 PVP: AUC 0.773 DP: AUC 0.773 Clinic-radiomics nomogram: AUC 0.920, Acc 90.0%, Sen 100.0%, Spec 71.4%
Li	2019	MaZda (v 4.6)	Differential diagnosis (NF-pNET vs. SPN)	119 (61 NF-pNETs, 58 SPNs)	RW (101 TS, 18 DS)	Histopathology	T2WI, DWI, T1WI, CE-T1WI	AP: AUC 0.925 DP: AUC 0.950
Cui	2021	MITK Software (v 3.1.0.A)	IPMN grading	202 (152 low-grade, 50 high-grade)	RW (103 TS, 48 VS1, 51 VS2)	Histopathology	T2WI, T1WI, CE-T1WI	SET 1 Radiomics signature: AUC 0.811; Nomogram: AUC 0.884, Sen 90.0%, Spe 79.0% SET 2 Radiomics signature: AUC 0.822; Nomogram: AUC 0.876, Sen 85.7%, Spe 83.7%
Jeon	2021	MEDIP	Prediction of IPMN malignancy	248 (142 Benign, 106 Malignant)	SW	Histopathology	MRCP	AUC 0.85 (Greater entropy and smaller compactness as independent predictors)
Guo	2019	Omni-Kinetics software (v 2.0.10)	pNET grading	77 (31 grade 1, 29 grade 2, 17 grade 3)	RW	Histopathology	T2WI, DWI, T1WI, CE-T1WI	Independent predictors of T2WI: inverse difference moment for G1 vs. G2 (AUC 0.833), energy+correlation+difference entropy for G1 vs. G3 (AUC 0.989), difference entropy for G2 vs. G3 (AUC 0.813); Independent predictors of DWI: correlation+contrast+inverse difference moment for G1 vs. G2 (AUC 0.841), maxintensity+entropy+inverse difference moment for G1 vs. G3 (AUC 0.962), maxintensity for G2 vs. G3 (AUC 0.703)

Table 3. *Cont.*

Author	Year	Radiomics Analysis	Task	N Pts	Data Split	Reference Standard	MRI Phase	Results
Kaissis	2019	Pyradiomics	PDAC prognosis	132	SW (100 TS, 32 VS)	Histopathology	T2WI, DWI, T1WI, CE-T1WI	AUC 0.90, Sen 87%, Spe 80%
Kaissis (1)	2019	Pyradiomics	PDAC classification	55 (27 KRT81+, 28 KRT81-)	SW	Histopathology	T2WI, DWI, T1WI, CE-T1WI	AUC 0.93, Sen 90%, Spe 92%
Taffel	2019	In-house software FireVoxel	Tumor diagnosis	42 (36 PDACs, 6 pNETs)	SW	Histopathology	T2WI, DWI, T1WI, CE-T1WI	ADC histogram differentiation NET-PDAC: AUC 0.88-0.92, Sen 94–97%, Spe 83–88%; Differentiation nodal status: AUC 0.80–0.82, Sen 87%, Spe 67–83%
Becker	2017	In-house algorithm (MATLAB R2015b)	Impact of b-values	8 controls	RW	Radiologist	DWI	Significant positive correlations with b-value: skewness, contrast, correlation, energy, LRE, GLN, RP; Significant negative correlations with b-value: kurtosis, entropy, homogeneity, LGRE, SRLGE, LRLGE
Lin	2019	IBEX	AcP classification	259 (142 mild AcP, 117 severe AcP)	SW (180 TS, 79 VS)	Radiologist	CE-T1WI	AUC 0.848, Acc 81.0%, Sen 75.0%, Spe 86.0%
Frokjaer	2020	SlicerRadiomics extension (v 4.10.1)	CP classification	99 (77 CP, 22 controls)	SW	Radiologist	T2WI, DWI, MRCP	Acc 98%, Sen 97%, Spe 100%

Acc—accuracy, ADC—apparent diffusion coefficient, AP—arterial phase, AcP—acute pancreatitis, AUC—area under the curve, CE—contrast-enhanced, CP—chronic pancreatitis, DP—delayed phase, DWI—diffusion-weighted imaging, IPMN—intraductal papillary mucinous neoplasm, MRCP—magnetic resonance cholangiopancreatography, MRI—magnetic resonance imaging, PDAC—pancreatic ductal adenocarcinoma, pNET—pancreatic neuroendocrine tumor, NF-pNET—nonfunctioning pancreatic neuroendocrine tumor, PVP—portal venous phase, RW—record-wise, Sen—sensitivity, Spe—specificity, SPN—solid pseudopapillary neoplasm, SW—subject-wise, T1WI—T1-weighted imaging, T2WI—T2-weighted imaging, TS—training set, VS—validation set.

Table 4. Applications of radiomics in pancreatic PET-MRI images.

Author	Year	Radiomics Analysis	Task	N Pts	Data Split	Reference Standard	Radiotracer	MRI Phase	Results
Gao	2020	LIFEx software	Prediction of metastatic disease	17 (11 metastatic PDACs, 6 non-metastatic PDACs)	RW	Radiologist and nuclear medicine physician	FDG	T2W HASTE, DWI, T1WI DIXON	SUV: AUC 0.818, Sen 72.7%, Spe 100%MTV: AUC 0.818, Sen 63.6%, Spe 100%TLG: AUC 0.848, Sen 72.7%, Spe 100%

AUC—area under the curve, DWI—diffusion-weighted imaging, FDG—fluorodeoxyglucose, HASTE—half-Fourier acquisition single-shot turbo spin-echo sequence, MRI—magnetic resonance imaging, MTV—metabolic tumor volume, PDAC—pancreatic ductal adenocarcinoma, RW—record-wise, Sen—sensitivity, Spe—specificity, SUV—standardized uptake value, T1WI—T1-weighted imaging, T2WI—T2-weighted imaging, TLG—total lesion glycolysis.

Table 5. Applications of radiomics in pancreatic CT and MRI images.

Author	Year	Radiomics Analysis	Task	N Pts	Data Split	Reference Standard	CT/MRI Phase	Results
Azoulay	2019	TexRAD	Differential diagnosis (G3-pNET vs. NEC)	37 (14 G3-pNETs, 23 NECs)	RW	Radiologist	CT: NECT, AP, PVP MRI: T1WI, T2WI, DWI, AP, PVP	CT histogram analysis AP skewness filter 4: AUC 0.736 AP skewness filter 5: AUC 0.758 PVP mean filter 0:AUC 0.712 PVP MPP filter 0: AUC 0.712 PVP entropy filter 0: AUC 0.719
Ohki	2021	NS	pNET Grading (G1 vs. G2–G3)	33 (22 grade 1, 11 grade 2/3)	RW	Radiologist	CT: AP, PVP MRI: ADC map	AP log-sigma 1.0 joint-energy: AUC 0.855 PVP log-sigma 1.5 kurtosis: AUC 0.860 ADC log-sigma 1.0 correlation: AUC 0.847

AP—arterial phase, AUC—area under the curve, CT—computed tomography, DWI—diffusion-weighted imaging, MPP—mean of positive pixels, MRI—magnetic resonance imaging, NEC—neuroendocrine carcinoma, NECT—non-enhanced CT, NS—not specified, pNET—pancreatic neuroendocrine tumor, PVP—portal venous phase, RW—record-wise, T1WI—T1-weighted imaging, T2WI—T2-weighted imaging.

4. Insights on CAD Applied to Pancreatic Imaging

In the last few years, multiple CAD software approaches have been developed and tested on pancreatic imaging to improve the accuracy of examinations and the clinical decision-making process [62–77]. They have shown promising results for segmentation [65–72,77], tumor diagnosis, and classification [63,64,73–75] (Figure 3).

4.1. CAD and CT

The use of CT is routine for the diagnosis and follow-up of patients with pancreatic cancer. The use of CAD can help doctors improve diagnostic efficiency and accuracy [63–65], which does not depend directly on the subjective judgment and experience of the single physician. Even so, the application of CAD in pancreatic CT imaging may be difficult due to a lack of contrast between pancreatic parenchyma and bowel, large variations in the size of the pancreatic volume, and large variations in peripancreatic fat tissue [62].

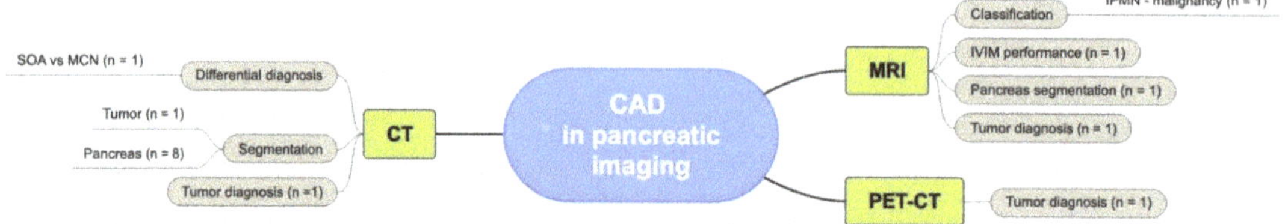

Figure 3. Summary of CAD applications in pancreatic imaging.

4.1.1. Oncological Applications

Liu et al. [63] aimed to diagnose pancreatic cancer using a convolutional neural network (CNN) classifier for CECT images. For this purpose, they used three different datasets. The first dataset had 295 patients with pancreatic cancer and 256 controls for training, and 75 patients with pancreatic cancer and 64 controls for validation. The second dataset consisted of 101 patients with pancreatic cancer and 88 controls, whereas the third dataset had 281 pancreatic cancer subjects and 82 controls. In all three sets, their model obtained an accuracy of more than 80%. The authors compared the use of the CNN in distinguishing pancreatic cancer from noncancerous tissue in CT to radiologist interpretation. Their CNN-based analysis achieved higher sensitivity than radiologists did (0.983 vs. 0.929, difference 0.054, $p = 0.014$). The CNN missed 3 (1.7%) of 176 pancreatic cancers (1.1–1.2 cm). Radiologists missed 12 (7%) of 168 pancreatic cancers (1.0–3.3 cm), of which 11 (92%) were correctly classified using the CNN. Finally, their CNN model obtained a sensibility of 92.1% for tumors smaller than 2 cm.

Cystic Lesions

Li et al. [64] assessed the effectiveness of a CAD scheme including tumor size, contour, location, and low-energy CT values in the differential diagnosis of pancreatic serous oligocystic adenomas (SOAs) from MCNs of PCNs using conventional and additional quantitative spectral CT features. The authors concluded that by combining conventional features with additional spectral CT features, the CAD scheme improved the overall accuracy from 88.37% to 93.02%. Reena Roy et al. [65] used a model for both an automated whole pancreas and PCN segmentation of CT images in oncologic patients using inter-/intraslice circumstantial instruction with preprocessing, segmentation, feature extraction, and classification. The authors found that the combination of various algorithms such as K-means, feature extraction using GLCM, and segmentation and classification using an artificial neural network (ANN) provides better results with increased efficiency, resulting in better classification of the pancreatic cysts.

4.1.2. Non-Oncological Studies

The main application of DL algorithms for non-oncological studies was the automatic segmentation of pancreas and pancreatic lesions, which can support diagnosis and treatment planning and reduce the workload. [66–72] Gibson et al. [66] used a deep learning-based segmentation algorithm for eight organs including the pancreas. Their model achieved a Dice similarity coefficient (DSC) of 0.78 vs. 0.71, 0.74, and 0.74. Similarly, Xue et al. [67] also worked on automated pancreas segmentation by using a cascaded multitask 3D fully convolutional network (FCN). Their method achieved a Dice score of 86.9. Zheng et al. [68] designed a 2.5D CNN in an automatic pancreas segmentation framework using 3D CT scans. Their method obtained a Dice similarity coefficient, sensitivity, and specificity of 86.21%, 87.49%, and 85.11%, respectively. However, some of the problems of automated DL segmentation performance in pancreas CT are poor gray-value contrast and the complex anatomy of the pancreas. To correct this situation, Boers et al. [62] developed a UNet they called iUnet to improve the quality of the colors. The performance for manual segmentation by a radiologist was 87% in 15 min, whereas the semiautomatic (radiologist + UNet) segmentation performance was 86% in 8 min.

Suman et al. [69] used the CTNVIDIA 3D slicer segmentation module, a DL model, for obtaining pancreatic segmentation. They used CECT scans that were previously reported as negative or unremarkable in the pancreatic region and obtained a DSC of 63%. Similarly, Nishio et al. [70] used CT images and a combination of DL and data augmentation to automatically segment the pancreas. The data augmentation method used included a mix-up, and random image cropping and patching (RICAP). Four-fold cross-validation was performed to train and evaluate these models with data augmentation methods and obtained a DSC of 0.703–0.789.

The interclass indistinction problem occurs as the density of the surrounding tissue is similar to that of the pancreas, resulting in the surrounding tissue being grouped with the pancreas, whereas the intraclass inconsistency occurs when the middle part of the pancreas is mistaken for the background, resulting in incomplete pancreas segmentation. Recently, Li et al. [71] focused on solving the issues of intraclass inconsistency and interclass indistinction in pancreas segmentation. To do this, they improved the contextual and semantic feature information acquisition method of the biomedical image segmentation model (UNet) based on a convolutional network and proposed an improved segmentation model called the multiscale attention dense residual U-shaped network (MAD-UNet). By using this new approach, the authors were able to reduce the effects of intraclass inconsistency and obtained a DSC of 86.10%.

Panda et al. [72] developed two-stage 3D CNNs for fully automated volumetric segmentation of the pancreas on CT. They also evaluated its performance in the context of intra-reader and inter-reader reliability at 1917 abdomen full-dose and reduced-radiation-dose CTs on a public dataset. Their 3D CNN obtained a DSC of 0.91 (0.03); they also obtained good reliability between model and R1 in both full- and reduced-dose CT (full-dose DSC: 0.81 (0.07), CCC: 0.83; reduced-dose DSC: 0.81 (0.08)).

Table 6 provides a summary of the papers included in the review, focused on the application of CAD in CT images.

Table 6. Applications of CAD in pancreatic CT images.

Author	Year	AI Model	Task	N Pts	Data Split	Reference Standard	CT Phase	Results
Li	2016	SVM	Differential diagnosis (SOA vs. MCN)	42 (23 SOAs, 19 MCNs)	RW	Radiologist	NECT, AP, PVP	Acc 93.2%
Liu	2020	CNN	Tumor diagnosis	690 local set 1(370 cases, 320 controls), 189 local set 2 (101 cases, 88 controls), 363 US test set (281 cases, 82 controls)	SW (412 TS, 139 VS, 139 test set 1, 189 test set 2)	Pathology	PVP	Local set 1: AUC 0.997, Acc 98.6%, Sen 97.3%, Spe 100% Local set 2: AUC 0.999, Acc 98.9%, Sen 99.0%, Spe 98.9% US set: AUC 0.920, Acc 83.2%, Sen 79.0%, Spe 97.6%
Roy	2020	ANN	Tumor segmentation	NS	NS	NS	NS	NS
Gibson	2018	Dense V-Network FCN	Pancreas segmentation	90 (43 public dataset 1, 47 public dataset 2)	SW	Radiologist	CECT	DSC 78%
Xue	2021	3D FCN	Pancreas segmentation	59	SW	Radiologist	CECT	DSC 86.9% JC 77.3%
Zheng	2020	VNet	Pancreas segmentation	82	RW	Radiologist	CECT	DSC 86.21% Sen 87.49% Spe 85.11%

Table 6. *Cont.*

Author	Year	AI Model	Task	N Pts	Data Split	Reference Standard	CT Phase	Results
Boers	2020	Interactive 3D UNet	Pancreas segmentation	100	RW (90 TS, 10 VS)	Radiologist	PVP	DSC 78.1%, average automated baseline performance 78%, semiautomatic segmentation performance in 8 min 86%
Suman	2021	NVIDIA	Pancreas segmentation	188 first batch, 159 second batch	SW	Radiologist	PVP	DSC 63%, JC 48%, FP 21%, FN 43%
Nishio	2020	Deep UNet	Pancreas segmentation	80	RW	Radiologist	CECT	DSC 70.3–78.9%, JC 0.563–0.658, Sen 64.5–76.2%, Spe 100%
Panda	2021	3D CNN	Pancreas segmentation	1917 internal dataset, 41 external dataset 1, 80 external dataset 2	RW (1380 TS, 248 VS, 289 internal test set, 50 external test set 1, 82 external test set 2)	Radiologist	PVP	Internal dataset: DSC 91% External dataset 1: DSC 83–84% External dataset 2: DSC 89%
Li	2021	MAD-UNet	Pancreas segmentation	363 (82 public dataset 1, 281 public dataset 2)	RW	UNet, VNet, Attention UNet, SegNet	CECT	DSC 86.10% JC 75.55% Sen 86.43% Spe 84.97%

Acc—accuracy, ANN—artificial neural network, AP—arterial phase, AUC—area under the curve, CECT—contrast-enhanced computed tomography, CNN—convolutional neural network, CT—computed tomography, DSC —Dice similarity coefficient, FCN—fully convolutional network, FN—false negative, FP—false positive, JC —Jaccard coefficient, MCN—mucinous cystic neoplasm, NECT—non-enhanced computed tomography, NS—not specified, PVP—portal venous phase, RW—record-wise, Sen—sensitivity, SOA—serous oligocystic adenoma, Spe —specificity, SW—subject-wise, TS—training set, VS—validation set.

4.2. CAD and PET-CT

Li et al. [73] extracted major structure and location information from the ROI on CT and PET images using a shape model-based algorithm. The algorithm used a collection of pancreas-shaped models. Li et al. achieved a 96.47% accuracy for PDAC classification in 80 cases with a 95.23% sensitivity and 97.51% specificity.

Table 7 provides a summary of the papers included in the review, focused on the application of CAD in PET-CT images.

Table 7. Applications of CAD in pancreatic PET-CT images.

Author	Year	AI Model	Task	N Pts	Data Split	Reference Standard	Radiotracer	CT Phase	Results
Li	2018	HFB-SVM-RF	Tumor Diagnosis	80 (40 cancer patients, 40 controls)	RW	Radiologist	FDG	NECT	Acc 96.47%, Sen 95.23%, Spe 97.51%

Acc—accuracy, AI—artificial intelligence, CT—computed tomography, FDG—fluorodeoxyglucose, HFB-SVM-RF—hybrid feedback-support vector machine-random forest, NECT—non-enhanced computed tomography, RW—record-wise, Sen—sensitivity, Spe—specificity.

4.3. CAD and MRI

The use of MRI as a soft-tissue contrast and noninvasive method is of great importance in the medical field, and even more now thanks to the use of CAD applied to oncological imaging [74,75].

4.3.1. Oncological Applications

Balasubramanian et al. [74] combined the response of ANN and support vector machine (SVM) techniques for pancreatic tumor classification. They used GLCM for extracting features from MR images of the pancreas and selected the best features using the JAFER algorithm. These features then were analyzed by five classification techniques: ANN BP,

ANN RBF, SVM Linear, SVM Poly, and SVM RBF. Their results showed that the ANN BP technique has a 98% classification accuracy.

Cystic Lesions

In a more recent study, Donofrio et al. [75] evaluated the diagnostic accuracy of dynamic MRI with DWI sequences in the identification of mural nodules of pancreatic IPMN by using pathological analysis as the gold standard. They performed a histogram analysis of the distribution of ADC and their results showed that entropy corresponded to the best J Youden index of 0.48 with a sensitivity of 68.75%, and a specificity of 79.25% in the distinction between a lesion with low-grade dysplasia and one with high-grade dysplasia. They also found that MRI with dynamic and DWI sequences was an accurate method for the identification of 5mm solid nodules of the IPMN, which correlated with the lesion malignancy.

4.3.2. Non-Oncological Applications

Barbieri et al. [76] prospectively assessed the feasibility of training a DNN for an intravoxel incoherent motion (IVIM) model fitting to diffusion-weighted MRI (DW-MRI) data. Two independent readers delineated regions of interest in the pancreas. DNNs were trained for IVIM model fitting using these data; results were compared to least-squares and Bayesian approaches to IVIM fitting. Their approach had high consistency between two readers (ICCs between 50% and 97%).

Chen et al. [77] developed a DL technique for fully automated pancreas segmentation. Their model took in multislice MR images and generated the output of the segmentation results, obtaining a DSC of 0.88. Their DL-based technique named ALAMO was found useful for fully automated multiorgan segmentation on abdominal MRI.

Table 8 provides a summary of the papers included in the review, focused on the application of CAD in MRI images.

Table 8. Applications of CAD in pancreatic MRI images.

Author	Year	AI Model	Task	N Pts	Data Split	Reference Standard	MRI Phase	Results
D'Onofrio	2021	NS	Prediction of IPMN malignancy	91	SW	Histopathology	T2WI, T1WI, DWI, MRCP	ADC map: entropy = 10.32, J Youden index 0.48, AUC 0.7288, Sen 68.75%, Spe 79.25%
Balasubramanian	2019	ANN, SVM	Tumor diagnosis	168 (68 with lesion, 100 controls)	RW (TS:VS = 7:3)	NS	NS	ANN BP 2 features (HOMO, CP): Acc 98%, Sen 100%, Spe 95%
Barbieri	2020	DNN	Evaluation of IVIM performance	10	SW	Radiologist	DWI	Dt: ICC 94–97% Fp: ICC 66% Dp: 50–51%
Chen	2020	UNet-based ALAMO	Pancreas segmentation	102	SW (66 TS, 16 VS, 20 test set)	Radiologist	T1WI-VIBE	Single slice: DSC 0.871 20 slices: DSC 0.880 40 slices: DSC 0.871

Acc—accuracy, ADC—apparent diffusion coefficient, ALAMO—automated deep learning-based abdominal multiorgan segmentation, ANN—artificial neural network, AUC—area under the curve, CP—cluster prominence, Dp—pseudo-diffusion coefficient, DSC—Dice similarity coefficient, Dt—pure diffusion coefficient, DWI—diffusion-weighted imaging, Fp—perfusion fraction, HOMO—homogeneity, IVIM—intravoxel incoherent motion, MRCP—magnetic resonance cholangiopancreatography, MRI—magnetic resonance imaging, NS—not specified, RW—record-wise, Sen—sensitivity, Spe—specificity, SVM—support vector machine, SW—subject-wise, T1WI—T1-weighted imaging, T2WI—T2-weighted imaging, TS—training set, VIBE—volumetric interpolated breath-hold examination, VS—validation set.

5. Discussion

For pancreatic pathologies, the use of medical imaging is essential for diagnosis, evaluation, and treatment planning [78]. The application of AI and radiomics is emerging and expanding, especially with regard to their applications for non-oncological pancreatic segmentation and tumor differentiation. In this review, we divided articles depending on their focus on CAD or radiomics, and further divided into two macro-categories based on their topic: non-oncological and oncological studies.

As concerns the non-oncological studies included in this review, the main application is DL segmentation, which is a useful step for training AI algorithms for detecting, characterizing, and classifying pancreatic lesions. As for the oncological studies included, AI is mainly used both for differential diagnosis and lesion segmentation. PDAC, which is the most prevalent neoplastic disease of the pancreas, has been extensively studied in the literature along with pNETs, especially in those studies focused on differential diagnosis.

Although great developments have occurred in recent years, it is important to address the obstacles that still need to be overcome before these technologies can be implemented into our clinical routines. However, despite the surge in publications on pancreas CAD and radiomics, there has not been a clinical translation of these applications.

Despite the use of large sample sizes in some studies and a large number of extracted features in radiomics, the limited heterogeneity of labeled training datasets may be one of the reasons that have precluded the clinical-grade performance and generalizability of the CAD and radiomics models. The articles reviewed were mainly retrospective with insufficient clinical data; for this reason, it is necessary to carry out more prospective studies that combine AI/radiomics and clinical data. Moreover, most of the articles included considered only the venous phase in CT for assessing pancreatic lesions, whereas only some of them included both arterial and venous phases in the study of lesion characteristics and showed better results than those who considered just the venous phase.

According to Chen et al. [78], there are three main challenges to the application of AI in pancreatic imaging. The first one is the inconsistencies and contradictions found in the results of the studies. For this reason, the authors proposed that there should be an initiative to standardize the development of quantitative imaging biomarkers. Second, there is a need for having more public annotated data on pancreatic imaging as the available data are not enough; this is due to the labor-intensive work that needs to be performed by experienced radiologists to label target lesions. Furthermore, the majority of the available studies are retrospective, with limited clinical, laboratory, and outcome data that prevent AI from being applied in clinical practice.

We are aware that the narrative nature of our review represents a limitation due to the absence of a systematic approach during the study selection process. We designed our study to provide only an overview of the available literature on the application of CAD/radiomics in pancreatic imaging.

6. Conclusions

This review demonstrated that AI applied to pancreatic imaging represents promising tools for a noninvasive diagnosis that will allow personalized approaches to patients. Up to now, the use of CAD and radiomics in pancreatic imaging has proven to be useful for both non-oncological and oncological purposes. There is much excitement and optimism about their applications; however, more multicenter, prospective, and large-scale studies need to be performed to introduce these tools into clinical practice.

Supplementary Materials: The following supporting information can be downloaded at: https://www.mdpi.com/article/10.3390/healthcare10081511/s1, File S1: Search strategy.

Author Contributions: Conceptualization, M.E.L., M.F., A.C. and V.S.; methodology, M.E.L., L.S. and M.A.O.; investigation, M.E.L., A.A. and L.L.; resources, A.A. and L.L.; data curation, M.E.L., A.A. and L.L.; writing—original draft preparation, M.E.L., A.A. and L.L.; writing—review and editing, M.E.L., A.A., L.M. and F.F.; supervision, M.E.L., M.F., A.C. and V.S.. All authors have read and agreed to the published version of the manuscript.

Funding: This research received no external funding.

Institutional Review Board Statement: This study did not require ethical approval.

Informed Consent Statement: Not applicable.

Data Availability Statement: No new data were created or analyzed in this study. Data sharing does not apply to this article.

Conflicts of Interest: The authors declare no conflict of interest.

References

1. Stevens, K.J.; Lisanti, C. Pancreas Imaging. In *StatPearls*; StatPearls Publishing: Treasure Island, FL, USA, 2022.
2. Chen, F.-M.; Ni, J.-M.; Zhang, Z.-Y.; Zhang, L.; Li, B.; Jiang, C.-J. Presurgical evaluation of pancreatic cancer: A comprehensive imaging comparison of CT versus MRI. *AJR Am. J. Roentgenol.* **2016**, *206*, 526–535. [CrossRef]
3. Xing, H.; Hao, Z.; Zhu, W.; Sun, D.; Ding, J.; Zhang, H.; Liu, Y.; Huo, L. Preoperative prediction of pathological grade in pancreatic ductal adenocarcinoma based on ^{18}F-FDG PET/CT radiomics. *EJNMMI Res.* **2021**, *11*, 19. [CrossRef] [PubMed]
4. Belli, M.L.; Mori, M.; Broggi, S.; Cattaneo, G.M.; Bettinardi, V.; Dell'Oca, I.; Fallanca, F.; Passoni, P.; Vanoli, E.G.; Calandrino, R.; et al. Quantifying the robustness of [^{18}F]FDG-PET/CT radiomic features with respect to tumor delineation in head and neck and pancreatic cancer patients. *Phys. Med.* **2018**, *49*, 105–111. [CrossRef]
5. Santos, M.K.; Ferreira Júnior, J.R.; Wada, D.T.; Tenório, A.P.M.; Barbosa, M.H.N.; Marques, P.M.D.A. Artificial intelligence, machine learning, computer-aided diagnosis, and radiomics: Advances in imaging towards to precision medicine. *Radiol. Bras.* **2019**, *52*, 387–396. [CrossRef]
6. Lambin, P.; Leijenaar, R.T.H.; Deist, T.M.; Peerlings, J.; de Jong, E.E.C.; van Timmeren, J.; Sanduleanu, S.; Larue, R.T.H.M.; Even, A.J.G.; Jochems, A.; et al. Radiomics: The bridge between medical imaging and personalized medicine. *Nat. Rev. Clin. Oncol.* **2017**, *14*, 749–762. [CrossRef] [PubMed]
7. Abunahel, B.M.; Pontre, B.; Kumar, H.; Petrov, M.S. Pancreas image mining: A systematic review of radiomics. *Eur. Radiol.* **2021**, *31*, 3447–3467. [CrossRef] [PubMed]
8. Kumar, H.; DeSouza, S.V.; Petrov, M.S. Automated pancreas segmentation from computed tomography and magnetic resonance images: A systematic review. *Comput. Methods Programs Biomed.* **2019**, *178*, 319–328. [CrossRef] [PubMed]
9. Yang, J.; Guo, X.; Ou, X.; Zhang, W.; Ma, X. Discrimination of pancreatic serous cystadenomas from mucinous cystadenomas with CT textural features: Based on machine learning. *Front. Oncol.* **2019**, *9*, 494. [CrossRef] [PubMed]
10. Yang, J.; Guo, X.; Zhang, H.; Zhang, W.; Song, J.; Xu, H.; Ma, X. Differential diagnosis of pancreatic serous cystadenoma and mucinous cystadenoma: Utility of textural features in combination with morphological characteristics. *BMC Cancer* **2019**, *19*, 1223. [CrossRef]
11. Shen, X.; Yang, F.; Yang, P.; Yang, M.; Xu, L.; Zhuo, J.; Wang, J.; Lu, D.; Liu, Z.; Zheng, S.-S.; et al. A Contrast-Enhanced Computed Tomography Based Radiomics Approach for Preoperative Differentiation of Pancreatic Cystic Neoplasm Subtypes: A Feasibility Study. *Front. Oncol.* **2020**, *10*, 248. [CrossRef] [PubMed]
12. Wei, R.; Lin, K.; Yan, W.; Guo, Y.; Wang, Y.; Li, J.; Zhu, J. Computer-Aided Diagnosis of Pancreas Serous Cystic Neoplasms: A Radiomics Method on Preoperative MDCT Images. *Technol. Cancer Res. Treat.* **2019**, *18*. [CrossRef] [PubMed]
13. Xie, H.; Ma, S.; Guo, X.; Zhang, X.; Wang, X. Preoperative differentiation of pancreatic mucinous cystic neoplasm from macrocystic serous cystic adenoma using radiomics: Preliminary findings and comparison with radiological model. *Eur. J. Radiol.* **2020**, *122*, 108747. [CrossRef] [PubMed]
14. Tobaly, D.; Santinha, J.; Sartoris, R.; Dioguardi Burgio, M.; Matos, C.; Cros, J.; Couvelard, A.; Rebours, V.; Sauvanet, A.; Ronot, M.; et al. CT-Based Radiomics Analysis to Predict Malignancy in Patients with Intraductal Papillary Mucinous Neoplasm (IPMN) of the Pancreas. *Cancers* **2020**, *12*, 3089. [CrossRef] [PubMed]
15. Chen, S.; Ren, S.; Guo, K.; Daniels, M.J.; Wang, Z.; Chen, R. Preoperative differentiation of serous cystic neoplasms from mucin-producing pancreatic cystic neoplasms using a CT-based radiomics nomogram. *Abdom. Radiol.* **2021**, *46*, 2637–2646. [CrossRef]
16. Hanania, A.N.; Bantis, L.E.; Feng, Z.; Wang, H.; Tamm, E.P.; Katz, M.H.; Maitra, A.; Koay, E.J. Quantitative imaging to evaluate malignant potential of IPMNs. *Oncotarget* **2016**, *7*, 85776–85784. [CrossRef] [PubMed]
17. Permuth, J.B.; Choi, J.; Balarunathan, Y.; Kim, J.; Chen, D.-T.; Chen, L.; Orcutt, S.; Doepker, M.P.; Gage, K.; Zhang, G.; et al. Florida Pancreas Collaborative Combining radiomic features with a miRNA classifier may improve prediction of malignant pathology for pancreatic intraductal papillary mucinous neoplasms. *Oncotarget* **2016**, *7*, 85785–85797. [CrossRef] [PubMed]
18. Attiyeh, M.A.; Chakraborty, J.; Doussot, A.; Langdon-Embry, L.; Mainarich, S.; Gönen, M.; Balachandran, V.P.; D'Angelica, M.I.; DeMatteo, R.P.; Jarnagin, W.R.; et al. Survival prediction in pancreatic ductal adenocarcinoma by quantitative computed tomography image analysis. *Ann. Surg. Oncol.* **2018**, *25*, 1034–1042. [CrossRef] [PubMed]
19. He, M.; Liu, Z.; Lin, Y.; Wan, J.; Li, J.; Xu, K.; Wang, Y.; Jin, Z.; Tian, J.; Xue, H. Differentiation of atypical non-functional pancreatic neuroendocrine tumor and pancreatic ductal adenocarcinoma using CT based radiomics. *Eur. J. Radiol.* **2019**, *117*, 102–111. [CrossRef] [PubMed]
20. Li, J.; Lu, J.; Liang, P.; Li, A.; Hu, Y.; Shen, Y.; Hu, D.; Li, Z. Differentiation of atypical pancreatic neuroendocrine tumors from pancreatic ductal adenocarcinomas: Using whole-tumor CT texture analysis as quantitative biomarkers. *Cancer Med.* **2018**, *7*, 4924–4931. [CrossRef] [PubMed]

21. Yu, H.; Huang, Z.; Li, M.; Wei, Y.; Zhang, L.; Yang, C.; Zhang, Y.; Song, B. Differential diagnosis of nonhypervascular pancreatic neuroendocrine neoplasms from pancreatic ductal adenocarcinomas, based on computed tomography radiological features and texture analysis. *Acad. Radiol.* **2020**, *27*, 332–341. [CrossRef] [PubMed]

22. Canellas, R.; Burk, K.S.; Parakh, A.; Sahani, D.V. Prediction of pancreatic neuroendocrine tumor grade based on CT features and texture analysis. *AJR Am. J. Roentgenol.* **2018**, *210*, 341–346. [CrossRef] [PubMed]

23. Reinert, C.P.; Baumgartner, K.; Hepp, T.; Bitzer, M.; Horger, M. Complementary role of computed tomography texture analysis for differentiation of pancreatic ductal adenocarcinoma from pancreatic neuroendocrine tumors in the portal-venous enhancement phase. *Abdom. Radiol.* **2020**, *45*, 750–758. [CrossRef] [PubMed]

24. D'Onofrio, M.; Ciaravino, V.; Cardobi, N.; De Robertis, R.; Cingarlini, S.; Landoni, L.; Capelli, P.; Bassi, C.; Scarpa, A. CT enhancement and 3D texture analysis of pancreatic neuroendocrine neoplasms. *Sci. Rep.* **2019**, *9*, 2176. [CrossRef]

25. Gu, D.; Hu, Y.; Ding, H.; Wei, J.; Chen, K.; Liu, H.; Zeng, M.; Tian, J. CT radiomics may predict the grade of pancreatic neuroendocrine tumors: A multicenter study. *Eur. Radiol.* **2019**, *29*, 6880–6890. [CrossRef] [PubMed]

26. Liang, W.; Yang, P.; Huang, R.; Xu, L.; Wang, J.; Liu, W.; Zhang, L.; Wan, D.; Huang, Q.; Lu, Y.; et al. A combined nomogram model to preoperatively predict histologic grade in pancreatic neuroendocrine tumors. *Clin. Cancer Res.* **2019**, *25*, 584–594. [CrossRef] [PubMed]

27. Guo, C.; Zhuge, X.; Wang, Z.; Wang, Q.; Sun, K.; Feng, Z.; Chen, X. Textural analysis on contrast-enhanced CT in pancreatic neuroendocrine neoplasms: Association with WHO grade. *Abdom. Radiol.* **2019**, *44*, 576–585. [CrossRef]

28. Ren, S.; Zhao, R.; Cui, W.; Qiu, W.; Guo, K.; Cao, Y.; Duan, S.; Wang, Z.; Chen, R. Computed Tomography-Based Radiomics Signature for the Preoperative Differentiation of Pancreatic Adenosquamous Carcinoma from Pancreatic Ductal Adenocarcinoma. *Front. Oncol.* **2020**, *10*, 1618. [CrossRef]

29. Kaissis, G.A.; Ziegelmayer, S.; Lohöfer, F.K.; Harder, F.N.; Jungmann, F.; Sasse, D.; Muckenhuber, A.; Yen, H.-Y.; Steiger, K.; Siveke, J.; et al. Image-Based Molecular Phenotyping of Pancreatic Ductal Adenocarcinoma. *J. Clin. Med.* **2020**, *9*, 724. [CrossRef] [PubMed]

30. Khalvati, F.; Zhang, Y.; Baig, S.; Lobo-Mueller, E.M.; Karanicolas, P.; Gallinger, S.; Haider, M.A. Prognostic value of CT radiomic features in resectable pancreatic ductal adenocarcinoma. *Sci. Rep.* **2019**, *9*, 5449. [CrossRef]

31. Yun, G.; Kim, Y.H.; Lee, Y.J.; Kim, B.; Hwang, J.-H.; Choi, D.J. Tumor heterogeneity of pancreas head cancer assessed by CT texture analysis: Association with survival outcomes after curative resection. *Sci. Rep.* **2018**, *8*, 7226. [CrossRef] [PubMed]

32. Xie, T.; Wang, X.; Li, M.; Tong, T.; Yu, X.; Zhou, Z. Pancreatic ductal adenocarcinoma: A radiomics nomogram outperforms clinical model and TNM staging for survival estimation after curative resection. *Eur. Radiol.* **2020**, *30*, 2513–2524. [CrossRef] [PubMed]

33. Kim, H.S.; Kim, Y.J.; Kim, K.G.; Park, J.S. Preoperative CT texture features predict prognosis after curative resection in pancreatic cancer. *Sci. Rep.* **2019**, *9*, 17389. [CrossRef] [PubMed]

34. Eilaghi, A.; Baig, S.; Zhang, Y.; Zhang, J.; Karanicolas, P.; Gallinger, S.; Khalvati, F.; Haider, M.A. CT texture features are associated with overall survival in pancreatic ductal adenocarcinoma—A quantitative analysis. *BMC Med. Imaging* **2017**, *17*, 38. [CrossRef] [PubMed]

35. Fang, W.H.; Li, X.D.; Zhu, H.; Miao, F.; Qian, X.H.; Pan, Z.L.; Lin, X.Z. Resectable pancreatic ductal adenocarcinoma: Association between preoperative CT texture features and metastatic nodal involvement. *Cancer Imaging* **2020**, *20*, 17. [CrossRef]

36. Li, K.; Yao, Q.; Xiao, J.; Li, M.; Yang, J.; Hou, W.; Du, M.; Chen, K.; Qu, Y.; Li, L.; et al. Contrast-enhanced CT radiomics for predicting lymph node metastasis in pancreatic ductal adenocarcinoma: A pilot study. *Cancer Imaging* **2020**, *20*, 12. [CrossRef] [PubMed]

37. Chen, Y.; Chen, T.-W.; Wu, C.-Q.; Lin, Q.; Hu, R.; Xie, C.-L.; Zuo, H.-D.; Wu, J.-L.; Mu, Q.-W.; Fu, Q.-S.; et al. Radiomics model of contrast-enhanced computed tomography for predicting the recurrence of acute pancreatitis. *Eur. Radiol.* **2019**, *29*, 4408–4417. [CrossRef] [PubMed]

38. Mashayekhi, R.; Parekh, V.S.; Faghih, M.; Singh, V.K.; Jacobs, M.A.; Zaheer, A. Radiomic features of the pancreas on CT imaging accurately differentiate functional abdominal pain, recurrent acute pancreatitis, and chronic pancreatitis. *Eur. J. Radiol.* **2020**, *123*, 108778. [CrossRef]

39. Zhang, Y.; Cheng, C.; Liu, Z.; Wang, L.; Pan, G.; Sun, G.; Chang, Y.; Zuo, C.; Yang, X. Radiomics analysis for the differentiation of autoimmune pancreatitis and pancreatic ductal adenocarcinoma in 18 F-FDG PET/CT. *Med. Phys.* **2019**, *46*, 4520–4530. [CrossRef]

40. Mapelli, P.; Partelli, S.; Salgarello, M.; Doraku, J.; Pasetto, S.; Rancoita, P.M.V.; Muffatti, F.; Bettinardi, V.; Presotto, L.; Andreasi, V.; et al. Dual tracer 68Ga-DOTATOC and ^{18}F-FDG PET/computed tomography radiomics in pancreatic neuroendocrine neoplasms: An endearing tool for preoperative risk assessment. *Nucl. Med. Commun.* **2020**, *41*, 896–905. [CrossRef]

41. Liberini, V.; Rampado, O.; Gallio, E.; De Santi, B.; Ceci, F.; Dionisi, B.; Thuillier, P.; Ciuffreda, L.; Piovesan, A.; Fioroni, F.; et al. 68Ga-DOTATOC PET/CT-Based Radiomic Analysis and PRRT Outcome: A Preliminary Evaluation Based on an Exploratory Radiomic Analysis on Two Patients. *Front. Med.* **2020**, *7*, 601853. [CrossRef]

42. Lim, C.H.; Cho, Y.S.; Choi, J.Y.; Lee, K.-H.; Lee, J.K.; Min, J.H.; Hyun, S.H. Imaging phenotype using ^{18}F-fluorodeoxyglucose positron emission tomography-based radiomics and genetic alterations of pancreatic ductal adenocarcinoma. *Eur. J. Nucl. Med. Mol. Imaging* **2020**, *47*, 2113–2122. [CrossRef] [PubMed]

43. Cui, Y.; Song, J.; Pollom, E.; Alagappan, M.; Shirato, H.; Chang, D.T.; Koong, A.C.; Li, R. Quantitative Analysis of (18)F-Fluorodeoxyglucose Positron Emission Tomography Identifies Novel Prognostic Imaging Biomarkers in Locally Advanced Pancreatic Cancer Patients Treated with Stereotactic Body Radiation Therapy. *Int. J. Radiat. Oncol. Biol. Phys.* **2016**, *96*, 102–109. [CrossRef]

44. Yue, Y.; Osipov, A.; Fraass, B.; Sandler, H.; Zhang, X.; Nissen, N.; Hendifar, A.; Tuli, R. Identifying prognostic intratumor heterogeneity using pre- and post-radiotherapy ^{18}F-FDG PET images for pancreatic cancer patients. *J. Gastrointest. Oncol.* **2017**, *8*, 127–138. [CrossRef] [PubMed]

45. Liu, Z.; Li, M.; Zuo, C.; Yang, Z.; Yang, X.; Ren, S.; Peng, Y.; Sun, G.; Shen, J.; Cheng, C.; et al. Radiomics model of dual-time 2-[18F]FDG PET/CT imaging to distinguish between pancreatic ductal adenocarcinoma and autoimmune pancreatitis. *Eur. Radiol.* **2021**, *31*, 6983–6991. [CrossRef] [PubMed]

46. Toyama, Y.; Hotta, M.; Motoi, F.; Takanami, K.; Minamimoto, R.; Takase, K. Prognostic value of FDG-PET radiomics with machine learning in pancreatic cancer. *Sci. Rep.* **2020**, *10*, 17024. [CrossRef]

47. Costache, M.I.; Costache, C.A.; Dumitrescu, C.I.; Tica, A.A.; Popescu, M.; Baluta, E.A.; Anghel, A.C.; Saftoiu, A.; Dumitrescu, D. Which is the Best Imaging Method in Pancreatic Adenocarcinoma Diagnosis and Staging—CT, MRI or EUS? *Curr. Health Sci. J.* **2017**, *43*, 132–136. [CrossRef]

48. Jeon, S.K.; Kim, J.H.; Yoo, J.; Kim, J.-E.; Park, S.J.; Han, J.K. Assessment of malignant potential in intraductal papillary mucinous neoplasms of the pancreas using MR findings and texture analysis. *Eur. Radiol.* **2021**, *31*, 3394–3404. [CrossRef] [PubMed]

49. Cui, S.; Tang, T.; Su, Q.; Wang, Y.; Shu, Z.; Yang, W.; Gong, X. Radiomic nomogram based on MRI to predict grade of branching type intraductal papillary mucinous neoplasms of the pancreas: A multicenter study. *Cancer Imaging* **2021**, *21*, 26. [CrossRef] [PubMed]

50. Guo, C.-G.; Ren, S.; Chen, X.; Wang, Q.-D.; Xiao, W.-B.; Zhang, J.-F.; Duan, S.-F.; Wang, Z.-Q. Pancreatic neuroendocrine tumor: Prediction of the tumor grade using magnetic resonance imaging findings and texture analysis with 3-T magnetic resonance. *Cancer Manag. Res.* **2019**, *11*, 1933–1944. [CrossRef] [PubMed]

51. Song, T.; Zhang, Q.-W.; Duan, S.-F.; Bian, Y.; Hao, Q.; Xing, P.-Y.; Wang, T.-G.; Chen, L.-G.; Ma, C.; Lu, J.-P. MRI-based radiomics approach for differentiation of hypovascular non-functional pancreatic neuroendocrine tumors and solid pseudopapillary neoplasms of the pancreas. *BMC Med. Imaging* **2021**, *21*, 36. [CrossRef] [PubMed]

52. Li, X.; Zhu, H.; Qian, X.; Chen, N.; Lin, X. MRI texture analysis for differentiating nonfunctional pancreatic neuroendocrine neoplasms from solid pseudopapillary neoplasms of the pancreas. *Acad. Radiol.* **2020**, *27*, 815–823. [CrossRef] [PubMed]

53. Taffel, M.T.; Luk, L.; Ream, J.M.; Rosenkrantz, A.B. Exploratory study of apparent diffusion coefficient histogram metrics in assessing pancreatic malignancy. *Can. Assoc. Radiol. J.* **2019**, *70*, 416–423. [CrossRef] [PubMed]

54. Kaissis, G.; Ziegelmayer, S.; Lohöfer, F.; Algül, H.; Eiber, M.; Weichert, W.; Schmid, R.; Friess, H.; Rummeny, E.; Ankerst, D.; et al. A machine learning model for the prediction of survival and tumor subtype in pancreatic ductal adenocarcinoma from preoperative diffusion-weighted imaging. *Eur. Radiol. Exp.* **2019**, *3*, 41. [CrossRef] [PubMed]

55. Kaissis, G.; Ziegelmayer, S.; Lohöfer, F.; Steiger, K.; Algül, H.; Muckenhuber, A.; Yen, H.-Y.; Rummeny, E.; Friess, H.; Schmid, R.; et al. A machine learning algorithm predicts molecular subtypes in pancreatic ductal adenocarcinoma with differential response to gemcitabine-based versus FOLFIRINOX chemotherapy. *PLoS ONE* **2019**, *14*, e0218642. [CrossRef]

56. Becker, A.S.; Wagner, M.W.; Wurnig, M.C.; Boss, A. Diffusion-weighted imaging of the abdomen: Impact of b-values on texture analysis features. *NMR Biomed.* **2017**, *30*, e3669. [CrossRef]

57. Lin, Q.; Ji, Y.-F.; Chen, Y.; Sun, H.; Yang, D.-D.; Chen, A.-L.; Chen, T.-W.; Zhang, X.M. Radiomics model of contrast-enhanced MRI for early prediction of acute pancreatitis severity. *J. Magn. Reson. Imaging* **2020**, *51*, 397–406. [CrossRef] [PubMed]

58. Frøkjær, J.B.; Lisitskaya, M.V.; Jørgensen, A.S.; Østergaard, L.R.; Hansen, T.M.; Drewes, A.M.; Olesen, S.S. Pancreatic magnetic resonance imaging texture analysis in chronic pancreatitis: A feasibility and validation study. *Abdom. Radiol.* **2020**, *45*, 1497–1506. [CrossRef] [PubMed]

59. Gao, J.; Huang, X.; Meng, H.; Zhang, M.; Zhang, X.; Lin, X.; Li, B. Performance of multiparametric functional imaging and texture analysis in predicting synchronous metastatic disease in pancreatic ductal adenocarcinoma patients by hybrid PET/MR: Initial experience. *Front. Oncol.* **2020**, *10*, 198. [CrossRef] [PubMed]

60. Azoulay, A.; Cros, J.; Vullierme, M.P.; de Mestier, L.; Couvelard, A.; Hentic, O.; Kusznewski, P.; Sauvanet, A.; Vilgrain, V.; Ronot, M. Morphological imaging and CT histogram analysis to differentiate pancreatic neuroendocrine tumor grade 3 from neuroendocrine carcinoma. *Diagn. Interv. Imaging* **2020**, *101*, 821–830. [CrossRef] [PubMed]

61. Ohki, K.; Igarashi, T.; Ashida, H.; Takenaga, S.; Shiraishi, M.; Nozawa, Y.; Ojiri, H. Usefulness of texture analysis for grading pancreatic neuroendocrine tumors on contrast-enhanced computed tomography and apparent diffusion coefficient maps. *Jpn. J. Radiol.* **2021**, *39*, 66–75. [CrossRef] [PubMed]

62. Boers, T.G.W.; Hu, Y.; Gibson, E.; Barratt, D.C.; Bonmati, E.; Krdzalic, J.; van der Heijden, F.; Hermans, J.J.; Huisman, H.J. Interactive 3D U-net for the segmentation of the pancreas in computed tomography scans. *Phys. Med. Biol.* **2020**, *65*, 065002. [CrossRef] [PubMed]

63. Liu, K.-L.; Wu, T.; Chen, P.-T.; Tsai, Y.M.; Roth, H.; Wu, M.-S.; Liao, W.-C.; Wang, W. Deep learning to distinguish pancreatic cancer tissue from non-cancerous pancreatic tissue: A retrospective study with cross-racial external validation. *Lancet Digit. Health* **2020**, *2*, e303–e313. [CrossRef]

64. Li, C.; Lin, X.; Hui, C.; Lam, K.M.; Zhang, S. Computer-Aided Diagnosis for Distinguishing Pancreatic Mucinous Cystic Neoplasms from Serous Oligocystic Adenomas in Spectral CT Images. *Technol. Cancer Res. Treat.* **2016**, *15*, 44–54. [CrossRef] [PubMed]

65. Roy, M.R.R.; Mala, G.A.; Sarika, C.; Shruthi, S.; Sripradha, S. Segmentation of pancreatic cysts and roi extraction from pancreatic ct images using machine learning. *Eur. J. Mol. Clin. Med.* **2020**, *7*, 2020.

66. Gibson, E.; Giganti, F.; Hu, Y.; Bonmati, E.; Bandula, S.; Gurusamy, K.; Davidson, B.; Pereira, S.P.; Clarkson, M.J.; Barratt, D.C. Automatic Multi-Organ Segmentation on Abdominal CT With Dense V-Networks. *IEEE Trans. Med. Imaging* **2018**, *37*, 1822–1834. [CrossRef] [PubMed]
67. Xue, J.; He, K.; Nie, D.; Adeli, E.; Shi, Z.; Lee, S.-W.; Zheng, Y.; Liu, X.; Li, D.; Shen, D. Cascaded MultiTask 3-D Fully Convolutional Networks for Pancreas Segmentation. *IEEE Trans. Cybern.* **2021**, *51*, 2153–2165. [CrossRef]
68. Zheng, H.; Qian, L.; Qin, Y.; Gu, Y.; Yang, J. Improving the slice interaction of 2.5D CNN for automatic pancreas segmentation. *Med. Phys.* **2020**, *47*, 5543–5554. [CrossRef]
69. Suman, G.; Panda, A.; Korfiatis, P.; Edwards, M.E.; Garg, S.; Blezek, D.J.; Chari, S.T.; Goenka, A.H. Development of a volumetric pancreas segmentation CT dataset for AI applications through trained technologists: A study during the COVID 19 containment phase. *Abdom. Radiol.* **2020**, *45*, 4302–4310. [CrossRef]
70. Nishio, M.; Noguchi, S.; Fujimoto, K. Automatic Pancreas Segmentation Using Coarse-Scaled 2D Model of Deep Learning: Usefulness of Data Augmentation and Deep U-Net. *Appl. Sci.* **2020**, *10*, 3360. [CrossRef]
71. Li, W.; Qin, S.; Li, F.; Wang, L. MAD-UNet: A deep U-shaped network combined with an attention mechanism for pancreas segmentation in CT images. *Med. Phys.* **2021**, *48*, 329–341. [CrossRef]
72. Panda, A.; Korfiatis, P.; Suman, G.; Garg, S.K.; Polley, E.C.; Singh, D.P.; Chari, S.T.; Goenka, A.H. Two-stage deep learning model for fully automated pancreas segmentation on computed tomography: Comparison with intra-reader and inter-reader reliability at full and reduced radiation dose on an external dataset. *Med. Phys.* **2021**, *48*, 2468–2481. [CrossRef]
73. Li, S.; Jiang, H.; Wang, Z.; Zhang, G.; Yao, Y.-D. An effective computer aided diagnosis model for pancreas cancer on PET/CT images. *Comput. Methods Programs Biomed.* **2018**, *165*, 205–214. [CrossRef]
74. Balasubramanian, A.D.; Murugan, P.R.; Thiyagarajan, A.P. Analysis and classification of malignancy in pancreatic magnetic resonance images using neural network techniques. *Int. J. Imaging Syst. Technol.* **2019**, *29*, 399–418. [CrossRef]
75. D'Onofrio, M.; Tedesco, G.; Cardobi, N.; De Robertis, R.; Sarno, A.; Capelli, P.; Martini, P.T.; Giannotti, G.; Beleù, A.; Marchegiani, G.; et al. Magnetic resonance (MR) for mural nodule detection studying Intraductal papillary mucinous neoplasms (IPMN) of pancreas: Imaging-pathologic correlation. *Pancreatology* **2021**, *21*, 180–187. [CrossRef] [PubMed]
76. Barbieri, S.; Gurney-Champion, O.J.; Klaassen, R.; Thoeny, H.C. Deep learning how to fit an intravoxel incoherent motion model to diffusion-weighted MRI. *Magn. Reson. Med.* **2020**, *83*, 312–321. [CrossRef] [PubMed]
77. Chen, Y.; Ruan, D.; Xiao, J.; Wang, L.; Sun, B.; Saouaf, R.; Yang, W.; Li, D.; Fan, Z. Fully automated multiorgan segmentation in abdominal magnetic resonance imaging with deep neural networks. *Med. Phys.* **2020**, *47*, 4971–4982. [CrossRef] [PubMed]
78. Chen, B.-B. Artificial intelligence in pancreatic disease. *AIMI* **2020**, *1*, 19–30. [CrossRef]

MDPI
St. Alban-Anlage 66
4052 Basel
Switzerland
Tel. +41 61 683 77 34
Fax +41 61 302 89 18
www.mdpi.com

Healthcare Editorial Office
E-mail: healthcare@mdpi.com
www.mdpi.com/journal/healthcare

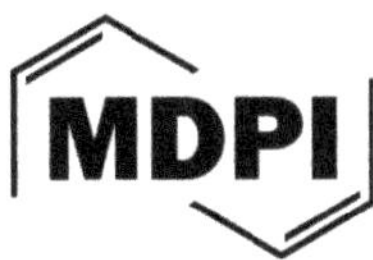